Steve [signature]

Wellcome Unit for the
History of Medicine

Manchester University

In this new synthetic history of American nursing, Susan Reverby contends that nursing's contemporary difficulties are shaped by the factors that created its historical obligation to care in a society that refuses to value caring. Building upon the questions being raised within women's history, the book provides insight into how a group of women could become so divided that their common oppression based on gender could not unite them. Nursing is thus used as a case history of the realities under which a particular women's work culture within the health-care industry became politicized in ways that often constrained its own efforts.

In this book Susan Reverby presents a history of nursing's development between 1850 and 1945 in the context in the changing health-care system. Beginning with a new analysis of nursing before the introduction of training, *Ordered to Care* describes the historical development of nursing ideology, work conditions, and efforts at reform and professionalization. With the insights from the new scholarship on the social history of health care, the author is also providing a retelling of the political history of the hospital from the vantage point of nursing.

As did women in other occupational settings, nurses created a "little world of their own." But, as the author argues, this was not always the familial and sharing culture so eloquently evoked by recent scholarship in women's history, or merely a heroic struggle as portrayed in earlier nursing histories. Rather, nurses were forced into an overcrowded, sex-segregated labor market where women of different backgrounds and education contended over an understanding of what counted as good nursing and the good nurse. The process of professionalization in nursing was fractured both by patriarchal constraints imposed from above by hospitals, physicians, and the broader culture, and by differences among women from within.

In keeping with the ongoing debate within women's studies over the meaning of caring and autonomy in women's lives, Susan Reverby describes how nursing developed within the cultural expectation that caring would be a part of a woman's duty to family and community. When training for nursing was introduced in the late nineteenth century, it was based upon understandings of women's duty, she argues, but not of women's rights. This gave trained nursing purpose but, when coupled with the growing economic and cultural power of the hospitals, limited nursing's ability to control or define its own future. The author concludes with a discussion of why nursing will have to find a way to move beyond the duty or rights framework to shape its own professional future and to provide a model for the care we all so desperately need.

Cambridge History of Medicine
EDITORS: CHARLES WEBSTER AND CHARLES ROSENBERG

Ordered to care

Ordered to care

THE DILEMMA OF AMERICAN NURSING, 1850–1945

SUSAN M. REVERBY

Women's Studies Program
Wellesley College

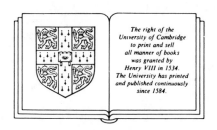

The right of the
University of Cambridge
to print and sell
all manner of books
was granted by
Henry VIII in 1534.
The University has printed
and published continuously
since 1584.

CAMBRIDGE UNIVERSITY PRESS

CAMBRIDGE
LONDON   NEW YORK   NEW ROCHELLE
MELBOURNE   SYDNEY

Published by the Press Syndicate of the University of Cambridge
The Pitt Building, Trumpington Street, Cambridge CB2 1RP
32 East 57th Street, New York, NY 10022, USA
10 Stamford Road, Oakleigh, Melbourne 3166, Australia

First published 1987

Printed in the United States of America

Library of Congress Cataloging-in-Publication Data
Reverby, Susan M.
Ordered to care.
(Cambridge history of medicine)
Bibliography: p.
Includes index.
1. Nursing – United States – History – 19th century.
2. Nursing – United States – History – 20th century.
I. Title. II. Title: Dilemma of American nursing,
1850–1945. III. Series. [DNLM: 1. History of Nursing
– United States. WY 11 AA1 R4520]
RT4.R45   1987   610.73'069   86–26815

British Library Cataloguing in Publication Data
Reverby, Susan M.
Ordered to care: the dilemma of American
nursing, 1850–1945. – (Cambridge history
of medicine)
1. Nursing – United States – History
I. Title
610.73'0973   RT4

ISBN 0 521 25604 6 hard covers
ISBN 0 521 33565 5 paperback

In memory of Anna Fox
and for Mariah and Micah

. . . Let the thought of the sore needs of the people who await your ministry fortify you, and let me speak if I may for the nurses of the country, and say that they stretch out welcoming hands to you as you enter the apprenticeship to duty to which you have dedicated yourselves.

M. Adelaide Nutting, "Apprenticeship to Duty,"
a speech before the students of the Vassar Training Camp,
September 9, 1918

Where there is one nurse with a missionary spirit . . . there are forty-nine others who are obliged to make the humiliating confession: "I am a nurse because I must earn a living for myself and those dependent on me, because my nursing is well-paid, honorable, and to me, interesting."

. . . Of course this spirit of self-immolation is very beautiful and lovely, but is it practical? Is it the motive power which had induced the army of sensible, practical women to take up this work? . . . Let us be honest, even at the sacrifice of sentiment. Let us not hesitate to do a good deed when opportunity offers, but let us not try to make people believe we are angels and that to do good is the chief object in our lives, with a small remuneration thrown in, to which we scarcely give a thought.

"Candor," Letter to the Editor
Trained Nurse Journal, April 1888

If we are to have self rule we must fight for it all the time.

Lavinia L. Dock to Mary M. Roberts, May 17, 1943

Contents

Tables and figures

FIGURES

Acknowledgments

This is the part that is fun. Ironically, it appears at the front of the book but is written at the end of a very long process. Without those acknowledged, however, there would have been no beginning or end.

Whenever I have given papers or talks on nursing history, I am inevitably asked if I am a nurse. Thus I have to start with an important confession: I am not a nurse but a historian. The usual queries about my training are almost as if some presumably hidden part of my occupational history has to explain this intellectual interest. I always find this question quite telling: After all, I usually respond, no one asks a political historian if her parents were in politics or inquires if a historian of textile workers ever worked in a mill. Nursing's supposed unimportance except to those in the field and a pervasive sexism appear to explain the questioning. I hope the book will make it clear why nursing history is important to us all.

This study's origins lie in the research I did as a staff associate of the Health Policy Advisory Center in New York in 1970. I was assigned to the areas of women's health care and later women health workers. Although I was responsible for articles on nursing's contemporary difficulties, my colleagues tolerated my historian's need to understand why things had ended up this way, even if they would not let me write about it endlessly.

Over the years, my contact with a number of nurses has sustained my sense that this kind of historical research was relevant to their struggles. I wish to thank Sondra Clark, Nancy Greenleaf, and Karen Wolf for their willingness to share nursing with an "outsider." Susan Sieber and Kate O'Connell were also helpful as guides to the nursing culture and its terminology. Nurse historians Karen Buhler-Wilkerson and Joan Lynaugh continually supported my efforts, asked probing questions, supplied me with additional "finds," and made me feel that it was all worthwhile. Other faculty members at the University of Pennsylvania School of Nursing gave me a second intellectual home.

Professor Emeritus Mary Ann Garrigan of the Boston University School of Nursing first introduced me to the Nursing Archives at Boston University that she started in 1966 and sustained over the years. Her insatiable curiosity and concern for nursing history have left both nurses and historians an invaluable resource. Margaret Goostray and her staff in the archives were more than helpful as I became a semipermanent resident. Richard Wolfe, curator of the Rare Books Collection at Harvard's Countway Library, gave me continual assistance and occasional relief with his acerbic wit. Somerville Hospital and Long Island Hospital nursing and hospital officials gave me complete access to their hospital and nursing student records, and the American Nurses' Association gave me permission to use restricted materials in their papers in the Nursing Archives. The librarians at Boston University and Wellesley College answered myriad small and large queries, introduced me to the wonders of interlibrary loans, and gave me a "room[s] of one's own" to work in. If only I could also have had a coffee pot!

Colleagues and friends sustained my efforts. Gerd Korman and Maurice Neufeld first taught me social and labor history and nurtured my interests when I was their undergraduate student at Cornell. Only now can I begin to appreciate the excellence of their efforts. Susan Bell willingly listened to endless parts of this study. Her broad knowledge of medicine's development, as well as her feminist sense of sisterhood, was invaluable at critical junctures. Lise Vogel provided me with a theoretical perspective I did not always share but which I always considered and learned from. My "informal work group" in graduate school shaped this book's earlier incarnation. I am grateful to Susan Porter Benson, Brian Gratton, Janet Golden, Linda Hansen, Barbara Hobson, Peter Holloran, Susan Porter, and Eric Schneider. Sam Bass Warner, Jr., pushed me to have faith in my own ideas. Diana Long and Janet Wilson James were my initial guides into health-care history and always my most important critics. They were the master "craftspersons" to emulate.

Other historians, also engaged in the rewriting of nursing and medical history, were continual points of reference. I wish to thank Susan Armeny, Darlene Clark Hine, Barbara Melosh, Jane Mottus, David Rosner, and Nancy Tomes for deepening my understanding of the complexity of our joint enterprise.

Others made the monumental effort to read and criticize earlier drafts. Charles Rosenberg always encouraged my efforts and made pithy and appropriate suggestions. His standards and commitment to scholarship guided my thinking. Unlike many other established scholars, he was never too busy to help, and his gifts of photocopies from obscure archives were very welcome. Allan Brandt, Nona Glazer, Mary Katzenstein, and Morris Vogel saw through the compilation of facts in earlier drafts to the critical questions. Joan Jacobs Brumberg raised the important women's history queries and broadened this study's relevance. My colleagues in the Department of Philosophy at Wellesley College, Katheryn Doran, Daniel Little, Ifeanyi Menkiti, Ken Winkler, and especially Owen Flanagan, guided my inquiries into the issues of duties and rights.

Financial support came in many different forms. The initial research was funded by the Milbank Multidisciplinary Program in Health Services, Research and Policy, the National Center for Health Services Research, DHSS, grant #RO 3 HS 02879-01, and the American Studies Program at Boston University. A Faculty Research Grant from Wellesley College made it possible for me to make the transition from fountain pens and paper to the computer. A number of Wellesley student typists were the laborers in this effort: Becki Ledbetter most of all and then, Gwin Wheatley, Robbin Evans, Dawn Fitzgerald, Kristin Powers, Catherine McKean, Faith Ferguson, and Carla Danella. At Cambridge University Press, Helen Wheeler, Rhona Johnson, and Janis Bolster guided the book through. Mary Byers caught my unconscious sexist language and struggled to clarify my writing.

Portions of several previous articles of mine have been revised and incorporated here, and I am grateful for permission to use these materials:

"The Search for the Hospital Yardstick: Nursing and the Rationalization of Hospital Work," which appeared in *Health Care in America: Essays in Social History,* ed. Susan Reverby and David Rosner (Philadelphia: Temple University Press, 1979), pp. 206–25

" 'Something Besides Waiting': The Politics of Private Duty Nursing Reform in the Depression," reprinted by permission of the publisher from Ellen Condliffe Lagemann, ed., *Nursing History: New Perspectives, New Possibilities* (New York: Teachers College Press, © 1983, Teachers College-Columbia University; all rights reserved), pp. 133–56

" 'Neither for the Drawing Room nor for the Kitchen': Private Duty Nursing in Boston, 1873–1914," which appeared in *Women and Health in America,* ed. Judith Walzer Leavitt (Madison: University of Wisconsin Press, 1984), pp. 454–66

"A Caring Dilemma: Womanhood and Nursing in Historical Perspective," *Nursing Research* 35 (January–February 1987)

I also thank the American Nursing Association for use of the "American Nursing Association Board of Directors Minutes," 1920–45, American Nursing Association Papers, Nursing Archives, Boston University.

My family did what one would hope: They tolerated my efforts. My children were born at the beginning and the end of this project, perhaps in my twentieth-century feminist's way of proving to Edward Clarke that women could use their brains and their wombs. Mariah and Micah made me want to stop working, and Pat Medeiros, Ann Harris, Tot Lot, and the Rosa Parks-Saundra Graham Alternative Public School of Cambridge made it possible for me not to worry about them when I was. Robert and Juanita Sieber accepted that this project kept me from longer visits to their home. My parents, Gertrude and Reuben Mokotoff, encouraged my foray into their medical world, even if they thought the form it took was peculiar. Tim Sieber shared equally in all the difficulties of running a two-career academic household and managed to listen to my midnight worries, correct my spelling and grammar, and remind me it was possible to finish. To all of them I am exceedingly grateful since their pride in my efforts sustained me.

My grandmother, Anna Fox, lived in a chronic-care hospital for over twenty years. She taught me much about the need for caring, and this book is dedicated to her memory and to my children she never lived to know or love.

Cambridge, Mass.

Introduction
The dilemma of caring

"Do not undervalue [your] particular ability to care," students were reminded at a recent nursing school graduation.[1] Rather than merely bemoaning yet another form of late-twentieth-century heartlessness, this
admonition underscores a crucial dilemma in contemporary American
nursing: the order to care in a society that refuses to value caring. This
book is a history of the creation of this dilemma and its consequences for
nursing. I will argue that nursing is a form of labor shaped by the
obligation to care. But its history, and ultimately its identity, cannot be
understood unless the bond that has wedded it to womanhood is also
unraveled and revealed.

Nurses, as do others who perform what our society defines as "women's
work," have always contended with the dichotomy between the duty and
desire to care for others and the right to control and define this activity.[2]
The balance between this duty and right has shifted over time as the circumstances of nursing have changed, but the obligation to care has been at
nursing's definitional core. When we become ill or injured, we expect to be
cared for as we hope for a cure. If our illness or injury is serious enough to
require help from those beyond our circle of family and friends, we turn to
some kind of nursing professional or worker for that care. Nursing as work
is thus based on our expectation and need for someone to take up the
obligation to care.

This caring is both an emotional and a material activity. In the words of
social-policy analyst Hilary Graham, "Caring touches simultaneously on
who you are and what you do."[3] Because of this duality, caring is an
unbounded act, difficult to define, even harder to control. Although much
has been written about caring from the perspective of individual nurse–
patient relationships, its historical consequences for nursing as a whole
have rarely been studied.[4]

This book examines the failure of our society to create the conditions
under which the desire to care can be valued. But on second thought, it is
more about limitations imposed upon nursing than failure. Nurses, whatever else can be charged against them, continuously try to meet their

obligations to care. Nurses have, however, confronted a series of limitations – of imagination, of cultural ideology, of economics, and ultimately
of political power – in their efforts to care. This book is really, therefore, a
study of constraints.

In nursing, these constraints took ideological, cultural, and structural
forms. At first nursing was grounded in the expectation that caring was
part of a woman's duty to her family or community. As some nursing
moved out of the realm of unpaid family labor into the marketplace, the
assumption that it would still be work of love, not money, remained. The
ideology of nursing, based on nineteenth-century understandings of
women's duties, but not of women's rights, gave trained nursing purpose
but limited its power to control or define its occupational or professional
existence.

Nursing as work was transformed in the context of the growth of our
contemporary health system. It is impossible to retell the story of nursing
without understanding its relationship to the development of medicine.
Furthermore, the political economy of the hospital as an institution is as
much a part of nursing's history as the political economy of nursing, in
turn, is integral to the history of the hospital and of medicine.

Under a conception of duty and within the hospital's walls, nursing
became the work of women who created, as much as possible, "a little
world of our own."[5] But this world was not always the familial and
sharing culture so eloquently evoked by recent women's histories.[6]
Rather, nurses were forced into an overcrowded, sex-segegated labor market where women of differing educations, classes, races, and ethnic origins
contended for the title of "nurse." Political unity became difficult to
achieve as differences undermined the basis for solidarity created by common gender. The process of professionalization and the creation of a common work culture were fractured both by patriarchal constraints from
above and differences among women from within.[7]

This historical study of the dilemmas confronting American nursing in
the nearly one hundred years between 1850 and the end of World War II is
structured in a narrative and chronological form. Before the 1870s, the
hospital was not a central institution for the provision of medical care, nor
was nursing an important form of paid labor for women. Medical care
was the work of a variety of lay healers and sectarian medical practitioners. It was provided mainly in a patient's home, although care could
also be sought in a physician's office, a dispensary, or a hospital outpatient
clinic. Nursing was the duty of female relatives or neighbors, assisted or
replaced, on occasion, by a hired, usually older, woman.

The hospital, in turn, was a marginal social-welfare institution for the
needy and the homeless, as well as the sick, whose clientele were more
inmates than patients. Minimal nursing care was provided either by ambu-

latory patients or a motley group of untrained attendants, labeled "nurses," whose abilities ranged from brute strength to self-taught skills developed during years of intelligent service.

The link between hospitals and nursing was forged in the context of post–Civil War social-welfare reform. Urban growth, changes in medical practice and education, and economic necessity exerted the pressures that led slowly, but inexorably, to the growth of hospitals as multiclass centers for the provision, and selling, of medical and nursing care. In 1873, elite social reformers, concerned with finding "respectable" service work for the daughters of the "middling classes," and with improving the hospitals, introduced the first hospital-based training schools.[8] These nursing schools provided the hospitals with a work force that made their institutional growth possible, while training provided women with a "secular ministry" within the expanding "benevolent empire" of Christian voluntarism.[9]

Training produced both a new hospital work force and a new hospital order. The pupil nurse was to exchange her practical labor in the hospital for her education in its school in the art and science of nursing. Genteel "good" women were to become disciplined soldiers in the war against disease and disorder, self-sacrificing mothers to the patients, efficient housekeepers for the hospitals, loyal and subordinate assistants to the physicians, and firm supervisors of the hospital's other workers. Upon graduation, a few trained nurses were to return to the hospitals as head nurses, supervisors, or superintendents; the majority sought work in patients' homes as private-duty nurses, or as "specials" for the hospitals' relatively few private patients. By the turn of the century, students, along with untrained attendants in hospitals without schools, became the hospital's nursing work force. It would not be until the 1930s that the majority of graduate trained nurses would find work on hospital staffs.

The hospital's need for a work force, and the nursing school's financial dependence on the hospital, led to training that was more work than learning. The nursing stress on womanly duty, submission, and practical labor gave hospitals the ideological justification for what quickly became outright exploitation. A reasonable and caring sense of order could barely be taught, as harsh discipline and practical work were necessitated by never-ending patient demands. Nor could the students learn the increasingly technical and administrative skills they needed when work demands, rather than an educational program, governed their training. Nursing superintendents were continually forced to choose between their responsibility to educate their pupils and the inevitable pressures to use them to complete the work.

What constituted training to become a "good" nurse, or the best way to perform nursing procedures, was an ongoing issue. Nursing became an occupation filled with women of diverse skills, training, abilities, education, class backgrounds, and work experiences. In the work world outside the hospital, trained nurses competed with other nurses, trained and untrained alike, for employment. The expansion in the number and size of training schools, but the failure of hospitals to hire graduates, created an oversupply of nurses and unemployment as early as the 1890s. Nursing became overcrowded, unstandardized, and disordered, despite efforts to bring the disorder under control.

The very factors that caused these problems also made it difficult to achieve accord. Nursing leaders, the educators and administrators who headed the national nursing organizations, saw the dilemmas as stemming from nursing's failure to obtain professional status and control of the occupation's open entry gate. They pursued a voluntary and legislative strategy to upgrade educational standards, obtain state licensure, introduce efficiency, and eventually sever the link between nursing education and the hospital's nursing service.

Many in the nursing work force, however, were less convinced that the problem stemmed from low educational standards and need for professional status. These women saw the difficulties as lack of work and respect for their individual skills and efforts. To them, the leadership's strategy was inappropriate, irrelevant, or threatening, and they often refused to follow it. In turn, hospital officials and physicians, who mainly saw the problems as caused by nursing's efforts to obtain professional autonomy, continually urged submission to their control.

Nursing's transition to paid and trained labor did not change the assumption that the work was based on womanly duty requiring service to others and acquiescence to the authority of physicians. The hospital, well after it became a service institution selling medical and nursing care as a commodity, continued the social relations appropriate to a charitable social-welfare institution. Thus by the 1890s many nursing leaders saw in the social relations of advanced capitalism – the reliance on wage labor, the separation of manual and mental work, the creation of the specialist-expert, and the development of a quantitative "scientific" rationality – the possibility for order and professional control in nursing. In such rationality, they believed, lay nursing's freedom from the paternalistic relationship to the hospitals and the patriarchal control of physicians.[10] Such rationality, however, also provided the basis for a new set of problems, as nurses quickly discovered.

Part I is a brief examination of the experienced, but untrained, nurse and her work in the years just before nursing schools were introduced. Chapter 1 is concerned with nurses and nursing in the home; Chapter 2 is about the hospital and its work force. Part II examines the ideology and structure of nurses' training and work as it developed and changed between 1873 and 1945. Chapters 3 and 4 explore the trained nursing model and its limitations in the hospital context, and Chapters 5 and 6 examine the backgrounds of the women who entered training and the factors that determined where they worked upon graduation. Although the focus is mainly on hospitals and nursing in Boston and New York, I have drawn upon national data and trends where appropriate.

Part III delves into the various political strategies nursing developed for reform and professional control that grew out of its ideology and place in the health-care industry. Chapter 7 lays out the main thrust, difficulties, and criticism of the nursing leaders' earliest efforts. Chapter 8 considers why the concept and schemes of efficiency, as they were being redefined and fashioned during the Progressive Era, held such promise, and trouble, as a basis for nursing reform. Chapters 9 and 10 suggest how the quest for reform came to depend on cooperation between nursing and the hospitals, an acceptance of division of labor within nursing, a credentials-based nursing hierarchy, and the graduate trained nurse as the "line manager" of the hospital's nursing work force.

Several terms warrant definitional clarity. The first part of the book concerns the untrained women called "nurses" by their contemporaries. The main focus is on the group originally called "trained" or "graduate" nurses, whom we would now refer to as RNs or registered nurses. After the introduction of training in 1873, untrained workers were variously labeled practical nurses, nurses' aids or aides, attendants, subsidiary nursing workers, or ward helpers. The term "nursing students" refers to those in the hospital training schools. The "nursing leadership" were the educators and supervisors who headed or advised the major professional nursing associations.

This book is both a study of nursing and hospitals in the area surrounding Boston and an attempt to widen its relevance to assess national reforms. The chronology of changes thus balances the historical specificity of one community's experience with its implications for American nursing as a whole. Similarly, I have limited the study to the history of white female nurses. I now regret that time, my circumscribed knowledge, and the racist blinders that limit so much of our education did not let me explore the relationship of race to gender and class in nursing. I am at least assured that such a history is being written by able hands. Similarly, the histories of the relatively few men who entered nursing and of the religious orders that nursed remain to be written.[11]

Ordered to Care is meant to be a contribution to the historiography of nursing, medical, labor, and women's history since nursing touches on all these areas of intellectual scholarship. In some ways my work is perhaps closest to JoAnn Ashley's *Hospitals, Paternalism and the Role of the Nurse* because we both examine the hospital–nursing relationship.[12] Ashley argued that the sexism of physicians and hospital paternalism kept nurses subservient and exploited. However, her anger toward the hospitals and physicians, and the determinism of her model, allowed her to see only the evidence of accommodation and passivity. She thus failed to explain under what conditions accommodation yielded to resistance and noncooperation on the part of some, or why others actively saw accommodation as salvation. In her effort to comprehend nursing's current dilemmas, Ashley too harshly judged and blamed its past. Nurses are neither the poor victims of hospital and physician oppression and the impotent descendants of a long line of women healers, nor the victors in a difficult and long struggle to gain professional recognition and status. Their history is more complicated than such simplistic analyses, built on either anger or romanticism.

The relationship between class and gender is also an essential element in the nursing story I tell. Ashley, among others, suggests that nursing stands as an example of a women's work culture that did not generate or share either an understanding of women's oppression or a feminist politics (although, I would add, it could become overtly and covertly anti-male).[13] Neither Ashley nor the older nursing histories have dealt with the ways class divisions within the nursing culture made a feminist politics difficult to achieve. Only Barbara Melosh's book, "*The Physician's Hand,*" provides a sophisticated analysis of the work culture of twentieth-century nursing and the tensions between the nursing leadership's quest for professional power and the rank and file's efforts to maintain control.[14] I share much of Melosh's perspective but have cast my study back into the nineteenth century and within a broader historical framework of the political economy of the hospital's development.

Nursing's history provides us with a specific example of a group of women so divided by class that their common oppression based on gender could not unite them. It examines the material realities under which a women's culture, crippled by ideology and social conditions, becomes politicized in a manner that constrains its own efforts. Nursing suggests the difficulty of trying to forge a basis for political unity when heterogeneous experiences, classes, and beliefs divide a group. It illustrates the limits of an antiquated and inappropriate political language and vision that increasingly could not mobilize a constituency.[15]

Finally, this book is part of a larger body of historical work attempting to expand our understanding of health-care history.[16] Many social historians are no longer dazzled by the scientific advances of modern medicine and nursing, or have focused solely on the heroic efforts, however inspiring, of the "great doctors" and nurses. Instead, they are trying to understand the complexity of the relationships among scientific developments, occupational and professional reform, and the broad ideological, cultural, and economic transformations in our society. I hope this study contributes both to this historical revision and to nursing's urgent need for a more realistic understanding of the roots of its contemporary dilemmas. The value of caring is too important for this to be ignored.

PART I

The nurse and the hospital before training

1

"Professed" nursing: from duty to trade

In the world of early nineteenth-century America, more defined by death and debility than our own, almost every woman could expect to spend some part of her life caring for the infirmities and illnesses of relatives or friends. Cultural expectation was formed in part by societal necessity since few institutions relieved a family of this inevitable burden. Within the domestic boundaries of antebellum women's lives, nursing played an important and inextricable part as caring and sacrifice became a poignant manifestation of female virtue.

As other forms of women's labor entered the marketplace, the care of the sick remained firmly rooted in the home. No great nursing factory transformed this work as the textile mills along the Merrimac River changed home weaving and spinning. The work was not, however, always performed alone. Although a family first looked to its female members in time of illness, this labor, as with other women's domestic work, could be shared. A neighboring woman or the minister's wife could be called on for "night watching" or to provide extra food and medicine, while a young girl could be hired to "help" with other household tasks to relieve the overall burden of work. Nursing thus remained a woman's duty, not her job.[1]

At the same time, women who had to find paid work often traded on their household or community experiences and entered the ranks of those who nursed for a living. In the country's burgeoning urban areas in particular, families of the growing "middling" and upper classes had the income to pay for such a service. Thus by the eve of the Civil War, although most nursing continued to be done by women for relatives in their homes, the "natural-born" or "professed" nurse became an increasingly familiar figure. Nursing, as women's domestic labor structured by duty and custom, was very slowly supplemented by nursing, as women's paid labor reshaped by market forces and cultural changes.

A WOMAN'S LABOR

Caring for family members was supposed to be central to a woman's self-sacrificing service to others. In a society whose deeply felt religious tenets assigned virtues on the basis of sex, Catherine Beecher declared that the sick were to be "commended" to a "woman's benevolent ministries." Such ministries often became a life's work as the needs of family shaped a woman's experience.[2] In her responsibility for the family "in both sickness and in health," a woman's skills and abilities were sorely tested. Out of serious concern with these duties, women flocked to lectures at the Ladies' Physiological Institutes or to hear the latest from itinerant healers of various medical sects. They sought help from the domestic manuals that provided special recipes for feeding the ill, guidelines for simple healing, suggestions for remedies, and general support for the anxious.[3]

The responsibility for nursing went beyond a woman's duty toward her children, husband, or aging parents. It fell to all available female family members. At any time the family's "long arm" might reach out to a daughter working in a distant city or mill, bringing her home to care for the sick, infirm, or newborn. No form of women's labor, paid or unpaid, protected her from this homeward pull. "You may be called upon at any moment," Eliza W. Farrar warned in *The Young Lady's Friend,* "to attend upon your parents, your brothers, your sisters or your companions."[4]

Caring for one's friends and relatives could become a joyful sharing, a time of intimacy and fulfillment, or an unending burden. The task of nursing was often physically and emotionally exhausting, requiring great patience, skill, and strength. It consisted of careful watching; the preparation of special foods and tonics; the changing of dressings; the application of plasters, poultices, and leeches; the giving of massages, as well as the emotional comforting necessary for recovery or a peaceful death. The nobility of such effort could be lost in the long hours of caring for a chronically ill patient while other household demands continued. Even when additional "help" could be found to take over other tasks, the accumulated exhaustion caused by the work of nursing was frequently overwhelming.[5]

Women often recorded the negative aspects of this duty in their journals and letters. Harriet Beecher Stowe bewailed the demands her son's illness made upon her life, and Susan Huntington, a Boston minister's wife, complained of the trials caused by her family's ill health. Louisa May Alcott, who nursed two sisters and both of her parents, saw this work as necessary but terribly disruptive of her writing.[6] Sympathetically, physician S. Weir Mitchell saw such sustained nursing care as one of the precipitators of women's nervous conditions.[7]

Obligation and duty were supposed to bind the nurse to her patient. Advice writer Dr. William Alcott urged women to provide nursing care as a charitable duty because:

If we do all the good we are able to do, with our hands we feel that we have better discharged our duty than if we had first turned our labor into money, and then applied the money to the same purpose.[8]

By the 1840s, however, Alcott's views were increasingly seen as a bit "old-fashioned." Pressures both internal and external had already reshaped domestic life. Women's obligations and work were transformed by the expanding industrial economy and changing cultural assumptions. Parenting took on increasing importance in middle-class families, as notions of "moral mothering" took hold and other productive labor became marketable outside the home. Female benevolence similarly moved outward as women's charitable efforts took increasingly institutional forms. Duty began to take on new meanings.[9]

In this context of a new calculation of women's obligations, William Alcott's advice-giving contemporaries, Catharine Beecher and Sarah Josepha Hale, stressed that a woman could fulfill her nursing responsibilities by *managing* competently those she hired to assist her. Female virtue could still be demonstrated as the balance of labor, love, and supervision shifted.[10] If a woman could find neither love nor joy in the self-sacrifice, exhaustion, and disorder that often accompanied nursing, she could discharge her responsibilities by carefully selecting a nurse for her loved ones. Under varying sets of circumstances, nursing could be added to the list of tasks that could be passed onto another woman to perform. And in the country's burgeoning urban areas it was often easy to find women to pay to take on this work.[11] Despite William Alcott's admonition, money, not just love, obligation, or charity, could tie a nurse to her patients. Caring as love could be separated, for some, from caring as labor.

A NURSE'S WORK

Even when nursing became paid labor, its definition remained vague and linked to a variety of women's duties. The very casualness with which the term "nurse" was used reflected its ambiguous, seemingly naturalistic, meaning as five distinct groups were classified as nurses. The "child nurse" or "nursemaid," for example, was the domestic servant who functioned in the household as the caretaker-maid for infants and young children. She might also care for her charges when they were ill, but this was not her primary duty. The "wet nurse" was responsible for suckling infants when their natural mothers would not or could not do so. Although often held responsible if the infant became ill, she was not expected to care for the baby under these circumstances.[12]

The midwife was an *accoucheur* and general healer rather than a nurse. Sent for when a woman entered labor, she stayed through the delivery and perhaps another day. The midwife was often a herbalist and healer, a kind of all-around general practitioner. As a "specialist" with distinctive skills, her primary responsibility ended with the birth of the child. Any additional nursing care or housekeeping work was provided either by relatives, neighboring women, or what became known as the "monthly" nurse. Hired to assist with, but not to perform, the delivery, she then stayed on in the household for approximately a month, as her title suggests, to help with the housekeeping and the care of the mother and newborn.[13]

Most commonly, the nurse was a woman summoned to aid in the care of the sick and infirm. In the colonial period such women were well-known figures in their communities and usually were called in on a casual basis when female relatives were not available. Women nursed the poor on behalf of town or parish benevolence societies, or received either goods or money from neighbors as part of a barter economy.[14]

By the early nineteenth century, nursing began to emerge in the more formal urban marketplace as a category in the expanding field of domestic service. Although a nurse might perform the same tasks as a family's female members, as a hired outsider she became the patient's servant, not just the neighborhood friend.[15] Her work varied and depended on who was sick and how much other help the family could employ. A bedridden mother might leave the nurse with the household chores in one family but not in another. In a wealthy household, a nurse could station herself by the patient and call for the food to be brought up and the bedding to be washed. In another she might find herself running between the cookstove, the laundry tub, and the bedside.[16]

As the nurse gained in experience, she often increased the sureness of her diagnosis, the certainty of proclaiming her abilities. If no physician had been called, or indeed if the nurse disagreed with the doctor's recommended regimen, she felt free to diagnose and to change procedures on her own. Although not specifically accorded the title of "healer," such nurses sometimes parlayed a kind of learned expertise into medical advice. Disagreements over what she ought to do and how she should do it were common. In the melange that characterized antebellum American medicine, physicians were not considered to have the monopoly on therapeutic wisdom.[17]

The social relations among nurses, physicians, and families varied considerably. In some communities, these women were highly respected and revered, known for their healing skills, and expected to prescribe for ordinary ailments. Others were remembered as haughty, demanding, stubborn, and unaware of their own ignorance. Some were meek and docile, willing to take any order a family or physician might give; others were impossible to manage or to discipline.[18] Massachusetts physician Alfred Worcester remembered fondly the orphaned girl who became a domestic servant, then a nightwatcher and nurse in his great-grandfather's home in the 1860s. "Miss Green," he recalled, became an "experienced nurse" whose "fame" matched her "efficiency."[19] In contrast, Louisa May Alcott, forced by her own ill health toward the end of her life to hire a nurse for her father, complained:

Much trouble with nurses; have no idea of health; won't walk, sit over the fire and drink tea three times a day; ought to be intelligent, hearty set of women. Could do better myself; have to fill up all the deficiencies and do double duty.[20]

The nurse was in an ambiguous position within the service hierarchy of a household, being neither as lowly as a simple domestic, nor as highly placed as a cook. Although she was expected to stay in the household on call twenty-four hours a day, sleeping in the patient's room, often for months at a time, it was assumed she was not as "permanent" as a regular domestic nor as "transient" as the outside laundress.[21] Paid both by the day and by the week, the nurse's wage rate placed her somewhere between a seamstress and a cook. Gratuities increased the pay and became expected.[22] One nurse declared that men were better patients because "they are sure either to pay better wages or make presents."[23] Wages and tips had to somehow compensate for the irregularity of employment and the necessity of keeping a room or flat for use between cases. With the uncertainty and unevenness inherent in the work, many women supplemented it with sewing or other domestic service.

Throughout the nineteenth century, increasing numbers of women slowly eased into the occupation. As domestic service became the domain of black and immigrant women toward the end of the century, nursing remained primarily the work of white, native-born, poor, and older women. A middle-class woman like Louisa May Alcott sometimes might serve as a companion-nurse to an invalid, but this was the exception. Despite occasional reminders of nursing's virtue as women's work, once in the marketplace it was too closely associated with domestic service to become the work of the more genteel woman in need of wages.[24]

Age and marital status, however, rather than class, race, or nativity, separated the nurse from domestic servants or other working women. In contemporary novels, histories, and advice books, the nurse is portrayed as an "old lady." Even the term "granny," primarily used synonymously or in connection with "midwife," was applied to the nurse. Such cultural expectation was reflected in the statistics: Most white women who sought wage labor were in their twenties, whereas nurses tended to be in their thirties or forties.[25]

Shifts in a woman's marital status often preceded her entry into nursing. Marriage to a very poor man, divorce or abandonment, or widowhood were often preconditions for nursing. Widowhood, in particular, appears to have been an important, if cruel, pathway into nursing. By 1890, the percentage of widows in nursing was more than twice that in all female occupations or in other domestic and personal service work.[26] With no need for formal credentials, a woman could offer her experience of caring for a dying husband as her qualification to nurse. For women in the precarious "state of affliction" that characterized widowhood, finding work as a nurse was often a positive alternative to the almshouse, keeping boarders, domestic service, or the uncertain dependence on grown children.[27]

Mehitabel Pond Knott Garside, a widow who turned to nursing, typified these statistics. Born in 1783 in Brookline, Massachusetts, she married Aaron Knott, a mechanic, and bore four children. When Knott died she married again, to James Garside, but outlived him as well. Widowhood introduced her to wage labor and nursing. She continued to nurse until her sixty-eighth year, when, unable to continue working and receiving no financial aid from her children, who by then had moved away, she applied for assistance to the Boston Home for Aged Women.[28] The case records of the home allow us to probe more specifically into the life course of a "professed" nurse like Garside and the other Boston women who shared her fate.

THE PROFESSED NURSE

In old age and poverty, Mehitabel Garside and her sister nurses turned to the Home for Aged Women as a viable alternative to the almshouse. Beginning in 1850, the home became one of the many benevolent institutions established by Boston's upper class for the respectable poor, in this case, for "retired" working women, primarily domestics. Caroline Doane, a wealthy Boston matron, left a bequest specifically for "a most deserving class, the Nurses of our city . . . [who] can look to us for a home and for the care and sympathy which they as a class so richly merit."[29]

Reflecting nursing's ambiguous meaning, Doane's bequest for "sick nurses" was used to provide for women who had cared for the sick, as well as the monthly nurse and nursemaid.[30] The limitations placed on women applying to the Doane Fund were similar to those for all women applying to the home: They had to be native-born and over sixty. In addition, two reputable Boston physicians had to vouch for "the respectability of their character, and the propriety of their conduct."[31]

Seventy-five percent of the nurses who ended their days in the home began life on the farms and in the small towns of rural New England (see Table 1.1). As with the former domestic servants in the home, a third of the nurses identified their father's occupation as farmer. The largest numbers were the daughters of skilled artisans – blacksmiths, masons, shoe-

Table 1.1. *Birthplace of nurses in Home for Aged Women, 1850–1912*

Birthplace	Number	%
Boston	35	26.5
Massachusetts (outside of Boston)	38	28.8
Maine	34	25.8
New Hampshire	19	14.4
Rhode Island	1	1.0
Vermont	3	2.3
Nova Scotia – New Brunswick	2	1.5
Total	132	

Source: Admission Records, 1850–1912, Home for Aged Women Collection, Box 11, Schlesinger Library, Radcliffe College, Cambridge, Mass.

makers, mechanics, and carpenters – as well as mariners, sailors, sea captains, and ship's carpenters. Mary Barker, for example, born in 1775, the daughter of a Gloucester shoemaker, came to Boston at the age of thirty-five, never married, and became a domestic servant in the Cambridge home of a Harvard professor. "In later life," she told the home's registrar, she became a nurse.

Marriage even to men in seemingly higher occupational categories than their fathers did little to protect these women in their widowhood from the vicissitudes of the economy (see Table 1.2). Mary Grace never left her Boston birthplace; she was the widow of a ship's carpenter and mother of fourteen children, only three of whom were still alive when she applied to the home. When her husband died, she turned to nursing work in patients' homes, alternating this with nightwatching at Massachusetts General Hospital.[32]

Marital status most clearly differentiated the nurses from other women in the home (see Table 1.3). In a study of the home's residents for the years 1850–80, Carol Lasser found that roughly half the women had never married. Those women who had done only domestic service were more likely to be single: The ratio of single to ever-married in this category was 70 to 30.[33] In contrast, for the comparable years, the nurses had almost the exact reverse in marital rates: More than 60 percent of the nurses were widowed, separated, or divorced, and only 40 percent had remained single throughout their lives.

Migration, age, and employment histories supply additional evidence of this age-specific characteristic of nursing. For daughters of farmers and artisans in declining trades, as Lasser has argued, migration to the city offered the opportunity for work and possible marriage. In contrast, more

Table 1.2. *Fathers' and husbands' occupation categories for nurses in Home for Aged Women, 1850–1912*

Occupational category	Fathers		Husbands	
	Number	%	Number	%
Professional – high white collar	3	2.4	3	3.9
Low white collar	15	11.9	16	20.8
Skilled	44	34.9	45	58.4
Semiskilled	21	16.7	3	3.9
Unskilled	3	2.4	2	2.6
Farmers	40	31.7	8	10.4
Total	126	100.0	77	100.0

Note: This table does not compare fathers' and husbands' occupations; for example, the three nurses whose fathers were high white collar are not necessarily the same three whose husbands were in this category.

Source: See Table 1.1.

Table 1.3. *Marital status of women in Home for Aged Women, by previous occupation, 1850–1912*

Marital status	Nurses		Women who did only domestic work		Women who did domestic and other work	
	Number	%	Number	%	Number	%
Ever-married	43	61.4	11	27.5	88	52.7
Single	27	38.6	29	72.5	79	49.3
Total	70	100.0	40	100.0	167	100.0

Source: See Table 1.1. and Carol Lasser, " 'The World's Dread Laugh': Singlehood and Service in Nineteenth-Century Boston," in *The New Labor History and the New England Working Class,* ed. Donald Bell and Herbert Gutman (Urbana: University of Illinois Press, 1984).

than half of the nurses as a group had migrated *after* they were thirty, at an age when there were fewer options for work and marriage.[34] The home's records do not reveal if these women were nurses before moving to Boston, or if the death of a spouse, in the case of the widows, drew them to

Table 1.4. *Occupational histories of nurses in Home for Aged Women, 1850–1912*

Occupations	Single		Ever-married		Totals	
	Number	%	Number	%	Number	%
Just nursing	17	36.2	39	47.6	56	43.4
Nursing & sewing	14	29.8	24	29.3	38	29.5
Nursing & domestic service	14	29.8	18	22.0	32	24.8
Nursing & sales-work or teaching	2	4.3	1	1.2	3	2.3
Total	47		82		129	

Source: See Table 1.1.

nursing and to the city. But they do provide further evidence of the age-specificity of nursing.

The nurses' migration ages by marital status and occupational histories suggest two slightly different patterns. When migration age was broken down by marital status, the single nurses tended to come to Boston before age thirty at a rate comparable to that of the domestics. Only the ever-married nurses were more likely to migrate later in their lives. Their occupational histories were different as well. Less than half of all the home's nurses reported that they had only done nursing, but of those who had, widows or abandoned wives made up nearly 70 percent, or 18 percent more than in the home's nursing population. The single women came to Boston at a younger age, had more varied occupational histories, and worked both as domestics and in the sewing trades before nursing. The widows, if they did work other than nursing, were slightly more likely to be in the sewing trades, a not uncommon pattern for older women (see Table 1.4).[35] Of the seventy women who had done other work in addition to nursing, 66 percent declared nursing their last occupation at about the same rate for single and ever-married women. Although single and ever-married nurses had slightly different occupational histories, both groups primarily entered nursing at the end of their working lives, even if they supplemented their meager nursing incomes with some sewing or other domestic work.

Alma Frost Merrill, for example, the daughter of a Maine wheelwright and justice of the peace, came to Boston in 1818 when she was nineteen years old to become a domestic servant. She worked as a nurse and seamstress, as she put it, "laterly." In contrast, Eleanor Young, also a spinster daughter of a Maine farmer, did not leave home until she was nearly forty and came to Boston to do both "house service and nursing." Elizabeth Bigelow, born on a New Hampshire farm, married a druggist and lived in New Hampshire, New York, and New Orleans. He died when she was forty-nine years old, and she moved to Boston and became a nurse.[36]

Necessity and cultural expectation met in the nursing marketplace. Older women did not so much choose nursing as slip into it through life experiences and lack of other options. Nearly 90 percent of the widows reported to the home that they were left with nothing when their spouses died. "Died poor," "was intemperate – did nothing for his family," and "left some property which was lost" are typical testaments to the hard world of nineteenth-century widowhood.[37] A widow who turned to nursing as a livelihood illustrated Virginia Penny's opinion that "to make a kind and sympathizing nurse, one must have waited, in sickness, upon those she loved dearly."[38] Others, having raised children, could also claim competence and experience in nursing the young. A domestic servant could also report experience with illness in the households she had served. A sympathetic physician or druggist willing to add a woman to his "lists," an ad placed in the city directory, or just word of mouth in a neighborhood, could begin to establish a woman as a nurse. With such ease of job entry, not surprisingly, nearly a quarter of all the women who applied to the home between 1850 and 1886 had been nurses at some point.

"Private nursing," a mid-nineteenth-century hospital nurse recalled, "was only considered suitable employment for elderly women." It was a position, a contemporary physician stated, for the "Widow Smith and Spinster Green."[39] There are several explanations for this cultural assumption. With no formal apprenticeship, a woman needed to claim some years of familial service to the sick to be accepted as a nurse. A younger woman might be allowed to do some nursing, but it was expected that her "natural-born" tendencies could not manifest themselves without practice and life experience.

Fears surrounding sexuality and contagion, as well as the demands of nursing, played roles in establishing this age-specific expectation. The exposure of an older motherly woman to naked bodies, especially those of men, was deemed neither shocking nor arousing. William Alcott's attempt to allay young women's fears of contagion, if they thought about becoming nurses, suggests that there were societal apprehensions about exposing such women to disease.[40] Finally, since it was assumed that nursing demanded twenty-four-hour attention, women were expected not to be burdened with their own families or children. Only an older widow without dependent children or an older spinster would be assumed to be able to give such concentrated attention.

Nursing remained confined to the household until the opening decades of the twentieth century because most sickness, birthing, and dying took place in the home. Considered part of a woman's natural work, nursing was an art practiced by women within their own families, or for other relatives or neighbors. But as notions of virtuous middle-class womanhood became more defined in emotional and maternal terms, nursing became a less important aspect of the parameters of such womanhood. Because it was also a skill a woman could learn in her own home or while a domestic servant in someone else's, it could easily become a trade to be "professed" in the marketplace.

Nursing became a trade because women were available to perform the work for wages, and urban middling- and upper-class families were willing and able to pay for this service. A fluctuating economy provided the cash for some women to pay for nursing, while it forced others to seek the work. By midcentury, physicians assumed a family might make use of both relatives and hired labor and tailored their advice accordingly.[41] Nurses became increasingly common figures as certain women had to cross the permeable boundary between household and market. By 1870, over 10,000 women practiced this trade in the United States; by 1940, the number had climbed to over 100,000.[42] Throughout these years paid nursing remained the province primarily of older women with no formal training or schooling. Even after training for nurses began in 1873, the professed or practical nurse (as she began to be called) remained a fixed member of the nursing work force. Those reformers who would seek to redefine the nature and status of nursing would continually have to contend with this cultural identification of nursing with both the caring and virtuous woman and the more truculent and older domestic servant.

2

Chaos and order in hospital nursing

An illness did not always confine patients to their own beds and to the care of loving relatives or hired household help. Circumstances, usually old age, isolation, or poverty, made household-based care difficult to pay for or to obtain. Under such conditions, patients might find themselves in hospitals under the "care" of a variety of men and women nurses, attendants or orderlies.

The nineteenth-century hospital in its appearance and social role, however, bore little resemblance to its modern equivalent. It was a marginal institution primarily for society's most marginal people: the sick, poor, or displaced members of the lower working class.[1] Most nineteenth-century Americans lived and died never entering, and perhaps never seeing, such places, for the country had only 120 hospitals when the first official national survey was taken in 1873.[2] The historical terms to define a hospital, a "hospice," or home for the destitute or sick, and a "spital," or foul and loathsome place, had real significance for Americans at that time. And such opprobrious terms for institutions left their marks on those who labored within them.

Within the hierarchy of paid labor, the hospital nurse was considered very near the bottom, caught in a degraded job in a fearsome institution. Unlike the professed nurse who became a household member only for the duration of a patient's illness, the hospital nurse was confined to the institution for both home and workplace. Many were partially recovered patients who were pressed into nursing duties. Before the 1870s, no nurses had any formal training or schooling for the work. Hospital nurses were considered the dregs of female society – mainly women who drank themselves into oblivion to endure their seemingly thankless and wretched labors of cleaning, feeding, and watching over the hospital's inmates. In the pejorative words of Florence Nightingale, hospital nurses were women "who were too old, too weak, too drunken, too dirty, too stolid, or too bad to do anything else."[3]

This description tells us more about Nightingale's reformer's rhetoric, however, than about the reality of institutional nursing. Within the close confines of the hospital's walls flourished a much more varied social order, created as much by the nurses as by those who tried to control them.

THE HOSPITAL AS A HOME

The hospitals that did exist were part of the complex of institutions for the dependent, deviant, and poor that began to be built at the end of the eighteenth century. Some hospitals grew out of public almshouses, but most were voluntary institutions established through the charitable efforts of the middling and upper classes. "Dependence as much as disease," a historian succinctly noted, defined the hospital's patients.[4] Social welfare, almost more than medical care, similarly defined the hospital's purpose. Hospitals were homes for the sick, dependent poor, many with long-term illnesses, rather than multiclass acute-care facilities.

Nineteenth-century medical etiology as well as social welfare structured the hospital's existence. Sharp lines between individuals and their environment, between moral behavior and illness, even between disease entities, had not yet been carefully drawn. For the majority of the hospital's patients, the regimen meted out discipline as well as beef tea and rest. Disease and dependence were intimately linked, and "moral treatment," "Christian nurturance," and exposure to proper discipline were all part of the curing and caring. Thus, in eulogizing Miss Sarah J. Wry, a midcentury nurse at the Massachusetts General Hospital, the hospital trustees noted "her moral influence over many a patient went further towards bringing about recovery than any other means she used. Remember her, in the way she would most wish to be remembered, as the *Good Nurse.*"[5]

Although most institutions served primarily a lower-working-class and semi-chronically ill population, the distinctions between public and voluntary institutions emerged in the eighteenth century. The public institutions, for the most part, became hospitals by increments as urban almshouses had to provide space for the care of the sick among their indigent inmates.[6] Voluntary hospitals were established by wealthy benefactors because of personal ties to physicians, a belief in moral stewardship, and a realization that some central location had to be found, outside the almshouse, for the "deserving and respectable poor" who were ill. Curability also distinguished the patients of the institutions. Chronically ill or consumptive patients, or those with venereal disease, were often barred from voluntaries. The public and voluntary hospitals were therefore attempts to build institutions that conformed to the nineteenth-century categories separating the deserving from the undeserving poor.[7]

Hospitals, whether voluntaries or public institutions, were primarily charity institutions supported by funds collected from church societies, donations and bequests, and governmental outlays, although patients were

encouraged to pay if possible. In most voluntaries some space was reserved for those who could pay extra for their care. Many hospitals had
one or two handsomely appointed rooms with damask drapes and heavy
cherry furniture for such "pay patients." But the very existence of such
rooms, and the differential treatment afforded these patients, only served
as a counterpoint to the institutions' more functional charitable nature.
Filth and neglect, rather than fancy drapes, characterized many of the
wards in institutions, particularly the larger public hospitals. The woodcut
of rats crawling over the comatose body of a young female Bellevue
patient that appeared in *Harper's Weekly* in 1860 drew attention to the
worst problems of hospitals. Dirt, vermin, and rampant cross-infection,
known as "hospitalism," were common. Benevolence did not necessarily
mean comfort or cleanliness.

The necessity for creating institutions for the centralized care of the
dependent sick came in part from the religious doctrine of moral stewardship. The doctrine held that divisions between rich and poor were natural
and inevitable but that the rich held their wealth in trust for the Lord.
Providing for the poor was part of this trust. Such endeavors were to be
rewarded ultimately by God and on earth by gestures of gratitude from
the lowly suffering patients. By the 1870s ideas of obligation were mixed
with the language of class relations of explanations of the hospital's mission. "The only sure way to reconcile labor to capital is to show the
laborer by actual deeds that the rich man regards himself as the steward of
the Master," Bostonians were reminded in a newspaper article on hospitals
in 1879.[8]

The attempt to enforce such class reconciliation was fostered by the link
between moral and medical cures and the continual metaphorical reference
to the hospital as a home. Patients were reminded that the hospital was a
home in which they were errant children in need of constant discipline.
The effort to create strict order and discipline, in the name of home life,
permeated the hospital as it did other nineteenth-century social-welfare
institutions.[9] Rigid rules for behavior were established to regulate daily
life; hours, visiting, and tobacco and liquor consumption were limited.
Those who transgressed the regulations faced dietary restrictions and even
punishment cells. The paternalism that pervaded the institutions sought to
define the boundaries of the patients' daily lives as much as the high walls
surrounding the institutions physically confined them.[10]

Patients did not always accept such charity, or disciplining and incar-
ceration, with deference and thankfulness. Most tried to avoid hospitalization. Others were willing to use the institutions, but only on terms that set
limits on the hospitals' jurisdiction. Massachusetts General Hospital surgeons, for instance, amputated the leg of a seven-year-old Irish girl after a
railway accident. In addition, the hospital could have extracted three hun-

dred dollars from the Maine Railroad in compensation if the girl would live in their institution, attend school nearby, and apprentice to become a hospital seamstress. Her parents refused this extra "help." At the Boston Lying-In Hospital, working-class women continuously circumvented the rules that allowed a woman only one illegitimate birth in the hospital by changing their names upon return visits. Rules prohibiting tobacco, food, and alcohol were constantly broken in the ongoing struggle between patients and those in control. Women at the Lying-In thought they could return whenever they wanted, leave their babies off while they went out looking for work, or use the hospital for lodging when nothing else could be found.[11]

Such behavior was possible because most patients were not acutely ill and could move around the institutions. Since most patient stays lasted weeks and months, not days, there was enough time to learn how to skirt the rules. Because most hospitals were relatively small, bureaucratic rules either did not exist or were easily ignored. The Massachusetts General in 1870 had only 137 patients in the "house" when it was full, and an average of only 120 on a normal day. On any given day in the 1870s, the Boston Lying-In housed only 14 patients. Some cities had large public hospitals, like New York's Bellevue with 1,000 beds in 1865, but the average hospital had less than 150 beds, with many providing space for only 10 to 20 patients at a time.[12]

The hospital's authority structure reflected the home as a model, modified to fit the division of labor typical for industries of the time. Trustees, usually male unless the hospital was built by women, controlled daily life in multiple ways.[13] As required by moral stewardship and general business practices, their main responsibility was financial, although deficits were expected and served as indexes of the hospital's usefulness and service. But these deficits had to be made up by collections by the "Saturday and Sunday" societies, church groups, bequests, the general public's donations, and, most important, by the trustees themselves. In addition, the trustees were concerned with admissions, rates of pay, extensions of free care, and the screening out of incurable patients. Complaints by patients and staff were listened to by individual trustees who made frequent visits to the wards and clinics. The position of hospital trustee, though limited to the elite, was hardly honorific. It was a serious and time-consuming responsibility.

The hospital superintendent or steward was just below the trustees in authority. Usually male, he ordered supplies, hired and fired servants and nurses, and in general oversaw the running of the institution. Frugality was expected and skimming from the hospital funds not uncommon. If the hospital was large enough, there was also a matron (commonly the superintendent's wife) who organized the daily work of the nurses and

servants and was responsible for supervising and for the cooking, washing, and cleaning of this enormous "household." In smaller institutions,
particularly those for women and children, the offices of matron and
superintendent were combined. Eliza Higgins, the matron and superintendent of the Boston Lying-In between 1873 and 1914, had responsibilities
that ran from worrying if the laundry would dry in the damp basements in
the winter to the keeping of the hospital's books. She spent much of her
summer and early fall, as would any genteel lady or head household
servant, overseeing the canning of fruits and vegetables and the making of
jams and preserves for the winter ahead. Her husband lived and worked
part of the time in the hospital; since he had another job, however, his
responsibilities were limited to caring for the ice and furnace in exchange
for his board.[14]

More than just the spokespeople for the trustees' policies, the superintendents or matrons were usually allowed a certain amount of discretion
and authority.[15] Higgins, for example, was consulted by both the trustees
and physicians before any major changes were made. When the housestaff
complained to the chief physician about the matron's restrictions on them,
he upheld her authority. Higgins often exerted her authority through her
alliance with the male chief of the medical staff, who made daily visits to
the hospital but did not live there.[16]

Most physicians never trained in, worked in, or brought their patients
to be cared for in hospitals. A small elite, concerned with gaining more
clinical experience or performing rare operations and treating unusual dis-
eases, sought hospital positions. But even for hospital physicians, medical
authority did not always translate into institutional power since the hospitals did not depend on the doctors for either their income or sense of
purpose.[17] A chief physician usually had some power and direct access to
the trustees. As did attending physicians, the chief physician lived outside
the hospital and made sporadic visits. If the institution had medical school
ties it might also have live-in housestaff responsible for the provision of
daily medical care. In this kind of setting, physician authority was often
problematic. Tensions and conflicts, therefore, existed between every level
of the hierarchy. In the interstices of such a fragmented authority structure, the life below of the patients, nurses, and servants flourished.

THE HOSPITAL NURSE

Hospitals had a very uncomplicated division of labor below the level of
physicians. Nightwatchers, as their name implied, came into the larger
institutions late in the evening to "watch" the patients until dawn. Head
nurses, along with their assistants and orderlies, lived in the institutions
and were responsible for whatever nursing care was given. Extra nurses

were sometimes brought in daily from outside when needed. A number of laundresses, cooks, and kitchen helpers made up the rest of the work force.

Class and position linked the hospital's patients and workers together as much as it divided them from the trustees, matrons, and physicians. Patient, nurse, and servant were often one and the same person since ambulatory patients were expected to do much of the nursing care. In public institutions, the use of inmates from the nearby almshouse as nurses was common. The role of the public hospital, in particular, as a workhouse for the city's marginal population continued well into the twentieth century. In 1913 a New York hospital survey noted: "In absence of other institutions where the periodic and semi-respectable drunks can live and work, they can, to the best advantage, both to themselves and to the City, be supported as workers in the City's hospitals."[18]

The line between nurse, hospital worker, and patient proved to be quite elastic. Margaret Gillis's relationship to the Boston Lying-In Hospital was not untypical. She gave birth to her first illegitimate child in March of 1874 at the hospital and then stayed on, first as kitchen help, next as a laundress. Within a year she was promoted to nurse. Feeling she had enough experience to work on the outside and physically run down from institutional nursing, she left early in January of 1875 to try nursing in patients' homes. She came back by the end of the month to help out with the night work and then quickly returned to home nursing. In March 1878 she was back in the hospital, this time to deliver her second child.[19]

Even when the nurses were not actual or former patients, they were drawn from the same sectors of the poor and working class that used the hospitals as patients. When not working as nurses they moved between the limited number of jobs for the increasing numbers of poor urban women forced into the labor market.[20] Sometimes they tried to do more than one job at once. In 1880, Eliza Higgins had to remind the nurses their time "belongs to the Hospital & no more dress-making or manufacturing of garments will be allowed in the wards. Darning a stocking, etc. wd not be objected."[21] As with home nursing, middle-class women, especially during the Civil War years, occasionally sought hospital employment or volunteered help, but they were far from typical.[22]

Hospital nursing drew from a much wider age range than home nursing because the hospitals were willing to hire almost anyone who would take the job. Furthermore, hospital work was more strenuous because of the numbers of patients to be cared for and more dangerous because of cross-infections. In June 1874, for example, the matron of the Lying-In Hospital placed this ad in the *Boston Evening Transcript:* "Wanted, a nurse at Boston Lying-In Hospital, 24 McLean Street. Experience not required. Age between 20 and 35." Four years later, she may have decided that twenty was a bit too young and the subsequent ad asked for women twenty-five to forty.[23]

In institutions that had the option to choose, not every warm body was accepted. At the Lying-In as elsewhere, Higgins often hired the sisters and sisters-in-law of nurses she already knew to be reliable. When word of mouth did not provide enough help, newspaper advertisements often resulted in a deluge of applicants. In November 1878, during one of the nineteenth century's worst depressions, Eliza Higgins again advertised for a live-in night nurse. Over a hundred women applied for the seventeen-dollar a month, room and board, position, in an age range from eighteen to seventy. She nevertheless had a difficult time finding the right woman since

> . . . the greater part were either washwoman style – or those who wd shortly consider themselves too nice for the place – being altogether too airy – others had husbands either out of work or earning low wages – whom it wd not be advisable to take as a night nurse to reside in the Hospital. Mrs. Selby is a widow with a child.[24]

It is not clear if Mrs. Selby's child also came to live at the Lying-In, although many other nurses at the hospital had children who were boarding elsewhere in the Boston area. But the hospital's paternalism did not extend to its employees' children. The institution was not always just a home.[25]

Higgins ideally sought women to nurse whom she variously described as having "courage," "self-possession," and "snap." Such women were often difficult to find. In June 1875 a nurse hired by Higgins in the middle of the month could not come to the hospital until the twenty-fourth. On the fourteenth she found a temporary nurse elsewhere. But on the sixteenth, "the temporary nurse who promised to come Tuesday am [A.M.] did not put in her appearance – tried to get four other persons – just did not succeed – finally decided to take laundress M. Hendron upstairs and hire a washwoman fr [from] outside." Higgins lamented several years later under similar circumstances, "It makes it very hard for the hospl [hospital] so many changes."[26]

There were constant personnel changes in the hospital as in other nineteenth-century industries and workplaces. The number of nurses at an institution at any given time varied with available funds, the acuteness of the patients' illnesses, the patient census, the mix between ward patients and the more demanding pay patients, and the illnesses and absences of the nurses. A considerable amount of time was spent scouring the city for extra temporary nurses – the hospital's equivalents of day laborers – needed to cover the institutions during a shortage. Higgins's entries for June and July 1879 give some hint of the frequency and reasons for the turnover:

June 3, 1879. Over 100 women have called about nurse position.

June 4. Hire Miss Alice Brown as night nurse.

June 7. Miss Ruth Appleton as day nurse. Now 4 day nurses.

June 11. Miss Brown not strong enough for the job and leaves.

June 19. Miss Sarah Hubbard enters as night nurse.

June 26. S. Glass leaves for private nursing. Mrs. Clara Brookes as day nurse.

June 28. Nurse Richberg leaving for illness.

June 30. Miss Mary Doyle entered as assistant nurse.

July 19. Nurse Mrs. Brookes is leaving at the end of the month.[27]

In her recollections of her life as a nurse and matron at the Massachusetts General between 1862 and 1895, Georgia Sturtevant claimed there were two different sets of nurses: the young ones, who were willing to do anything else if it came along, and a more "determined group who were willing to dedicate their lives to the institution."[28] Similarly, at the Lying-In there were groups of temporary nurses who worked, on average, only about eleven days and a more permanent group who stayed approximately two years and two months.[29] Promotions often came quickly to those who stayed more than a few weeks. After two months' probation as an assistant nurse, Georgia Sturtevant was put in charge of a twenty-one-bed male surgical ward at the Massachusetts General, "with about as much knowledge of nursing as one usually has after that length of service in a hospital ward," she recalled. Similarly, Linda Richards, before she had the schooling that bestowed on her the title of "America's first trained nurse," was offered a head nurse position at Boston City Hospital after three months as a lowly assistant.[30]

Rules concerning patients' language, use of alcohol and tobacco, visiting, general behavior, sexual activity, and the right to leave the hospital were all extended, with very little change, to cover the hospital's workers. All the nurses and servants, except for the nightwatchers, were similarly expected to live in the hospital itself, usually shunted off to the corners of the institutions in attic garrets or in very small rooms off the wards. Some hospitals paid wages only quarterly, but monthly wage payments were common with room, board, and some laundry service also being provided. The nurses and patients usually shared the same physical space and conditions. But nurses were frequently indignant over the hospital's refusal to provide them with food or lodging that separated them from the patients. Complaints ranged from the use of solid-silver spoons for the patients and pewter for the nurses to the extreme temperatures in windowless attic rooms. Although subjected to the hospital's charity, they argued, they did not benefit from it.[31]

Although nurses felt they deserved better treatment, the similarity between patients and nurses was reinforced by the very nature of nursing work as much as by class and institutional position. Much of nursing was sheer drudgery: cleaning and enormous amounts of washing. At the Massachusetts General, the day began at about 5 A.M., when the nightwatchers left, and ended around 9:30 P.M., when they returned. Fouled cotton and gauze dressings were washed first in the ward bathroom and then sent on to the hospital laundry for further cleaning. Heavy wooden trays were carried upstairs from diet kitchens, the patients fed, and the dishes washed. Sweeping, dusting, and the continual washing followed. Nurses also did some assisting at operations and were frequently responsible for changing and washing surgical dressings. At the Lying-In before the 1880s, nurses also had to do all their own personal laundering and ironing, clean their bedrooms, mop the upper stories of the hospital, and wash all the poultice cloths. In the years before knowledge of germ theory and antiseptic and aseptic techniques, incessant attempts to scrub the hospitals and launder the dressings were the institutions' major weapons against infections. Patients were given medications and had their dressings changed, but this was often done only by the head nurse or the matron. Teaching institutions often limited the nurse's work so that interns could learn to take vital signs.[32]

The hours of nursing work were long and often difficult, but unevenly paced. In her so-called off hours, Sturtevant sat with the other nurses in their rooms and "*patched* the hospital linen" (her emphasis). At the Lying-In, Higgins had the nurses reclean the wards or overstitch the blanket edges whenever things were quiet.[33] Her attempt in 1880 to stop nurses from doing outside sewing suggests that nurses sought ways to spend their time in more personally advantageous and remunerative ways. Many spent the hours drinking and visiting with the patients. Those who stayed on at the hospitals, often for years at a time, could and did make the institutions their homes. Both patients and nurses could turn a spital into a hospice, but neither group easily assented to the order the trustees, physicians, and matrons sought.

AN ORDER OF THEIR OWN

Varying degrees of order prevailed in different hospitals as nurses organized their work and accepted and rejected the authority of those nominally above them. In smaller institutions, matrons tried to watch over and direct the nurses' work as would a housekeeper in a home with many servants. In larger institutions, the head nurse on a ward, however quickly she obtained that title, determined the pace and nature of daily life. Sturtevant's account suggests that establishing procedures and caring for patients were important parts of the nurses' work at Massachusetts General. Richards claimed, however, that the wards at Boston City were badly kept by

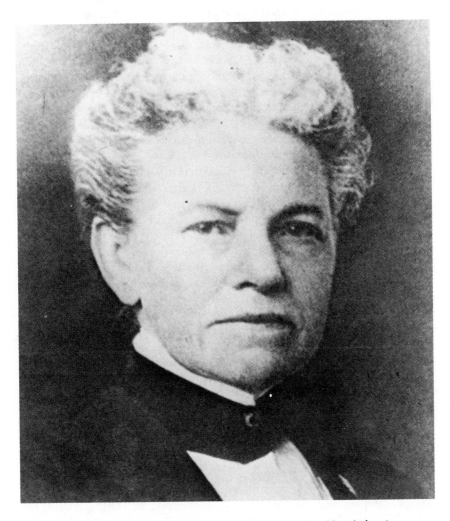

Eliza Higgins, matron of the Boston Lying-In Hospital, 1873–1913.
Source: Countway Library

nurses who did not know the names of medications they administered, how to understand a patient's symptoms, or how to respond humanely to a patient's needs. At the Lying-In, Higgins had to continually remind the nurses about the untidiness and slovenliness of their wards and bedrooms.

Although physician authority was not established or accepted, implicit norms governed both nurse and physician behaviors. Nurses, the physicians believed, were supposed to defer to their authority and to keep the institution orderly and clean. Physicians, the matrons and nurses thought, were to be reasonable in their demands, gentlemanly, and responsible for the patients under their care. But those nurses who stayed any length of time, and had the initiative and interest, could and did learn how to do more than merely the domestic chores. In certain situations they often acted on their own expertise, even when it countered physician authority. Physicians clearly expected deference from the nurses, but it was not often forthcoming. Such normative expectations, or what Eliza Higgins sarcastically referred to as "M. E." or "Medical Etiquette," were frequently violated, especially in situations where the nurses and matrons felt aiding a patient in distress was more important.[34]

Such violations of "etiquette" were particularly common at the Lying-In when emergencies arose and physicians could not be found. Both of the hospital's house officers, despite nurse and matron objections, frequently went out together for dinner, leaving the institution with no medical coverage. Nurses often managed entire labors and deliveries on their own. For example, a patient arrived in convulsions one evening in 1888 when both house officers were out. A physician was sent for, and the nurses administered ether before his arrival. The house officer later objected, claiming, " 'at the MGH [Massachusetts General Hospital] no treatment cd be given without Drs. orders.' " When the particular case was finally discussed with the chief physician, the matron supported the nurse's actions and nastily queried the doctors, " 'If a patient shd unexpectedly start up hemorrhaging either nurse shd not go [unclear] uterus – or one to fall on the floor – she cd remain just in that position until the House Dr. arrived.' " The head physician quickly assured her that, of course, this was not the idea he wished to convey. "It was a case," Higgins admitted diplomatically at the end, "of omission of duty in one and commission of fault in the others."[35] The physicians resented, however, any initiatives taken by the nurses, even when the physicians themselves were clearly either at fault or being unreasonable.

Nurses, as did other nineteenth-century workers, expected to be able to manage the pace and content of their own work. In 1885, nurses at the Lying-In Hospital isolated a typhoid patient and sent for a special nurse to assist in her care. This was normal procedure, especially when nurses felt they were too busy to provide the extra care such a patient needed. A house officer objected to this, primarily, Higgins maintained, "because he had not suggested it himself." Another physician complained when the nurses did not follow his order to give two patients "interuterine douches" during a very busy supper hour when afternoon temperatures and pulses also were being taken. Nurses also clearly followed their own discretion on more serious issues such as when to give extra doses of morphine or to apply a poultice to control a patient's lochia. At the same time, one nurse was bedridden with lameness and complained it was caused by helping a physician carry a patient. This was something, she maintained, " 'the Dr. ought not to asked a nurse to do.' "[36]

A pattern emerges from Higgins's reports of these conflicts. The physicians most likely to run into difficulties with the nurses, and whose authority the nurses were most willing to ignore, were those whose behavior was described again and again as "ungentlemanly."[37] These instances appear to fall into two categories: *behavioral* lapses such as smoking a pipe, yelling at the nurses, or being too physically attentive to them, and *professional* failings, such as leaving the hospital while on duty, not following proper procedures, and making unreasonable demands. It is not clear if the physician's failure to live up to established norms allowed the nurses to violate the behavioral rules, or if the nurses used such failures post hoc to justify having taken initiatives. Certainly the physicians' complaints about the nurses' "inefficiency and inexactness," and the nurses' insistence on setting their own priorities in terms of work, suggest that nurses used the physicians' behavioral violations to justify their own actions. In either case, balance and reciprocity, based on gender-defined behaviors, were expected on all sides.

Some physicians learned that a nurse with excellent observation skills and the willingness to report honestly on all she saw was of critical importance to a patient's recovery. Oliver Wendell Holmes noted that the Massachusetts General nurses quickly learned that Dr. James Jackson, for example, would not tolerate anything less than the truth in their verbal reports. Holmes recalled that Rebecca Taylor, a much-praised nurse, had a "clinical dialogue" with Jackson that "was as good questioning and answering as one would be like [*sic*] to hear outside of the court-room."[38]

Deference rituals were practiced, however, as a means of symbolically asserting physician and trustee control. Physicians' rounds at Massachusetts General, for example, were made with enough regularity so the nurses could plan their daily schedules around them. Sturtevant recalled:

Though the nurses received no special training, were given no systematic instruction, everything impressed me as being exceedingly systematic, and the smallest details important. At a certain hour the heavy counterpanes, which were used at that time, were carefully folded back and extra blankets substituted in their places. The strips of bedside carpet were swept and shaken and laid away till morning, the linen-stand covers were also removed at night, and were not put on again until after the dressings were done and the last touches given to the ward. Everything must be in order before the "visit." This ceremony or putting in order impressed me so much, I began to regard its observance at the exact time of as vital importance as the administering of the gttxxx [*sic*] of "Smith & Melvin's" to the restless patient. I would say by way of explanation, that the doctor's "visits" could be pretty correctly timed in those days, and the nurses could arrange this work accordingly.[39]

Sturtevant's emphasis on system and regularity revealed how the very emphasis on preciseness and order made it possible for the nurses to always *appear to be* in compliance with the normative behavior. She perceived the making of order as a "ceremony." She used similar language when she related the importance of the trustees' major quarterly meeting visit. She called it an "*event*" (her emphasis) and an "impressive ceremonial." She then described the extent to which her failure to follow the exactness of the rules of the ceremony brought her enormous disgrace. Her comments emphasized the extent to which nurse–trustee and nurse–physician relations were highly ritualized with all the participants fully aware of their roles and responsibilities.

In the case of trustee visits the rules required that a patient be either in bed or in a bedside chair for examining and questioning. When "No. 21" in Sturtevant's ward grew weary of this whole procedure, he abandoned his post and ambled over to converse with "No. 15" at the precise moment when the trustee entourage strode into the ward. Sturtevant was immediately held responsible for this violation of the ceremony.[40] Her failure emphasized the extent to which rigid rules were known and regular visits expected. Since the nurses could arrange their work to have everything in order for these checks, they could then have other times to do their work as they wished.

Such rituals, as in other settings and societies, had dual functions. They reasserted at the symbolic level the social hierarchy that was more ambiguous in daily life. They also used verbal punishment and shaming to remind nurses of the necessity for deference, though such deference was rarely practiced during the normal course of hospital life.[41]

On the day-to-day level, nurses both fought and used the hospital's authority structure to their individual and group advantage. They clearly expected to be able to pace their own work and to do what they pleased. Massachusetts General nurses were allowed to organize their time off and to change it at will as long as the hospital floors were covered in sufficient numbers.[42] But Eliza Higgins at the Lying-In, as did increasing numbers of other employers in the late nineteenth century, tried to take this power away. Early in October 1873 she noted:

The nurses are getting so now that they will not accept any recreation time that is offered them – but take just such occasions as suits their pleasure – they were at liberty to go out 3 afternoons this week, but neither wd accept either. – Yesterday Mrs. Hew remarked "I suppose I can go out this evening." She was told it was uncertain at that time whether she cd go or not – and she replied "Well – I shall go whether you say I can or not even if I leave this place thro' it" and she went accordingly.

Almost two weeks later, Higgins tried to assert her authority again by suggesting to the nurses that they have a regular afternoon and evening off as did the hospital's domestic help. The nurses clearly objected on several grounds: They did not want to be classed with either the help or the patients and they resented any intrusion on their individual and collective right to decide when they would work. They had their own ethic about how their work should be paced and controlled. They told Higgins: "They were not like children —. Neither were they as common help for possibly on their appointed afternoon they might have no inclination for going out." They were aware of the Massachusetts General nurses' schedules and argued that such rules should apply at the Lying-In. Higgins insisted this was not possible and the nurses, in turn, threatened to take their complaint over her head to the chief physician. By the next day, they had clearly discussed the matter among themselves and decided not to take the conflict to the physician and agreed to abide by Higgins's rules. But her continued entreaties about their taking "French leaves" (staying out beyond their allotted times) suggested the nurses' acceptance of the rules was merely an attempt to placate her.[43] In subsequent years she was forced to give the nurses explanations for why she requested changes in their recreation time, to reissue orders that they could not stay in the dining room more than half an hour, or leave their wards without permission.[44] The nurses were clearly successful in resisting an order not of their own making.

Ultimately Higgins, as do all employers, resorted to the power to fire. In May 1879 she dismissed virtually the entire nursing force for their use of "coarse expressions and slang phrases and . . . profane words." The firings were forced not because of the nurses' language but because tales of such behavior were being discussed at Massachusetts General.[45] Behavior that was known beyond the hospital's walls and threatened its reputation as a responsible charitable institution was out of bounds. The lines that surrounded the nurse's world could be stretched only so far.

THE RIGHTS OF CARING

Behind the established rules and rituals, the daily life of the hospital, as in any workplace, was constantly being shaped and reshaped by the nurses' own understandings of their rights and obligations as hospital workers. Nurses fought the hospital's attempts to regulate their entire lives, and yet wanted to use the institutions as homes as well as workplaces. They resisted encroachments on their own time, and then returned to use the hospital as a home when out of money or ill. They insisted on their own definition of obligation and duty between hospital and nurse. Within their shared occupational community, informal yet enforced norms were established.

Certain conditions made this kind of implicit bargain possible. Nurses did not spend their entire lives locked into one institutional setting. If the work was miserable, they could quit and try to find something else. Hospital nurses moved back and forth between institutions, family, or other work. Lucy Hubbard Kendall had a typical work pattern. A thirty-seven-year-old spinster, she was brought into the Lying-In by her sister as a substitute nurse for four months in the winter of 1879–80. The next year she did intermittent private-duty home nursing and then married a Boston shopkeeper. With marriage she left nursing to share in the burdens of running a dry goods store. Three years later, she was widowed and was either unable or unwilling to keep up the store. She moved into a downtown Boston hotel and for the next twelve years continued to do both private duty and hospital nursing.[46]

Nurses also brought many of the mores and behaviors of their own class and cultural milieu into the hospitals. Higgins constantly complained that she had to remind the nurses not to laugh or talk loudly and to reprimand them for bringing men into the hospital, staying out beyond their allotted times, or wearing pin curlers.[47] It was the nurses' particular combination of seeming insouciance and insolence that appalled the genteel women and bourgeois gentlemen who tried to run the hospitals. Middle- and upper-class standards of behavior and morality were rarely achieved in the demi-world of hospital life as the shape of work and caring took more working-class forms.

Every nurse was not, of course, belligerent or prone to keeping pin curlers in her hair. Georgia Sturtevant angrily defended her sister nurses, claiming many were "sweet-faced, intelligent women, refined and gentle in manner, who ministered to the wants of those under their care with devotion and sacrifice."[48] Whether or not the nurses as a group fit Sturtevant's *ladylike* descriptions, they clearly resisted as best they could being defined, as they told Higgins, as the hospital's *children*. With this kind of language the nurses were taking the working-class stance of "womanly" behavior in front of a boss, the sex-specific analogue to the "manly bearing" historian David Montgomery describes as integral to male working-class culture.[49] Such statements were both an assertion of individual rights and an acknowledgment of a shared mutualistic ethic.

Within the diffuse culture of the hospital, nurses were frequently able to create an authority of their own. Their sensibility of caring, sometimes barely existent, other times highly developed, structured much of the hospital's daily life. Drunkenness and dissolution were often a way to survive the hospital's horrors and demands. But the right to provide what seemed to be appropriate care could also be expressed in the struggle for autonomy. It was this kind of hospital culture and order that the introduction of trained nursing was designed to transform.

PART II

The trained nurse: an apprentice to duty

3

Character as skill: the ideology of discipline

A Georgia Sturtevant may have been impressed by hospital order and the gentleness of the nurses, but charity reformer Elizabeth Christophers Hobson was overwhelmed in 1872 by the "unspeakable" dirt, foul smells, and disorder she encountered when touring New York's Bellevue Hospital. It was women like Hobson who were, at first, to introduce training for nurses as a way to begin what she called the hospital's "reformation and purification."[1] Indeed, the "invention of the modern hospital," as historian Morris Vogel labeled the post–Civil War period of the institution's change, depended, in part, on the invention of the trained nurse.[2]

After the Civil War, as the pace of urbanization and industrialization quickened, a number of converging changes called forth this dual invention. In time of illness, hospitalization, rather than home-based care, became a necessity for more working-class Americans, as families were increasingly separated by migration or had their financial resources strained by the uncertainty of the economy. With transformations in medical thinking and therapeutics coupled to the reorganization of medical practice, the hospital slowly became an acute-care, rather than a chronic-care, facility. By the end of the century, with more serious economic depressions, municipal government reorganization and declines in charitable donations, the increased financial strain on the institutions forced further internal reorganization.[3] As a result of these pressures, a different kind of hospital work force became necessary.

As an upper-class charity reformer, Elizabeth Hobson became aware of these needs as she, and thousands of other women like her, expanded their institution-building efforts begun in the antebellum years. With a consciousness that reflected both their class and their gender, the reformers' focus was often on the increasing difficulties of native-born women who were migrating to the cities for work.[4] In hopes, therefore, of both reordering the hospitals *and* providing suitable employment for respectable women, training for nursing was introduced in 1873.

Under this new schema, nurses were to be selected, properly trained, and differentiated from patients and domestics alike. The nursing student

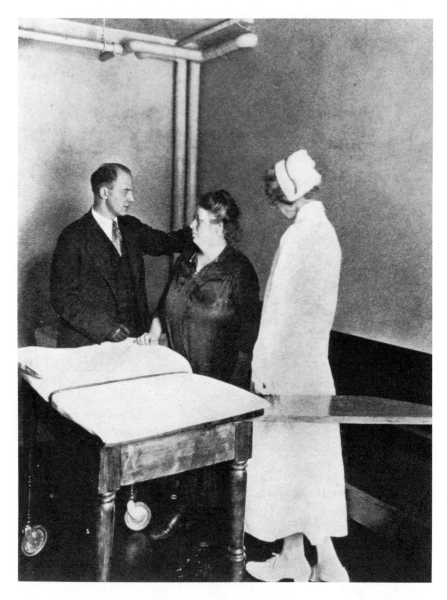

"The Hospital Trinity–Doctor, Nurse and Patient" was the caption beneath this photograph in the pamphlet *The Free Hospital for Women: 52nd Anniversary of the Founding, 1875–1927* (Boston, Massachusetts, 1927). *Source:* Countway Library

ideally was to be younger than the professed nurse of the community, more disciplined than the untrained nurse of the hospital, and more animated than either by concepts of order and caring. The domestic order created by a good wife, the altruistic caring expressed by a good mother, and the self-discipline of a good soldier were to be combined in the training of a good nurse.

As were many other forms of labor in the nineteenth century, nursing was thus "feminized." But in this particular case, the change was in the *behavior* of the work force, not its gender. Conceptions of female obligation and caring, formed in the antebellum years, were reshaped to create the ideology of training. Recent feminist critics of nursing have charged that the emphasis in training was on "character not skills."[5] Comprehending the meaning of training, however, necessitates understanding that *character was the skill* deemed critical to the "reformation" in both nursing and hospital care. With the introduction of training, a woman's duty to nurse took on new forms but kept its older ideological mantle.

LADY WITH A VISION

Florence Nightingale never set foot on American soil, yet she profoundly influenced the model for the training of American nurses. Her accomplishments and methods became well known in the United States as her books, papers, letters, and personal emissaries shaped the thinking and efforts of several generations of American hospital and nursing reformers.[6]

Nightingale was an extraordinarily powerful upper-class reformer who sought to bring efficiency and moral order to the world around her from military procurement and civilian hospitals to the Indian sanitation system.[7] Facing the disasters she perceived in military and civilian health care, she fought for the training of "proper" nurses. Women with the appropriate character and discipline, she believed, honed by careful training, would impose the nursing order needed to restore health in both homes and hospitals. The funds, donated by a grateful nation after the Crimean War, and her formidable political skills and connections made possible the opening of a training school to test her vision at St. Thomas's Hospital in London.

Nightingale's model for nursing's revitalization, and the hospital's re-ordering, was built on an uneasy alliance among concepts drawn from the sexual division of labor in the family, the authority structure of the military and religious sisterhoods, and the link between her moral beliefs and medical theories.[8] As did other midcentury reformers, such as Anna Jameson in the United Kingdom and Caroline Dall and Virginia Penny in the United States, Nightingale accepted as "natural" a sexual division of labor based on biological characteristics used to justify the employment of women in occupations close to their domestic labors. These reformers shared the assumption that a woman's nature and moral superiority destined her for a special role in society. Furthermore, Jameson, Dall, and Penny used the tenets of natural-rights philosophy to argue that women had a right to employment that suited their nature.[9]

Nightingale shared their belief in women's special nature and work but not their concept of rights. She accepted that a good nurse first had to be a good woman. But she also agreed with American domesticity advocate Catharine Beecher, who spoke in the language of women's *duties and obligations* rather than *rights*. Beecher asserted that a respectable woman's greater moral character and sense of order, if properly channeled and disciplined through education, could bring an end to social chaos. Similarly, Nightingale believed that women entering training were answering a secularized calling, not demanding their rights. Nightingale sought order and health through women's special endeavors as Beecher hoped to create social cohesion through women's self-denial.[10]

Although Nightingale thought nursing was an art, she nevertheless felt that practical and liberal training were necessary. To the public and physicians alike she asserted that mere womanhood did not qualify someone to nurse. The laws of life, death, and health, she argued, were not intuitive. They did not come "by inspiration to the lady disappointed in love nor to the poor workhouse drudge hard up for a livelihood."[11]

Nightingale believed that such learning and order had to take place within the hospital training school under the control of a female hierarchy that was equal to, but separate from, that of the men. Nursing did not present a direct challenge to physicians' authority because it was structured around a hierarchy of its own, with a separate arena of concern. The nurse was to be loyal to the physician, but not servile. "True loyalty to orders," she declared, "cannot be obtained without the independent sense or energy of responsibility, which alone secures real trustworthiness."[12]

Her beliefs about female duty and authority meshed with her environmentalist ideas on disease etiology. As a nineteenth-century sanitarian, Nightingale believed the proper moral, environmental, and physical order made the restoration of health possible. She never accepted the ideas of germ theory and disease specificity. "Hospital morale" had to be created through order, ventilation, clean drains and sewers, and decent diets, so that nature's healing processes could take place.[13] Medical therapeutics and surgical care played only small parts in this drama of curing or in the hospital's function. More broadly, it was nursing that was to be responsible for making the environment clean and conducive to healing. She even rejected Elizabeth Blackwell's proposal for joint nursing and medical training in part because she perceived medicine as too narrow a realm for women's skills.[14]

Nightingale also expected the nurse to be the kindly, if strict, disciplinarian of the patients. Training was to separate nurses from personal and social contact with patients and to prepare them to act as household mistresses disciplining their servants. Nightingale even redesigned the ward (she advocated a barracks arrangement with two rows of beds and a nursing station at its head) to allow the nurse to survey the condition of her charges and to move quickly to discipline the unruly.[15]

Training had to elevate and shape all the essential characteristics of the controlled and sympathetic, but nonsentimental, woman. It had to eliminate any hint of eroticism and its apparent concomitants: disorder, dirt, and immorality. In the words of one of her biographers, Nightingale sought "to prove that the woman can be sunk in the nurse."[16] More appropriately, sexuality was to be replaced by motherly authority and skill. Nightingale's abiding concern with the pristine nurse was not the fixation of a sexually repressed Victorian, but rather an attempt to limit any male claim on a woman through the sexual exchange. Furthermore, she sought to place nurses above the suspicion that sexual interest motivated their desire to care for male patients.

The Nightingale model thus emphasized character training and strict discipline, a distinct field of work for nurses separate from physicians, and a female hierarchy with deference and loyalty to physician authority. In combining the sexual division of labor, military and religious sisterhood models, and sanitarian ideals, Nightingale's format for nursing reform linked duty, obligation, and order. Although Nightingale sought to free women from the bonds of familial demands, in her nursing model she rebound them in a new context. It was within these boundaries that nursing reformers sought to implement training in the American context.

"ALL OUR WOMEN ARE FLORENCE NIGHTINGALES"

As the opening salvos of the American Civil War were fired, Nightingale's experiences, at Scutari in the Crimea and at her training school at St. Thomas's Hospital, were not lost on elite Northern charity reformers. The initial outpouring of male volunteers, the chaos of the military procurement and medical systems, and the eagerness to help of women perceived as inexperienced created fears that the disorder and terrible mortality of the Crimean War would find its American equivalent and endanger the war effort.[17] Within days of the bombardment of Fort Sumter, women's relief associations (which later would become the backbone of the U.S. Sanitary Commission) and the Army Nurse Corps, under the direction of Dorothea Dix, began to be organized. The Civil War brought to the attention of the American public, as the fighting in Crimea had to the British, not only the dangers of a disorganized military hospital and sanitary system but also models for their reform.

The more personal and romanticized image of Nightingale as the virtuous savior of the British army reached thousands of American women just as the war began. *Godey's Lady's Book* lionized her in 1860 when an American edition of her *Notes on Nursing* was published. When their male relatives and neighbors went off to war, thousands of American women on both sides of the conflict rushed to hastily established army hospitals to offer their services, both as volunteers and as paid nurses.[18] This was the first major U.S. war in which women as nurses were to play a significant role.[19] Many were working-class women – domestics, laundresses, or nurses – for whom hard physical work and even some nursing were not new experiences. Others were middle-class women who had nursed family members or neighbors, but who never had worked for wages, seen the inside of a hospital, or been responsible for the physical care of strangers. Yet they hoped that the special skills of "respectable" women, proper housekeeping and mothering, could be put to useful and patriotic ends.

Middle-class women entered the ranks of Civil War nursing for a variety of reasons. Many responded to reports that a son, father, or husband lay wounded in an army hospital. Others volunteered in an effort to break out of the chains of domesticity. "I want something to do," Nurse Periwinkle asserted in Louisa May Alcott's semiautobiographical account of Civil War nursing. "Good-bye! *This is life.*" Katharine Wormeley cheerfully wrote her family as she embarked on a Sanitary Commission ship loaded with hospital supplies and staff. In an enthusiastic editorial in 1864, the *New York Herald* declared: "All Our Women Are Florence Nightingales."[20] Whether motivated by patriotism, familial duty, or a search for meaningful work and adventure, these women did not face the relative ease of nursing a grateful brother or relative in the comfort of their homes. Rather, they confronted the overwhelming filth and stench of the barracks' hospitals, the disorder of the military procurement system, the cries of wounded and dying strangers, and the intransigence and hostility of physicians unwilling to accept the aid of "meddling" women. In despair, many women were forced to give up their romantic images of themselves as ministering angels in the horror, extreme temperatures, and disorder of wartime medical care. Many found truth in wound dresser and nurse Walt Whitman's comment that "it is a natural faculty that is required, it is not merely having a genteel young woman at a table in a ward."[21]

Many who gave up the nursing role directly, or who never tried it, worked through the Sanitary Commission to see that better care was provided for soldiers and to press the government to live up to its responsibilities for the wounded. Many women, whose skills in dealing with

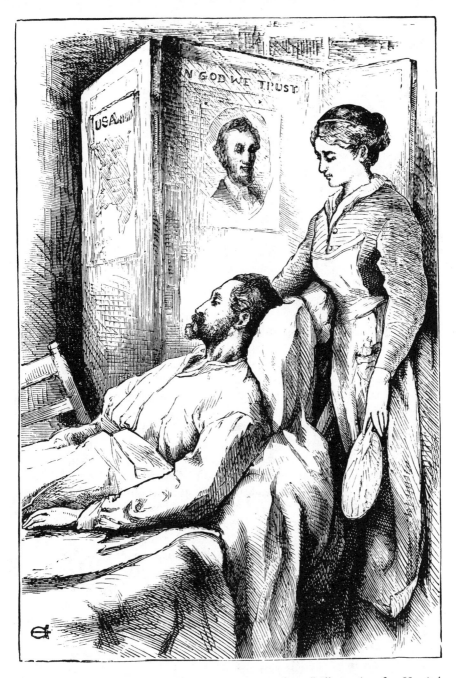

" 'John.' The manliest man among my forty." Illustration for *Hospital Sketches*, Louisa May Alcott's 1869 fictionalized account of her experiences as a Civil War nurse. *Source:* Louisa May Alcott, *Hospital Sketches* (Boston: Roberts Brothers, 1883 ed.), frontispiece both strangers and official indifference had been honed in prewar reform and missionary organizations, fought tenaciously to forge a role for women in the army's medical system. This role was intimately linked in their minds with the necessity for organized benevolence by the elite, careful planning, and unsentimental action. Writing to her mother in 1863, Katharine Wormeley, by then associate manager of the Sanitary Commission's New England branch (and, later in the war, superintendent of nurses at the Portsmouth Grove Hospital in Rhode Island), declared: "You *can't conceive* what it is to stem the torrent of this disorder and utter want of organization. We are all well, and can only thank God that we are here, with health, strength, and *head*."[22]

Such women perceived the authority of the physicians and the surgeons as their biggest problem. Looking beyond the expected formality and rules of the hospital culture to its effects, the women continually expressed anger and dismay. The worst enemy, declared New York reformer Georgeanna Woolsey, was "that sublime, unfathomed mystery – 'Professional Etiquette' [an] . . . absolute Bogie . . . which puts its cold paw on private benevolence . . . which keeps shirts from ragged men, and broth from hungry ones."[23] With such feelings, some women quickly replaced their meekness with indignation and outrage. In such a context, tensions between the physicians and nurses often ran high.[24]

In search of a mode of behavior that would bring them a certain degree of power, some women turned to what one historian has characterized as a "womanly professionalism" based on gender, class upbringing, and the authority of the mother. The belief in the saving grace of a loving and serene mother figure could counter the authority of male surgeons. "I . . . doubt," nurse Jane Swisshelm recalled, "if a dozen of them [men she nursed] ever knew me by any other name than that of 'Mother.' "[25] But in the absence of any meaningful support and orders from higher authorities, such qualifications did not give women the basis for an organized assault on male power in the army hospitals.[26] Disdain and abuse rather than "courtesy and kindness" were more often the nurse's fare.

The women were the first to admit the disorder of Civil War nursing. Georgeanna Woolsey's sister Jane wrote in her memoirs of the conflict: "Was the system of Women-nurses in hospitals a failure? There never was a system." Similarly, Katharine Wormeley believed that a more orderly system for the recruitment and training of nurses, along with firm discipline, could have overcome the surgeon's suspicions of gentlewomen as nurses. In a tract written for the Sanitary Commission in 1863, she urged other women to understand that they would find their "true work" in nursing and gain the "power of benevolence" only through obedience and discipline.[27] The lessons of the war – the necessity for organized private benevolence in the systematization of hospital care and for organized training of respectable women in nursing – would be remembered after the war when the attention of reformers turned to civilian hospitals.

"AT LAST OF GREAT USE IN THE WORLD"

In the immediate postwar years, little changed in hospital nursing: It continued to be the work of untrained women or almshouse inmates. But a small coterie of urban upper-class women, who either had nursed during the war or actively participated in the Sanitary Commission or other relief activities, returned from their war efforts eager and confident that feminine virtues and organizational skills had a larger role to play in society. Awareness of their importance to the improvement of military hospital care deepened their commitment to such endeavors in civilian life. They harnessed their considerable talents and social connections to overcome two glaring social problems: the perceived disorder and disreputable conditions in hospitals, particularly in large municipal institutions, and the increasing numbers of daughters of "respectable" small-town families who, because of the deaths of male relatives in the war and desperate economic conditions in the early 1870s, were entering the cities in search of work.[28]

With their Civil War experiences freshly behind them and the Nightingale model for hospital and nursing reform already in place in England, the efforts of a number of elite reformers thus turned toward hospitals and nursing. The Civil War campaigns had given these women a political education in organizational battles as they became skilled in the intricacies of infighting and pressure politics. Some believed, as one historian has suggested, "that the very presence of women on the wards would promote reform . . . [that] virtue would transform the institution." Others knew their class position and kinship ties to the hospitals' boards of trustees and physicians gave them important leverage in introducing change.[29] Carefully, and fully aware of the difficulties that lay before them, they laid plans that led to the opening in 1873 of the first Nightingale-inspired training schools in New York, Boston, and New Haven.[30]

In theory, the nursing school was to be part of the hospital but supported by separate funds. Students were to replace the untrained hospital nurses and provide care for patients as they received practical and theoretical training. Upon completion of the two- or three-year program, the better graduate nurses were to help establish and run schools in other hospitals, whereas the majority were to become private-duty nurses in patients' homes.

Challenging the position of army surgeons was almost simple compared to the difficulties of introducing a permanent change in the hospital. Physicians were frequently reluctant to accept another trained person in the sickroom. The doctor's authority rested primarily on gentlemanly behavior and carefully constructed relationships with patients.[31] Furthermore, many physicians still trained in apprenticeship to other doctors and never saw the inside of either a hospital or a medical school. In this context, the existence of a hospital-trained gentlewoman could easily be perceived as quite threatening. Just as many physicians feared "medical women," they saw trained nurses as yet another female intrusion into a male domain.[32]

Yet many physicians, rooted in concepts of sanitation, quickly understood the importance of a trained nurse to patient recovery and health. Others, with European training, had seen the differences trained nursing had made. Even when knowledge of antisepsis and asepsis began to make safer surgery possible, the physicians' materia medica remained limited. Patients' lives continued to depend on the food they ate, care in the cleaning of their dressings, careful watching for dangerous hemorrhaging, and provision of ice bags or baths to control their fevers. All of this was to come within the purview of the nurse.[33] Thus if her role and status were clearly limited and demarcated, much of her threat to physician authority could be eliminated.[34]

Nurse's training, in turn, promised the prospective student both independence and dependence, a slow easing into the world of work, not unlike the state of "semiautonomy" that domestic service had provided generations of young women. For primarily rural and small-town "respectable" native-born families, who earlier in the nineteenth century might have sent their daughters "to help" in another family or to the mills at Lowell, the nursing school provided a new potential haven. As both service and mill work became the domain of the immigrant, nursing was one of the few occupations that could promise white native-born parents that their daughters would receive both a moral *and* an occupational apprenticeship. "A purposeless, listless girl," Waltham, Massachusetts, Training School founder Alfred Worcester stated in Svengalian tones,

after she joins a training school will bend to the work with noble, womanly enthusiasm, and at once become a new being. Her face brightens, she makes hosts of grateful friends, she has the supreme happiness of knowing that she is at last of great use in the world. No other occupation, excepting that of making a home for her own family, can better bring out all that is best in womanhood.[35]

Not unlike educators of the mid-nineteenth century, nursing school advocates saw their training programs as "social incubators" for a particular class of respectable young working women. In the protected environment of the nursing school, within the hospital family, the innocent young woman would be nurtured, they hoped, through a combination of moral uplift and hard work. Ideally, the nursing school was to take a woman of "character" between the ages of twenty and thirty-five, old enough to accept the regimentation and young enough to do the strenuous labor.

Thus, the nursing school was potentially similar to other post–Civil War institutions such as YWCAs, Working Girls' Clubs, and boarding houses, organized by middle- and upper-class reformers to "save" the native-born young rural woman who had come to the city. Unlike these organizations that depended on the working woman's voluntary acceptance of proselytizing, the nursing school, once it had acquired its students, had a more captive audience.[36] A nineteenth-century son might have been sent off to sea to become a man, but his sister, it was argued, could safely cross over into womanhood by way of nursing training.

Nursing was to become, as one nursing leader aptly called it, an "apprenticeship to duty."[37] Behavior and demeanor as much as bed-making skill were to become the hallmarks of the trained nurse. "Respectability" had to separate the trained nurse from her predecessor, even if the nature of her labors had not changed.

A WOMAN OF CHARACTER

In the Nightingale schema, the essential element that differentiated the trained nurse from her untrained predecessors was her character. The new nurse's very skill – in gaining acceptance from hospital authorities and physicians, as well as compliance from her patients – depended on the nature and force of her character as it was molded through training. Furthermore, love of humanity manifested in a dignified and controlled manner was to transform drudge work into almost consecrated labor. As the Massachusetts General Hospital's training school rules for probationers promised, "If you love to help others and if you work with your heart as well as your head and hands, you will have compensation all along the way that will make you forget weariness and discouragement."[38]

For early nursing educators, as for other nineteenth-century educators, character was inherent in an individual. Louise Darche, a New York nursing superintendent, explained in a popular women's magazine in 1894: "It should never be forgotten that the woman herself – what she is morally and personally – counts as the largest factor in the question of success in nursing."[39] A nurse was to be a "gentlewoman" with all the virtues and qualities that defined idealized middle- and upper-class womanhood in Victorian America.

The list of virtues ran from attentive to trustworthy, but none was evoked more often than the general adjective "womanly." As one nursing leader declared, "The true trained nurse [is a] womanly woman who . . . inspired hope and confidence in all around her." In the Victorian vocabulary, words like "womanly" and "manly" carried the burden of holding all the essential values necessary for a distinguished and accomplished individual of each gender. For many Victorians, such terms became almost "incantations" used to stave off disorder and change. To be womanly then was to be virtuous and stable.[40]

These innate "womanly" qualities had long been idealized in the image of the neighborhood "natural-born" nurse. But as Nightingale's dictum made clear, much more was necessary than inherent goodness. As with a fine piece of metal whose qualities are properly tempered in the heat of the furnace, the leaders of the nursing schools sought to forge the ideal nurse out of the natural qualities of the good woman. Nightingale used a similar metaphor and referred to the return of a nurse for further education as "retempering."[41] "Scientific" evidence was also used to justify a woman's fitness for nursing and the necessity for training. Physician William Draper told a Bellevue nursing student audience in 1876: "Today science recognizes that woman is indeed the only material from which nurses can be formed, yet teaches that nurses are made not born."[42]

Most nineteenth-century educators were preoccupied with the molding of character. By midcentury, character formation, rather than the conversion experience, became the essential *rite de passage* into adulthood. Historian Thomas Le Duc noted at Amherst College in the 1880s that "as [the] evangelical fervor subsided men came to place less emphasis on conversion and more on conduct." Similarly, the nursing school, to paraphrase influential theologian Horace Bushnell, was to control the nursing student so that she would learn to control herself. As concern over the family's and church's inability to provide such training deepened, the special responsibility of the educator grew.[43] The women who rose to nursing leadership felt a special pedagogical concern for the character of those they trained. As one nursing educator noted, "We assume a moral responsibility for the character of the nurses we send out."[44]

The man and woman of character were very different beings. The nineteenth-century middle-class man of character, unlike his colonial counterpart, no longer answered primarily to the call of his God or developed himself through "habits of industry and frugality" and harsh external discipline alone. Rather, an "earnest and manly" individual sought through his own efforts and mental aggressiveness to develop his own innate sense of moral values and obligations and to become independent, self-contained, orderly, and sure of purpose.[45] Debates over appropriate behavior, and therefore professional authority, extended into medicine as well. By the post–Civil War years, collegiality and social skills no longer served as the basis for professional control as confusion over the importance of scientific skills reigned. Character, even for the doctor, took on myriad new meanings.[46]

For the woman of character, submission and self-sacrifice, rather than independence and individualism, were stressed. As with the middle-class man of character, behavior rather than piety became the measure of a moral being. In a woman, however, it was altruism rather than individualism that defined her moral state. Such altruism and morality thus provided the justification for middle-class women's entrance into the public arena, whether in voluntary associations or in "respectable" paid labor. For many of the early nursing reformers and educators, nursing was therefore a secularized religious and moral occupation. As Isabel Hampton Robb, the first superintendent of the Johns Hopkins Hospital nursing school and a leading nursing educator, declared, "The nurse's work is a ministry; it should represent a consecrated service."[47]

Yet neither Nightingale nor the American nursing reformers desired a mindless supplicant. Nightingale wanted women who were neither self-immolating religious martyrs expecting only the thanks of the Lord nor hardened working women whose motivation for nursing came from their hunger rather than their hearts. The nursing reformers were trying to define a role for women in the service of humanity in which women trod softly and tactfully between the equally dangerous poles of total deference and outright defiance to accomplish their tasks. One superintendent commented: "Modesty and a proper deference to the medical authority does not mean self-abnegation. Such a one has no confidence in herself and cannot be expected to inspire it in others."[48] Similarly, nursing leader Lavinia Dock declared in 1893: "This obedience to orders, founded in principle and animated by an intelligent interest, is the dominant characteristic of the new system of nursing and is the secret of its success in its professional work."[49]

In practice, however, loyalty and deference to the physician, rather than independence, were stressed. The hospital equivalent of ministers' sermons on woman's role was the physician's speech, frequently made at nursing graduation exercises. Endless homilies about loyalty and paeans to the moral good of deference sent the nursing student into her occupational world. "Always be loyal to the physician," Dr. William Richardson bluntly told the graduating students at the Massachusetts General Hospital in a widely reprinted speech. "What error can be more stupid," he rhetorically queried, "than the nurse attempting to impress the doctor with her knowledge?"[50] Equally directly, Lavinia Dock commented that these annual talks were "wearisome, perennial rubbish and . . . platitudes already taught."[51] "Rubbish" or not, such lectures were a given on the nursing school agenda. An important hospital administration text even admonished that such lectures on behavior were not enough: "It must be a constant drilling."[52] The insistence on drilling in conduct was not out of place. Drill and discipline, as well as character, became the hallmarks of training.

THE DISCIPLINE OF THE *GARDE-MALADE*

The models of hierarchy, duty, and discipline taken from the military and from the Victorian family that shaped Nightingale's vision were similarly interwoven to form both the art and science of American nursing. Nurses in a training school were likened, in their starched uniforms, to an army of disciplined soldiers sweeping away disorder and death. Lavinia Dock told an international gathering of nurses in 1893: "The organization of a training school is and must be military. It is not and cannot be democratic . . . to this end complete subordination of the individual to the work as a whole is as necessary for her as for the soldier."[53] Anna M. Fullerton, a physician concerned with nursing education, presented a similar argument when explaining the "science of nursing" to the annual Conference of Charities in 1890.

Discipline, organization, and drill make of each man in the army a mechanical instrument by which his every act becomes a living organism, affecting the end desired. Thus should it be in the Nurse Training School. The emergencies of disease are as sudden and serious as those of war. The *garde-malade* should, therefore, never be found napping.[54]

The discipline, as in an army, had to be constant. Fullerton argued that the nurse's quarters had to be spartan and the rules rigid so that the nurse learned "to endure hardness as a good soldier."[55] Behavior that Eliza Higgins had tolerated at the Boston Lying-In Hospital became the grounds for dismissal. Furthermore, there was very little organized respite from the rules. "The average nurse rarely goes outside the hospital except on her afternoon off," reported the Massachusetts General Hospital's nursing superintendent in 1909.[56]

Alongside the analogy between nursing and army life lay the insistence that the nursing student in the hospital was joining a family. Although the Lying-In's nurses may have insisted they were not children, in 1917 the Chicago Hospital Association could comfortably declare: "Nurses in training are not employees in the sense that they are wage-earners. They are a part of the hospital family, and are cared for as a father cares for his children." A Brooklyn hospital considered each training school student "a member of the Matron's family." Similarly, an Iowa hospital superintendent asserted: "A Happy Congenial 'family' will Graduate Loyal Nurses."[57]

The fact that the students were fed, clothed, and cloistered within the hospitals, which were often only redesigned large Victorian houses, or in an adjacent nurses' *home* (as they were labeled), reinforced the sense of "family" living. In addition, since the hospitals were competing with the private home as the site for the delivery of medical care, they attempted to stress the "homelike" qualities of the institutions. When a Massachusetts nursing student was on a rotation in another hospital, she wrote back to the nursing superintendent, referring to her own school as "home." Similarly, the letters of other nursing students to their superintendents read very much in the vein of reports home to parents.[58] Thus the demand that the nursing students accept the discipline of the older authorities in their "new" family, either as fathers, mothers, or older sisters, accorded with earlier familial patterns. It also helps to explain why nursing educators constantly wanted students who had "good home training" in domestic skills and proper socialization as dutiful daughters.

The rigid hierarchy of the military and familial model reinforced both distance and harsh discipline. A leading nursing textbook justified the harshness in terms of the need for omnipresent discipline: "We rarely obtain unquestioning, prompt obedience from those with whom we are too familiar, and we respect less the judgements and the decisions of our superiors if they are familiar to us."[59] As in the military, special uniforms, badges, pins, and caps, as well as elaborate ceremonies to acknowledge or deny advancements, served to reinforce the disciplinary aspect of the hierarchy. When two sisters in training at Boston City Hospital signed out for an afternoon picnic one warm July day, for example, they were denied their six-month chevrons by the school authorities because they overstayed their allotted time off.[60] Public humiliation, through the removal of the coveted nurse's cap, was also done.

Strict discipline was the essence for Nightingale of moral training and nursing education. Thus, moral order, ethical rules, and technical competence were confounded. Individual ideas on order and method were to be replaced by those ordained by the nursing educators interpreting the laws of nature and God. "Calmness," "self-control," "reconciliation to duty," would come through self-discipline exercised by the nurse at all times, both on and off the wards. There must be, argued American nursing leader Isabel Hampton Robb, "implicit unquestioning obedience." Lavinia Dock similarly asserted that such "absolute" obedience "must be the foundation of the nurse's work."[61]

Continual monitoring of behavior characterized the training. Almost in the custom of eighteenth-century pietism and self-scrutiny, Nightingale required nursing students to keep daily diaries that their matrons read. In addition, a "monthly sheet of personal character and acquirements of each nurse" was kept. The accounting measured the nurse's moral record by her "punctuality, quietness, trustworthiness, personal neatness and cleanliness, and ward management" as well as her technical skill in observation and bed making.[62] The American schools did not require the diaries, but similar constant reporting on the nurse's moral and intellectual developments followed her through training. Every aspect of her life served as a potential discipline lesson.

Thus, several mutually reinforcing strands of thought were interwoven to justify the discipline. It was necessary to ensure that the nurse learned both idealism and proper ethical behavior toward her patients. It was to forge a woman of forceful yet tactful character, with instinctually proper behavior and skills, who was able to accomplish her ordained destiny of bringing about both order and health.

Whereas the *ideology* of training justified the hierarchy and discipline, the reality of the *work* demanded of the nursing student made it necessary. Hospitals soon realized that the opening of what could be labeled a "nursing school" made it possible for them to obtain a younger, more ordered, and cheaper labor force. As nursing students increasingly became a hospital's only nursing staff, they were frequently placed on the wards long before their technical skills and nursing judgment had matured.[63] Independent decisions made by the neophyte nurse might have serious consequences for the patients. Hospital and nursing officials therefore sought to minimize the chance that an arbitrary action or broken rule would cause a patient harm.

The learning of technical and moral skills was thus fused by both ideology and necessity. Repeating procedures until they became automatic became one of the essentials of training. "There is a right way and that is the one and only one she must learn," Isabel Hampton Robb warned. "Only by constant repetition can you become really familiar with the work." Another nursing superintendent explained: "The essence of a nurse's training is the forming of right habits so that the performance of her duties becomes second nature and technical mistakes be reduced to a minimum."[64] George H. M. Rowe, the judgmental superintendent of Boston City Hospital, noted on a student's report: "Miss Stewart has undoubted faults but I think it is because she is English, only a short time here. I have told her that if it proves to be conceit she will have to abandon her own ideas."[65] Individual identity and thought were to be vanquished in the *garde-malade*.

THE MONITORING OF STUDENT BEHAVIOR

Nursing students were given lectures on medical and nursing techniques by both physicians and nurses, but the crucial lessons of training focused on behavior. As in any family or institution, behavior varied widely from the expected norms. But it was precisely behavior as an index of the student's character that so concerned nursing and hospital authorities. At the Massachusetts General Hospital, for example, a student, admonished for incorrectly performing a task, was rebuked in terms of character failure: Forgetting to record a temperature correctly was labeled "unscrupulous" rather than the result of ignorance or inaccuracy.[66]

In general, behavior that suggested the student nurse had qualities associated with the untrained nurse was seen as a serious transgression. These were defined variously as crudeness in manners, displays of sexual interest or activity, and any real show of comradeship with the "help." In 1888 the physicians at the New England Hospital for Women and Children in Boston rebuked a student, saying that she "was 'too much of a servant' and that she showed it by associating with the servants of the house (one of whom she had known before entering) than with the nurses."[67] Similarly, in 1905 a Boston City Hospital head nurse reported a student who "allowed herself to act in a 'common' manner and talk in a way that would be more becoming to a domestic than a nurse." Flirtation or any sexual liaison with men, if known about, was considered "unnurse-like" behavior. Two students were dismissed at the end of their probation period at the City Hospital for bringing a male caller through the halls of the nurses' home after hours for, they claimed, "the fun of it." There was, of course, the cultural double standard. A nursing student at Boston's Long Island Hospital caught with a physician was dismissed, but the doctor was allowed to continue his training.[68]

Even worse was the student who was both flirtatious and too friendly to patients and domestics. The student reprimanded for being too "common" was also disciplined for raising her voice, treating ward maids and patients as her equals, and lacking "tact and firmness" in dealing with the "help." Other students were criticized for talking "too freely with orderlies and patients," or "coquettishness and showing feelings too plainly on the ward." A Montreal father was informed by Boston City Hospital authorities that his daughter was suspended for "not obeying the rules, going to a ballgame with an orderly, spending time playing with men and neglecting patients." Another student was put on probation for walking on the street in her uniform and for having an open friendship with an orderly. In addition, her head nurse reported: "She is inclined to be familiar with ward maids and on one occasion I have observed her talking to mine in a very friendly manner."[69] At the Massachusetts General the training school authorities even went as far as separating the students' laundry from that of the other hospital workers, perhaps in fear of some kind of behavioral contamination from the soapsuds.[70]

The students, in defense, claimed that their talking to patients and other help was not overstepping the boundaries of propriety. But the right to define these limits belonged to the head nurses and nursing administrators. Such norms could be used either to praise a student for her ability to achieve compliance from her patients and other hospital workers or to damn her for "servantlike" qualities.[71] Above all, such norms taught the nursing student that her future depended on separating herself from the hospital's domestics and patients.

Quietness, poise, and maturity were also expected. A student was suspended from the City Hospital school for several months because "her manners are somewhat crude and countrified . . . talking too loudly . . . loses her self-possession."[72] It was lack of composure and presence of mind rather than lack of sophistication that was of concern. A nursing superintendent wrote of a student in 1904: "Agnes Bell's manners at times may be said to be unsophisticated, but never undignified."[73] At Somerville (Massachusetts) Hospital's training school, nursing students were reported to "lack refinement" but to still be "good workers." At the same time, students who were "too nervous" were asked to leave. Similarly, students were expected to lose their "frivolous, noisy and youthful ways" or their "abrupt and unattractive personal manners."[74]

An innate sense of "refinement," however undeveloped, was considered essential, especially at the better schools. George Rowe, at Boston City Hospital, noted: "Miss Moore was seen by me and told she could not be accepted for her second six months until she showed a marked improvement in her manners, language and dropped her social solecisms." It seemed the student's head nurse claimed she used "slangy expressions . . . rather uncultivated ones, such as 'yes M'am,' or when told to do anything would reply 'sure.' "[75] Youthful pranks also were frowned on. Two students were suspended for hanging a sheet from their windows one evening proclaiming "Night nurses sleeping – please do not disturb," and another was dismissed for riding down the hospital's corridors on an orderly's hand truck.[76] Smaller institutions placed less stress on this, although superintendents did bemoan students who had "unfortunate manners." Similarly, a training school like the one attached to Long Island Hospital, Boston's almshouse hospital in the harbor, had difficulty attracting students and thus placed less emphasis on the students' manners and speech.

Appearance and body type took on grave importance as spirit and body were assumed to be intertwined. George Rowe commented on a new student's records: "She is by no means an ideal probationer, is heavy in body and mind. Not refined in face or manner . . . looks like a servant." Another student, whose middle-class credentials were more apparent since she was the niece of a Boston physician, was described by Rowe as having "good 'blood,' good figure, good face and a pleasing manner."[77] A "handsome" face and pleasing manner were equally important in nursing students, and such women often received a variety of accolades from their sister students as much as from the authorities.[78]

Gross violations of the rules were punished by suspensions or dismissals. Drunkenness or pregnancy usually resulted in the nursing student being asked to leave. Physically abusing unruly patients, recording temperatures or other vital signs not really taken, giving incorrect amounts of drugs or the wrong medications, refusing to follow physicians' orders were all dangerous transgressions worthy of dismissal, or at least suspension.[79] The severity of the punishment varied, however, depending on how much the student readily admitted to her errors and appeared contrite, whether the failures were cumulative, or inherently dangerous or fatal to the hospitals' patients.

Not every young woman entering training developed deference. Many learned the difference, as Nightingale had hoped, between supplication and a caring strength. In the better nursing schools, superintendents saw their roles as reshaping and "finishing" the unsophisticated but good-hearted young woman into a virtuous woman of service. Emma Nichols, assistant superintendent at Boston City Hospital Nursing School, wrote to her superior in 1910, describing a student who "when she entered our School was rather crude, having had few advantages. . . . Her gain was so great we take considerable pride in her attainments." When another student's lack of dignity and responsibility was commented on, Lucy Drown, the nursing superintendent, wrote that the woman "believes" herself to be "on a level with her patients and the ward maid." However, on further reflection, Drown crossed out the more definitive "believes" and wrote "allows herself to be etc." Change was possible.[80]

After a period of time, however, proper nursing behavior or spirit had to be demonstrated or the student might be dismissed. A Connecticut woman was asked to leave Boston City Hospital in 1911 because "her reports all show that she did not plan her work well and that her head never saved her feet." Another was let go for not carrying out "the spirit of the hospital rules in her relationships with other hospital personnel."[81] At Long Island Hospital, in contrast, nursing students who clearly did not live up to the standards were allowed to graduate, mainly as a result of political pressures from the trustees. Instead, the nursing superintendent refused to write them letters of recommendation when they applied for jobs.[82] Thus the criticism, disciplining, and even dismissal of nursing students centered on their behavior.

THE DILEMMAS OF SELF-SACRIFICE

Many nursing superintendents lived the Nightingale ideals as best they could and infused them into their schools. The authoritarian model could and did "retemper" many women. It imparted to nurses idealism and pride in their skills, began to differentiate the trained from the untrained nurse, and helped to protect and aid the sick and dying. It could provide a way for virtuous women to contribute to the improvement of humanity.

Nursing could become a way to empower a young woman by giving her meaningful work, a sense of accomplishment, and a group identity. Nursing school was, for many, the place they came as girls and left as women. As one nursing superintendent reminded a graduating class in

1904, "You have become self-controlled, unselfish, gentle, compassionate, brave and capable – in fact, you have risen from the period of irresponsible girlhood to that of womanhood."[83] Nursing thus became, for some women, a less elite equivalent of an education in womanly virtue and female solidarity afforded their richer sisters in the women's colleges.

But for many, as nursing historian Dorothy Sheahan noted, the training school "was a place where . . . women learned to be girls."[84] Training narrowed, not widened, the range of permissible behaviors for respectable women. And unlike students in the women's colleges, nurses were strongly discouraged from developing either independent thinking or autonomy.

Women or girls, the idealism and discipline could also make nurses vulnerable to exploitation. The nursing model's elements worked only if the spirit that absorbed the discipline and behavioral codes did not become worn down so that only a stark, harsh, and hollow shell remained. "Self-abnegation" rather than "tact" was often the result when institutional norms weighed in favor of submission. The emphasis on "the one right way" could standardize behavior and technical skills, but it could, and did, often stifle initiative and freeze attempts for change. Ritualistic behaviors, devoid of thought and caring, were often all that remained.[85]

The conception of nursing as an occupational sisterhood built on caring and the demand for rights, rather than the need to accept obligations and duties, might have provided some of the ideological material necessary to guard against exploitation. As historian Nancy Cott has argued, some nineteenth-century women made the transition from "women's sphere to women's rights" through "Quakerism, Unitarianism, radical sectarianism or de-conversion" experiences.[86] The nursing equivalent of this would have been some kind of powerful alternative idea and context for understanding service to humanity without self-sacrifice. In the institutional framework of the hospital nursing school and within the ideological stance of nursing and Victorian womanhood, such radical thoughts were occasionally planted but were hardly nurtured. Furthermore, given the stress on separating the nursing student from contact with the hospital's other workers, trained nursing began with an elitist ideology that precluded alliances across occupational categories.

The nursing model was also built on environmentalist theories that stressed the importance of the nurse in the creation of physical and moral cleanliness and order. The model assumed relatively separate but equal responsibilities for nurses and physicians. But as scientific medicine became more important, the number of medical tasks defined as necessary for good patient care increased. Physicians came to expect that nurses, as their assistants, would take on these increasingly technical and administrative tasks. Similarly, the theoretical and moral power behind the basis of nursing theory was devalued. Cleaning became more a domestic chore than a scientific and moral one. Separate became unequal and less important.

Finally, the model assumed that the doctrine of spheres would give equal power to nurses and physicians. But the economic difficulties that confronted American nursing schools undermined this tenet as well. In their hopes of making the hospital into a proper Victorian home, the reformers succeeded only too well.

4

Training as work: the pupil nurse as hospital machine

The model for trained nursing stressed discipline, self-sacrifice, order, and a separate sphere for nursing within the hospital structure. The caring and order-making nurse was to be neither a physician's assistant nor a hospital drudge. She was to exhibit both autonomy and altruism. As part of a vital female-headed hierarchy, she was to be protected from inefficiency and the political and sexual corruption of the hospital. From within the safety of the nursing structure, she was to transform the institution around her.

The hopes of nursing reformers and educators that this uniformly well-trained and properly behaved "new lady" nurse would be shaped in the Nightingale mold foundered, however, in the political economy of the hospital–nursing school relationship. Despite the wealth, position, and bureaucratic skills of the women responsible for the establishment of the first American nursing schools, there was no outpouring of funds sufficient to endow training schools on the Nightingale model, attached to, but not part of, the hospitals. Unlike colleges established for women's higher education, nursing attracted neither the endowments nor the cultural interest that supported such separate women's institutions.[1]

Beginning with the founding of the school at Boston City Hospital in 1878, most nursing schools were the creations of hospital boards and were fully integrated into the work of the hospitals. The demands of the hospital for a work force often overcame the nursing school's abilities to educate its students. Autonomy was sacrificed and altruism was sanctified. In the course of developing the training schools, the female nursing hierarchy remained (probationers, junior nurses, senior or head nurses, and a nursing superintendent or matron as head), but its independence was undermined. With an ideology that stressed discipline, self-sacrifice, and order, an institutional context that weakened the idealistic aspects of this ideology, and the removal of a mediating autonomous female power structure, trained nursing became infamous for its drudgery and machinelike students. Nursing education was called training; in reality it was work. Training introduced a new order within the hospitals and provided a new justification for the exploitation of the nursing work force, as well as engendering new conflicts and divisions. In this context, the ability to care was often hard to sustain.

TRAINED TO WORK

The introduction of training for nurses transformed the hospitals in ways the early reformers could not have expected. In 1873, when the first nursing schools were established, there were 178 medical and mental hospitals in the United States. By 1923, there were 6,830 hospitals (an increase of over 3,700 percent), and every fourth one included a nursing school.[2] Nursing superintendent Isabel Hampton Robb commented in 1897: "With the advent and success of the trained nurse, the question of providing for the proper care of the sick in hospitals was solved."[3] Before the early 1900s, however, a hospital opening a nursing school had no minimal standards to meet and proper care could become problematic. In 1895, even a hospital with a dozen beds, and a patient census of one, could purport to have a "school" with two pupil nurses.[4] By 1910, in Massachusetts, for example, hospitals with training schools outnumbered those without them nearly two to one. Melrose Hospital and the New Bedford Emergency Hospital, with 18 and 16 beds respectively, had training schools. In contrast, Boston City Hospital had nearly 1,000 beds and a training school of 183 pupils.[5] "Uniformity," Mary Riddle, the assistant superintendent at Boston City Hospital, stated in 1898, "is conspicuous by its absence."[6]

The "training school" could provide a hospital both with a cheap labor source and additional income from fees collected when students were sent out to patients' homes on private cases. Somerville Hospital, located in a working-class suburb of Boston, opened a training school within two years of admitting its first patients in 1891. The hospital's board of trustees assured the community that the nursing school was a good investment: "They are paid a small salary, but the amount received by the hospitals for their services outside more than equals their salaries, so that the cost of the nursing service in the hospital is practically nothing."[7] Similarly, Boston City Hospital officials declared that even increasing the number of nurses by establishing a school had not increased costs.[8] More than one hospital superintendent admitted that "it would be impossible financially . . . to maintain [the] hospital if they did not have pupil nurses."[9]

Once training was introduced, the hospitals theoretically had three options in terms of staffing: continue to use untrained women, establish a school with pupil nurses, or hire trained graduate nurses. The advantages of the school were numerous. Expenses to the hospital were low. Nursing students were "paid" what was frequently called an "allowance," that is, money for personal expenses, rather than wages. At rates of about eight to twelve dollars a month in addition to room and board for a thirteen-hour day (or night), a six-day week and a fifty-week year, they were a cheaper work force than were women without training who, moreover, might leave on a moment's notice.[10] Dr. Abner Post, a consulting surgeon at Boston's Long Island Hospital, summarized the advantage of using student labor: "It keeps a constant – I believe it allowed the employment of a larger number of nurses than would otherwise be employed. It certainly brings to the service of the hospital a more intelligent class of nurses than under the old regime."[11]

A graduate nursing staff presented the hospitals with certain disadvantages. Few graduates were willing to return to the drudgery of institutional work with, as one nurse complained, "very little prospect of learning anything new, and none whatever of advancement."[12] Some of the larger hospitals hired graduate nurses as head or operating room nurses, but most graduate nurses were expected to find work in private duty in patients' homes. When such work was available, it paid fifteen dollars a week during the 1890s, more than four times what the hospitals paid a pupil nurse.[13] Because nursing schools emphasized "the right way" of doing work, graduate nurses also brought to the institutions their own schools' ideas of proper procedures. "Your best plan," Dr. Alfred Worcester sagely advised those considering different staffing arrangements, "is your own training school."[14]

By the turn of the century the nursing schools, with few exceptions, served almost like hiring halls where the hospitals obtained their nursing work force. Nursing students often entered training every two months or were allowed to enter individually from an "emergency list" if a dropout occurred. Ironically, there was no sick leave. If the pupil nurses became ill, the hospital usually cared for them, but their "allowances" were stopped and the time they lost had to be made up before they could graduate.[15]

The hospital's control and use of students as a work force were most evident in the procedures for recruitment and monitoring. At Boston City Hospital a prospective nursing student wrote to the nursing superintendent for the application forms, but her filled-in papers and letters of recommendation were sent directly to the hospital's superintendent. He also had the final word on student evaluations. At Somerville Hospital in the 1890s the right to appoint pupil nurses lay with an executive committee of the trustees, upon the recommendation of the medical board. At Long Island Hospital, as in many municipal institutions, the political patronage power of trustees undermined the nursing superintendent's control. She reported that incompetent students were allowed to graduate because the trustees were more concerned with the "fairness" of granting diplomas in exchange for hard work than nursing standards.[16]

Selectivity in recruitment varied considerably. In the Massachusetts

Table 4.1. *Application and drop-out rates for training schools in Massachusetts, 1897*

Hospital bed size	Number of schools	Average number of applicants	Average applicants taken (%)	Drop-out rate (%)
0–50	15	19	53	26
51–100	7	78	21	22
101–250	5	65	39	25
251 +	3	*a*	*a*	*a*

[a]The number of applicants to the three schools varied so considerably (35, 50, and 644) as to make an averaging meaningless.

Source: Calculated from raw figures in Jane Hodson, ed., *How to Become a Trained Nurse* (New York: William Abbatt, 1898), pp. 133–49.

training schools in the late 1890s, the average percentage of applicants taken varied from 20 to 50 and depended in part on the size of the school (see Table 4.1). The 700-bed Boston City Hospital accepted only seventy-three students in 1897, 11 percent of those applying, and kept on only fifty-seven, or 78 percent of those who entered. In contrast, the 35-bed Fall River Hospital received six applicants for its nursing school and accepted and graduated them all.[17]

The use of nursing students as the hospital's work force was evident in their titles. As nursing educator Adelaide Nutting shrewdly noted:

The habitual use in hospitals of the word "nurse" in speaking of a student nurse by physicians, patients and the public, is a correct indication of her status, showing where the emphasis lies, and how little she really is looked upon as a student. In this connection it is interesting to note the scrupulous care with which we withhold the title of "doctor" from medical students until they have completed their work leading to it in Medical Schools.[18]

The woman entering nursing school may have expected to *train;* what she did primarily, however, was to *work.*

A HOSPITAL MACHINE

Hospital nursing remained work that entailed hard physical labor and a good deal of drudgery. Anna Fullerton's *garde-malade,* exorcising the dreaded enemies of death and disorder, became an army of mechanical women bent on incessant cleaning. As late as 1920, scrubbing of bathrooms and floors and the washing of laparotomy pads, operating sheets, and towels was still a pupil nurse's daily task.[19] Despite the rhetoric, much of the actual work of the nurse in training differed very little from that of her predecessors, except that she was to do it cheerfully and with more precision. With students on duty ten or more hours, the time for lecture or lab when the students were not half asleep was difficult to find.[20] Exhaustion, at the very least, was the usual outcome from such herculean efforts.

In many cases, exhaustion was followed by illness. Stella Goostray, in recalling her days as a probationer at Children's Hospital in Boston, was once asked to assist on a typhoid fever ward before she had adequate training or any immunization against the disease. Required to clean up some spilled stools, she subsequently contracted the disease. At the New England Hospital for Women and Children, physicians became so alarmed by the illness rate among their students in 1893 that they counseled the nursing superintendents to admit only very healthy women into the training program. They did not suggest, however, that she lighten their work load or cut their hours.[21]

Surveys revealed that the danger of typhoid and scarlet fevers, pneumonia, and diphtheria could be measured in the high morbidity and mortality rates among students. Tuberculosis felled or permanently disabled many. Under the press of work, students were often required to return to service before they were completely recovered. Sick leaves were rare, and "exhaustion" was the leading reason for student withdrawals.[22] Poor living conditions compounded the problem as nursing quarters were more barracks than homes. As one witty student noted, she and her roommate labeled their barren space the "orphan's home."[23]

In theory, the actual educating of the students took place on the wards amid all the necessity of caring for patients. This learning-by-doing was supplemented by lectures. These were usually given in the evenings, after a ten- to twelve-hour workday. In the 1880s and 1890s much of this lecturing was done by the hospital's physicians, when they remembered to show up, who frequently pitched their talks either too high or too low for the students. Nursing students were expected to take careful notes and to be able to recite what they had "learned." The practical training was to be in steps from simpler duties of cleaning to the dispensing of medications and the teaching of other students.[24]

Such order, however, continually broke down. Emergencies and understaffing were the rule rather than the exception. Students frequently had to provide care in situations for which they were ill prepared. The necessity for order and discipline, coupled with the hospital's chronic understaffing, forced the students to realize that the priorities were to finish the overwhelming number of tasks as quickly as possible, with no questions asked. "It was often my lot as well as of many of my fellow pupils," a graduate nurse identified as "O. K. B." wrote in *The Trained Nurse,* to be repulsed in such a way as to discourage any repetition of questions as to the How, Why and Wherefore of things put to those from whom we had a right to expect reasonable answers, leaving us to find out as best we could with our limited time and means, what was necessary we should know.[25]

Given these conditions and the nursing ideology, it is not surprising that by 1900 terms like "hospital machine" and "industrial slave" began to be used to describe the student nurse.[26] The image of the student as a drudge, devoid of individuality, mechanically following orders, reverberated in the wider culture. Thus in a 1913 novel entitled *The White Linen Nurse,* a nursing student, Rae Malgregor, is about to graduate when she decides to quit because, she tells the nursing superintendent, "Don't you see that my face doesn't know anything?" she faltered, "except just to smile and smile and smile and say 'Yes, sir – No, sir – Yes, sir.' " Later, the senior surgeon inquires why she does not want to be a trained nurse. Malgregor replies, "Because – my – face – is – tired." The author, in order to make the identity problem even clearer, has the surgeon realize after several exchanges who Rae is. "Excuse me for not recognizing you," he apologized gruffly, "but you girls all look so much alike!" To this, the novel's heroine replied:

Yes! Yes, sir! . . . That's just exactly what the trouble is! That's just exactly what I was trying to express, sir! My cheeks are almost sprung with artificial smiles! My eyes are fairly bulging with unshed tears! My nose aches like a toothache trying never to turn up at anything! I'm smothered with the discipline of it! I'm choked with the affectation! I tell you – I just can't breathe through a trained nurse face any more! I tell you, sir, I'm sick to death of being nothing but a type. I want to look like *myself!*

The nursing superintendent's response to this soliloquy is sadness: "There goes my best nurse! . . . Oh, no, not the most brilliant one, I didn't mean that, but the most reliable! The most nearly perfect human machine that it has ever been my privilege to see turned out."[27] Order was indeed created, but by repressing the humanity and innovative and caring skills of the students.

THE POWER OF THE HEAD NURSE AND STUDENT REBELLION

Turning out such human machines was primarily the responsibility of each ward's head nurse. She organized the work and supervised the pupil nurse on a day-to-day basis. The role of the head nurse was in part a holdover from the division of labor in the hospital before the introduction of training schools; Nightingale redefined the position, added the chain of nursing command, and provided a clearer justification for the head nurse's power. Such head nurses, whether graduate nurses (in some of the better

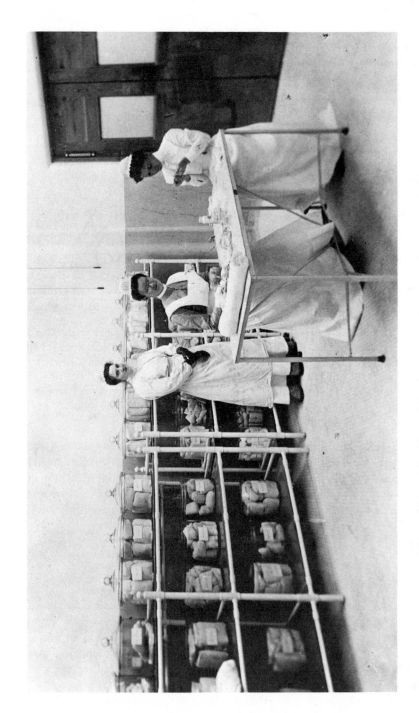

The making and rolling of bandages was often part of a nurse's work. Massachusetts General Hospital, circa 1900. *Source:* Countway Library

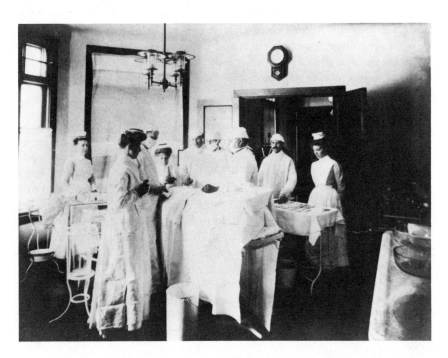

A not uncommon hospital operating room sight: female nursing students, male surgeons, and a nurse anesthetist with an ether cone, a possibly posed photograph. Somerville Hospital, Somerville, Massachusetts, circa 1900. *Source:* Somerville Hospital President's Office

hospitals) or, more commonly, senior nursing students (in the smaller institutions), became the hospital equivalent of a factory's line supervisor. It was the head nurse's demands that did much to shape the nature of the training experience.

The ideology of discipline and the stress and pressure of the work converged on the head nurse, investing her with grave responsibilities and often arbitrary control. Lucy Drown, a superintendent of nurses at Boston City Hospital, wrote a senior nursing student who was fearful of holding such a trustworthy position: "Head nurses are expected to be ready to take responsibility. One learns in the doing and I cannot guarantee that you will have some position in which there is no responsibility."[28] Some pupil nurses did learn and grow from being placed in such positions. But many others, as the letter from the nervous senior to Drown indicates, were frightened by the responsibilities. In such a situation, absolute control could become absolutism, and arbitrariness a way to cover insecurity and uncertainty.

Although the textbooks contended that "no nurse is fit for her position who will sacrifice to any narrow jealousies or disputes the working order of her department," such disputes and divisions constantly occurred.[29] The capriciousness and harshness of the discipline codes and the strain of the work all converged to make them inevitable. The pressure from the hospitals on the nursing superintendents, in turn, forced them to press the students to keep in line and accomplish the necessary work.[30]

Such a form of authority encouraged students to conform to the norms. Those who chose to question the arrangements were often severely reprimanded. In June 1918, for example, a pupil nurse at Boston City Hospital was reported by her head nurse for shirking responsibilities. Her transgression, it appears, was her refusal to obey the rules established by the head nurse on how much work had to be done, especially when a supervisor was visiting. The student tried to defend herself on the grounds that her only offense was an inability to "camouflage down to a science" the fact that there was little to do after 2 A.M. on a particular ward. Her plea to the nursing superintendent fell on deaf ears.[31]

A student's failure to conform to the school's informal norms often brought swift retribution. In a long, rambling, and plaintive letter, an Irish-born nursing student wrote to the Boston City Hospital nursing superintendent in 1908 to question her dismissal from the school. The head nurses had faulted her "determined manner," labeling her "an neurasthenic with introspection pronounced." In response, Minnie Callahan accused the Canadian-born head nurses of discriminating against her for being Irish and using "savage" expressions to upbraid her in front of patients. She reported numerous examples of their flirtations and sexual behavior with orderlies and doctors at the expense of patient demands. Aware that acquiescing to the head nurses' "whims" was required, she declared, "It is not my notion to kiss and hug my head nurses and rub them over with flattery so as to escape my duty, and get along serenely." Finally in deference to the expectations of "good" nurse behavior, she stated her willingness to do her "duty" to patients, but not "to tramp the streets evenings with other nurses and talk in their rooms after duty is over."[32]

Callahan's letter suggests the difficulties faced by a student who would not accept the school's informal norms or join the "homosocial network" of female relationships.[33] Callahan's unhappiness also illustrates the negative aspect of female bonding that could lead to the isolation of those unwilling to conform. "The formation of cliques," nursing educator Isabel Hampton Robb warned, "is to be discouraged."[34]

Other issues could have been at work here, of course. Writing in 1908, Callahan's sexualized language may reflect merely typical female discourse of the nineteenth century, or the more modern anger of a rebuffed lover.

Certainly by this time many nursing educators worried that the intense "smashes" and relationships of students could indicate sexual interests ("forms of perverted affection," as Robb labeled them), rather than just social needs.[35]

The nature of the hospital social system and the nursing work culture engendered such cliques and supported the arbitrary use of power. Most students had to agree when they entered the school that the hospital could dismiss them "at its own discretion." The hospitals were under no obligation to explain the reasons for dismissals or to allow the students to face their accusers.[36] The fears expressed in the letters written to Lucy Drown reflect this reality, as do the charges in the nursing journals that there was "favoritism" within the schools.

Despite the pressures for conformity and submission, however, nursing students were not merely mechanical hospital machines. The very existence of so many rules, and the incessant efforts to discipline, suggest the very tenuous hold nursing authorities had over their charges. As in any family or military establishment, rules and reality differed widely. Close friendships could lead to enduring camaraderie and personal support as well as the isolation a Minnie Callahan would experience.[37]

Rebellion was also a possibility, even if only on the level of wishful thinking. In November 1890, a Boston graduate nurse wrote the editor of *Trained Nurse:*

While completing my course of two years training in the Hospital I often rebelled against those long hours and thought that a strike would be the very thing, but it is hard to do this among women as there are too many nurses, "favorites" to the Hospital, who take the work easy and let thing [*sic*] go undone rather than put themselves to any inconvenience to have the work done up, or in other words work together and not apart.

But, she concluded, she herself put in overtime "many a time and done it gladly and cheerfully for the *sick patients,* but not for the Hospital or the Superintendent of Nurses; only for the patients who would otherwise have been neglected."[38] Similarly a pupil nurse in 1908 anonymously declared her sadness at being forced to

. . . devote my energies to perfecting myself in the art of letting the patients wait while I take time to make empty beds in the orthodox way . . . but I here confess that I sometimes think there is just a little too much stress tied upon the things that count only for appearance and not quite enough upon other things that tend more directly to make the patients comfortable and happy.[39]

Even in fantasy, however, patients' needs came first.

Other nursing students put such thoughts of rebellion into actions. During the 1910s, the period historian David Montgomery has labeled the "strike decade," nursing students, like other workers across the United

States, took up this weapon.[40] Nursing and hospital journals reported a rash of strikes but condemned such actions and discussed few details.

The pressure to conform, coupled with exploitation, could thus help to build alliances within nursing work groups. In the majority of strikes, for which there is evidence, the walkouts were instigated by the students or head nurses *against* the nursing superintendent because of harsh conditions, bad food, overwork, assignment to dangerous wards without proper training, or in sympathy against the arbitrary disciplining of a student. In several strikes, however, where exploitation was less of an issue, the students struck in sympathy *with* their nursing superintendent over her disagreement with higher authorities.[41]

Such strikes were mainly the ephemeral and desperate actions of women angered by overwork and the abuse of power. They did not result in lasting, formal organizations. For most nursing students the moral dilemma of leaving ill patients, the professional dilemma of classing oneself with workers, and the psychological dilemma of openly thwarting authority were overwhelming. Instead they sought survival through more subtle tactics on a day-to-day basis, or simply quit. For nursing students, at least during this period, an overt assault on their institutional home and their hospital family was too difficult to make.

INSTITUTIONALIZED SUBORDINATION

Nightingale and the other nursing reformers had not anticipated the necessity for such an assault. They had seen the exploitation and degradation of untrained nurses by male hospital authorities and physicians. Nightingale believed that the school's departmental independence from the hospital and the power of the nursing superintendent and her female hierarchy would protect the integrity and education of the students. As with other nineteenth-century female reformers, nursing leaders understood the importance of separate women-controlled institutions. But the nursing school–hospital arrangement was not one of separateness. It constrained the nursing superintendent to demand conformity and work, but gave her little power or incentive to defend her students.[42] Nevertheless, conflict between the nursing and hospital authorities was not uncommon.

As soon as training was introduced, American hospital superintendents and physicians recognized that an administratively distinct nursing department headed by a powerful nursing superintendent, who reported directly to the hospital's trustees, would be an ever-present threat to their own positions and to the use of pupils as workers. Such a bureaucratic division of authority could undermine in practice whatever apparent ideological deference nurses were taught to give to physicians and administrators.

Hospital superintendents therefore sought to assure the departmental dependence of nursing.

The question of the power of the nursing superintendent was just one of the conflicts over authority that characterized hospitals in the years between 1873 and the opening decades of the twentieth century. As both medical care and, subsequently, paying patients became increasingly important to the hospitals, the power of physicians began to grow. Administrative decisions once made primarily on moral grounds by trustees (e.g., patient admissions) began to be made on medical grounds by doctors.

Trustees also relinquished more day-to-day decision making to the increasingly powerful hospital superintendent. Trustees, while retaining their role in theory as the institution's moral guardians, in practice became its financial guardians. While tensions between trustees, hospital superintendents, and physicians continued to exist, by the early 1900s the hospital's dual authority structure – a lay one controlled by a superintendent or administrator and a medical one controlled by the medical or surgical chief – began to emerge.[43]

As this authority structure was being worked out, the superintendents, often in alliance with the physicians, moved to assure that the nursing school and its female superintendent remained dependent on *both* physician and hospital superintendent authority. Although nursing superintendents often yielded to pressures and conformed, there was inherent conflict in this administrative arrangement as nursing superintendents tried to balance the hospital's demands with the educational needs of their students.

In 1902, Dr. George H. M. Rowe, superintendent of Boston City Hospital, made the clearest statement of the necessity for nursing's subordination. In a speech before the National Association of Hospital Superintendents, he called for what he characterized as a "unal" plan that would centralize authority in the hospital superintendent's hands. Such a plan would minimize "warfare in the hospital family" and lead to the "best discipline," he contended. In contrast, a school with a separate training school administration was, he argued, "illogical, unbusinesslike, conducive to friction, shifting the various responsibilities. . . . Sometimes the result is 'open war.' " Similar sentiments in equally strong language were expressed by "war-weary" superintendents at other meetings.[44]

Some nursing educators and superintendents were well aware that the loss of independence for their schools was the death blow to their original hopes of developing nursing training on the Nightingale model. Lavinia Dock, for example, called the relationship between hospitals and nursing schools "dispiriting . . . with a formlessness, a lack of tradition, an adoption of hasty and tentative methods, and an acceptance of imperfect results."[45] The basis of her argument and that of other nurses was to question the soundness of such structures in the interest of both nurses' training *and* the hospital. The link between nursing and hospital reform was continually evoked. But underneath their arguments lay nearly a century of "female institution building" and the political sensibility that understood the necessity for separate institutions run by women.[46]

In response to the argument that the medical board of a hospital should have final authority over the nurses, it was contended that the nursing superintendent, rather than the physicians, had the interest of the whole institution at heart. Lillian Wald, the director of the Nurses' Settlement in New York, offered a minority report on hospital–nursing relations at the second New York State Conference of Charities and Corrections, when the majority report favored giving final authority to a medical board. Wald argued that the nursing superintendent's responsibility was to manage the "household economy" and moral reputation of the hospital, the carrying out of medical orders, and the proper education and protection of the nursing students. If appointed by the doctors, Wald contended, the nursing superintendent would "almost inevitably overdo her responsibilities to them and slight her other . . . equally grave responsibilities."[47]

Lavinia Dock, on clear feminist grounds, furthered this argument by directly attacking Rowe's "unal plan." Dock, the most overtly feminist of the first generation of nursing educators, attacked him for what she saw as his old-fashioned patriarchal ideas, likening his views on hospital organization to that of the traditional vision of the family as headed only by a man. She noted:

The orthodox conception of the family in many countries and many centuries was of course on the "unal" plan, the man being the unit. But modern states are abolishing by legislation this "unal" form and are replacing it by a dual institution of the family. . . . With the disappearance of patriarchalism the modern family is seen to have two heads, – on the principle, I suppose, that two heads are better than one.[48]

Dock's attack did not, however, conclude with a call for an egalitarian structure or a "symmetrical" family. Rather she cleverly appealed to the authority of the trustees, investing them with the crucial power in the hospital. She placed her hopes in their ability to see that the broader goals of the hospital could best be obtained with power invested equally in the hands of the nursing superintendent and the hospital superintendent.

Dock was not unaware of a critical flaw in her argument: "It may be said," she queried rhetorically, " 'Will she be better off with the Trustees?' " "Yes," Dock answered because here in front of the board of trustees at least she would be on an equal footing with the hospital superintendent. As would the hospital superintendent, she would have a chance to educate the trustees to accept her viewpoints and to allow her to work out the specific details. She could not have a similar relationship with the superintendent because he did not possess "the final power." Further, Dock contended, the superintendent "must himself go to the trustees for his authority and if, overburdened with his own claims and problems, hers are lost in the transition, who can wonder?"

Finally, Dock placed the blame for the "friction" in the hospital family on the shoulders of the blundering and interfering men who failed to understand women's work. She concluded that such "friction" was necessary because

in a disorderly business, or home, or hospital, where no one knows exactly what another one ought to do or has the rights to do, there *ought* to be friction, for otherwise there would be dull acquiescence in all sorts of improper arrangements – one of the worst of conditions.

Lavinia Dock, in language more overly anti-male than that of other nursing educators or of Nightingale herself, nevertheless was articulating a position common to them all: the work of women through properly organized trained nursing could bring moral and technical order to the hospitals. As with other workers, in particular engineers, who took on the role of bringing structure and order to enterprises, nursing educators like Dock saw their role and the mission of the institutions as inexorably intertwined.[49] Although her argument about the essential nature of the trustees was built more on rhetoric than facts, it appealed to traditional conceptions of both the hospital and of community. It countered the growing view that the hospital was merely a scientific workshop for physicians. Rather, Dock was arguing, the importance of medicine to the hospital did not undercut the continual necessity for the trustees' moral stewardship. The argument assumed that the advice of women would be taken as equal to that of men; in a sense, Dock was rejecting the notion that women had to be subordinate either at the bedside or in the boardroom.

Appeals to boards of trustees were not usually successful, however, as physician and administrative power grew. In 1905, for example, Francina Freese, a former student of Adelaide Nutting's, wrote to her mentor about her difficulties as superintendent of nurses in a small western Maryland hospital.[50] Her antagonist was the chief surgeon and the issues concerned what constituted proper nursing procedures and who had the right to decide. The surgeon wanted the students to learn to catheterize male patients, a procedure Miss Freese, along with other nursing educators of her time, thought was improper for young women since it entailed the handling of male genitalia.[51] The surgeon accused Freese of being a "prude" and asserted that it was essential for nurses' education. Further, he wanted the students to write patient histories. This Miss Freese believed to be his attempt to foist off clearly medical responsibilities on the student nurses.

The battle was finally brought before the board of trustees, in part because Miss Freese went directly over the physician's head to a prominent member of the board. Nutting counseled her to show restraint, to discuss her feelings with no one, and to argue her case before the board. Despite her appeals, however, the board remained divided and the one female board member supported the surgeon. It was assumed he knew best what the nurses should do.

Such "friction" may have seemed necessary to a fighter such as Lavinia Dock, but to many nursing superintendents it was frightening and difficult. Clearly uncertain of herself, Francina Freese queried Nutting: "Do all superintendents keep running into things like this, or am I a quarrelsome sort of person that can't get along smoothly?" In an article on institutional positions, a nurse warned: "One must be of heroic stuff and infinite tact to endure the certain vexation and surmount the certain difficulties which present themselves."[52] But most women were made of human stuff. The pressures of daily life in the institutions necessitated continual compromises in their ideals. Many learned to follow Lucy Drown's advice to one of her students who tried to impose Boston City Hospital's nursing standards on a hospital in Halifax: "One hospital cannot set the standard for another hospital. My advice in the matter would be to proceed very slowly and cautiously about making any marked innovations in the management of hospital and nursing affairs."[53]

Even when the trustees were willing to support the nursing superintendent, however, the growing power of the physicians in the hospitals undercut the value of that alliance. At the New England Hospital for Women and Children, where the nurses, doctors, and trustees were women, disputes that underscored the physicians' power were common. Common gender did not necessarily lessen the conflict between doctor and nurse since the power structure, not the specific sex of the individuals, shaped the encounters.

At a meeting of the medical board on April 2, 1886, Dr. Marie Zakrzewska, the leading power at the hospital, criticized a ruling by the nursing committee that allowed the superintendent of nurses to accompany the physicians when they made their rounds. Dr. Zak, as she was known at the hospital, believed this somehow placed too much authority in the nursing superintendent's hands.

A month later, the nursing committee backed down and agreed to abolish this custom. The superintendent, Miss Billings, insisted that this decision "degraded" her position to such a degree "that it would with difficulty be filled." As a result of her arguments, the nursing committee wavered but voted to let the physicians have the final say. The compromise allowed the superintendent to follow *after* the physicians' visits but "to see that the nurses promptly carried out the orders given."[54]

Similar problems continued to plague the New England Hospital, and its rapid turnover in nursing superintendents reflected these difficulties. The newly hired nursing superintendent in 1897 lasted less than four months because she felt it was impossible to put "the school into shape" since the physicians held so much power and "on account of her hands being tied." In a curious argument that recognized the difficulties but refused to make any real changes in the arrangements, the medical board tried to cajole her into staying on the grounds that "if she gets a reputation for bringing order out of confusion here they could help her later get a better position with a larger salary because of her 'fitness for a greater position.' "[55] Apparently unmoved by such remonstrations, she left the New England Hospital to its own chaos.

Such problems were not uncommon, and one commentator warned: "It is a fundamental truth in the management of small hospitals that a transient personnel deals a death-blow to efficiency."[56] At some of the larger institutions, more powerful and heroic women were able to extract a greater degree of authority from trustees, superintendents, and physicians.[57] But the average nursing superintendent, as Wald had warned, found herself constantly pressured to serve the institution's and physicians' demands before the needs of her students. Ultimate control over nursing was out of her hands.

THE RESULTING DILEMMAS

Nightingale and the American nursing reformers had expected nurses in training to learn their practical skills by working on the hospital's wards. But the demands of the hospital for a work force meant that pupils' education was continually sacrificed to the exigencies of hospital work. The growing needs of increasingly acutely ill patient populations and the continual financial pressures on the institutions made certain the ever-present demand for such sacrifices. Furthermore, since nursing theory emphasized training in discipline, order, and practical skills, the ideological justification explained the abuse of student labor. And because the nursing work force was made up almost entirely of women, altruism, sacrifice, and submission were expected and encouraged. Exploitation was inevitable in a field where until the early 1900s, there were no accepted standards for how much work an average student should do or how many patients she could successfully care for. Nor were there any mechanisms through which to enforce standards.

If there had been a nursing authority structure with an independent power base, it might have protected the students from some of the exploitation. But as Adelaide Nutting bluntly pointed out in 1912, "Under the present system the school has no life of its own."[58] In some of the larger hospitals, such as Johns Hopkins, powerful superintendents like Isabel Hampton Robb were able to carve out a better educational program. But Hopkins was not an "average" hospital, nor was its training school average. Most nursing superintendents, as Lillian Wald warned, were expected to show economy in the nursing department and to meet the hospital's labor demands; thus, they had to place nursing education as a low priority. Those who did not found themselves in inevitable conflicts, or out of a job. Submission was rewarded; innovation, experimentation, and advocacy were not. The nursing superintendent, because of the subordination of women, the hospital's authority structure, and growing physician power, was thwarted in her efforts to become an advocate for nursing. Instead the nursing authority structure, rather than protecting the student, became the mechanism through which she experienced her oppression.

Economic exploitation coupled with a nursing ideology that stressed strict discipline subverted the very hopes nursing reformers had for the trained nurse. Character was threatened by demands for conformity, order continually slipped into rigidity, and caring was given a subordinate position. Rebellion and questioning, although inevitable and ever present, were punished or led to dismissals. Nursing superintendents' pleas to boards of trustees, in the name of better patient care or the hospital's moral duty, fell on ears more closely attuned to arguments made by doctors in the name of science and medical care. Within this structure, conflict and divisions were inevitable. Nursing was continually at loggerheads with the hospitals, physicians, and, inescapably, within itself.

5

"Strangers to Boston": who becomes a nurse

Despite the rigors and drudgery of training, nursing remained an occupation that attracted women searching for a way to serve both humanity and themselves. In the cultural matrix of late nineteenth- and early twentieth-century womanhood, nursing appeared to link altruism to autonomy. It also offered young women geographic mobility. Because most schools were located in cities, nursing seemed to be a way for a woman to participate safely in the excitement, independence, and opportunity of the urban working world.

Those entering training shared similar needs and desires, but little else. By the end of the nineteenth century, the ideal of a united band of respectable women nurses reforming the hospitals became an extremely uneven army whose training, skills, and work experiences varied. Furthermore, as the reality of nursing training and work became more widely known, and other opportunities opened for women in the sales and clerical fields, nursing schools found it more difficult to attract the respectable and educated daughters of the middling classes so prized by reformers.[1] By the 1910s and 1920s, the nursing school, which could ease well-brought-up small-town and rural women into the urban work world, looked more and more like a reformatory. For the sophisticated young urban woman, nursing offered more limitations than opportunities, whereas her suburban or rural counterpart continued to be attracted by its promise.

IN SEARCH OF A WOMANLY OCCUPATION

Untrained nursing was an occupation into which older, urban, native- and foreign-born women, often widows, drifted toward the end of their lives. In contrast, *trained* nurses were younger, native- and rural-born, single women who were "selected" by the nursing schools. Within these broad categories, there was a good deal of heterogeneity reflecting both the differences among the schools and the changing place of nursing in the hierarchy of available women's work.

For many women, nursing school was the portal to the freedom of the

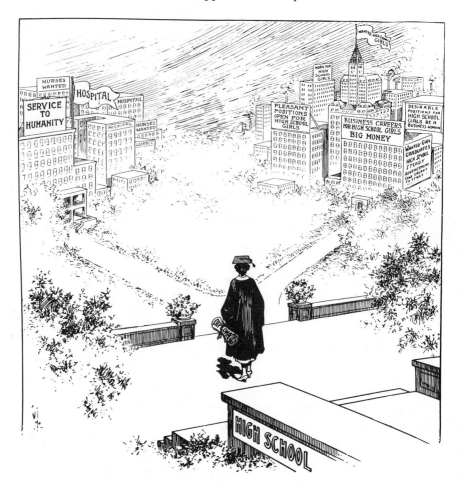

Acknowledging the difficulty of attracting high school graduates to nursing, hospital managers still emphasized nursing's "service to humanity." The caption read: "Help her to decide." *Source: Hospital Management* 10 (July 1920)

urban working world. "I am a stranger to Boston . . . am accustomed to work and have to earn my own living and so I like nursing, have a tact-for-it," wrote a prospective nursing student to a Boston City Hospital superintendent in 1881. Equally direct, another potential student declared: "I consider myself fitted for the work by inclination and consider it a womanly occupation. It is also necessary for me to become self supporting and provide for my future." The sentiments of Flora Jones reflected those of many of her sister students when she stated in her application: "It is my firm belief that every person should have a trade so they can be independent and nursing has *always appealed to me.*"[2] The necessity of working, "a preference for independence," and the attraction of a "womanly occupation" all motivated women to apply for training.

Missing from applicants' letters is any hint, however, of the embarrassment and shame of having to find employment that frequently characterized the applications of nineteenth-century women seeking clerical positions.[3] Nursing seemingly offered both a livelihood and a state of grace. As an educator noted in 1890, "Young strong country girls are drawn into the work by the glamorer [sic] thrown about hospital work and the halo that sanctified a Nightingale."[4]

Nursing and hospital superintendents considered women ideal who had these attributes and expressed similar motives.[5] Class and upbringing, as much as inclination, health, character, and education, also affected a woman's chance for acceptance. Nightingale, in her own school, had insisted that the training be given to "any woman, of any class, of any sect, 'paid or unpaid,' who had the requisite qualifications, moral, intellectual and physical, for the vocation of a Nurse." Although Nightingale believed nursing should not be limited to the "lower middle class," the early English schools acknowledged that their best candidates were the "daughters of small farmers who have been used to household work – and well-educated domestic servants."[6]

Although many American schools were closed to domestic servants, woman similar in background to the British nurses entered training. At the turn of the century, an American nursing school superintendent succinctly compared those attracted to nursing with other women's occupations.

The college-bred woman takes up teaching, or music or art, or seeks to adorn society. The high school graduate either goes to college or enters the field of office-work, bookkeeping, stenography, or other work which takes a comparatively short time for preparation. Where, then, do our candidates come from? They come from the small towns or the country, where the education has been that of the district or small high school. The parents of such girls are people of moderate means, usually with large families to support, who can give their daughters but few advantages. The training school for nurses affords an opportunity for such girls to fit themselves for lucrative work with very little outlay or expense during the time of training.[7]

Through national census and nursing school data it is possible to assess the truth of this statement. A selected sample was drawn of 509 nursing students' applications to three Boston-area training schools. The schools were chosen because they represented, for different reasons, typical hospital programs: Boston City was a large urban municipal hospital; Long Island, an almshouse and small chronic-care institution; and Somerville, a medium-sized community voluntary hospital.[8] The more elite program at Massachusetts General Hospital was not studied precisely because more work has been done on this kind of school by other historians of nursing, and it was indeed less typical.[9]

Nursing was overwhelmingly entered into by native-born women. Throughout the first half of the twentieth century, trained nurses were much more likely to be native-born than the average in the female working population as a whole. They were also white. In 1910 and in 1920, for example, less than 3 percent of the trained nurses in the United States were black, whereas black women made up 17.6 and 24.0 percent, respectively, of the female working population. Nurses were thus part of the vast influx of native-born white women into the labor force in the decades around the turn of the century.[10]

There was one important exception: Canadian women of English, Scottish, or Scotch-Irish descent were the most important minority in American training schools. Nursing schools in Canada developed around the same time as those in the United States, but at a somewhat slower rate. With less competition for more places, the U.S. schools were a logical choice for a Canadian woman seeking training. The Canadian presence was quite noticeable in the Boston training schools because proximity to eastern Canada, particularly the Maritime Provinces, drew many women as part of the wider out-migration of men and women of working age that began in the 1860s.[11]

In many ways women entering training in Boston typify the national data (see Table 5.1). Native-born women predominate, although nearly one-third of the women came from the Maritimes, as did over half of those women who trained at Somerville Hospital. The only significant shift over time was the increasing number of Irish-born women who entered Long Island Hospital's school in the 1910s and 1920s and the overwhelming numbers of Maritime-born women at Somerville in the 1920s.

These changes were not accidental. The Long Island figures most likely reflect the growing ascendancy of Irish politicians in Boston. As Long Island was a small municipal hospital, "political pull" no doubt was an important criterion in determining both who was admitted and who was allowed to graduate. In turn, Somerville, which was having difficulty in the 1920s attracting local women to its school, effectively advertised in the Halifax, Nova Scotia, newspapers for students throughout these years.

Mary Elizabeth McLaughlin, a 1915 nursing school graduate, was typical of the rural-born women who entered training in Boston. The second of eight children of a sea captain father, McLaughlin was born on a farm near Sydney, Cape Breton. When she was still young, her family moved into Sydney. Her father's death when she was a teenager prompted her to

Table 5.1. *Foreign and native-born nursing students in Boston training schools sample (in %)*

	Birthplaces			
Period entering training	United States	All Canadians	Maritimes only	Other foreign born
1878–99	62.7	27.4	18.6	9.8
1900–19	53.6	33.2	27.6	13.2
1920–39	53.5	41.9	40.0	4.5
	Birthplaces			
Nursing school	United States	All Canadians	Maritimes only	Other foreign born
Boston City	65.8	20.4	18.2	7.8
Somerville	40.8	52.8	51.1	6.3
Long Island	56.9	22.5	18.6	20.6
All (N = 507)	55.4	34.7	29.6	9.9

Source: Nursing Student Records from Boston City, Somerville, and Long Island hospitals, 1878–1939.

apply for training in a nursing school in Montreal. When she failed to gain admission, she came to Boston and found work as a nursemaid in a private home. McLaughlin continued to be interested in nursing and took a Chautauqua nursing correspondence course, but still wanted to enter formal training. Her acceptance to a Boston-area school finally came in 1911, in part through the personal connections of her employers. Their letter of recommendation listed McLaughlin's regular church attendance, her lack of interest in parties, her childlike character, and her earnest desire to become a nurse as qualities that would suit her for nursing. A typical final comment summarized McLaughlin's main attributes: "She comes of sterling people, entirely superior to the class whose daughters in our country go out to domestic service . . . sound stock and country childhood."[12]

Rural-born women like Mary Elizabeth McLaughlin, from "sound country stock," whether American or Canadian, were actively sought by the nursing schools. Such women were assumed to have the proper disci-

Table 5.2. *Birthplace of nursing students in the Boston training schools sample, by size of birthplace (in %)*

Birthplace	Period entering training			
	1878–99	1900–19	1920–39	All
Rural/small town (2,500 or under)	49.0	53.2	45.8	50.1
Medium towns (2,501– 9,999)	24.5	22.8	23.2	23.3
Urban (10,000 or over)	26.5	24.0	31.0	26.6
N = 507				

Source: See Table 5.1.

pline from home training and the experience with difficult labor to withstand the rigors and petty tyrannies of nursing school life. "Our Iowa girls," Boston City's superintendent George H. M. Rowe commented, "always do well." Another Boston City nursing superintendent added that such rural-born women had the proper nursing qualities "almost by instinct." The words "she comes from a very respectable country family" were thus frequently found in the letters of recommendation of successful candidates for admission.[13]

In nursing, the meaning of "country" was complex. Not unexpectedly, in the Boston sample, 50 percent of the students had been born in rural areas or small towns with populations under 2,500, and nearly 25 percent came from towns between 2,501 and 9,999 in population.[14] About one-quarter were from more urban areas, although only 6.7 percent were born in Boston proper (see Table 5.2). There was no statistically significant shift in this distribution over time, although Long Island and Somerville had a slightly more urban draw beginning in the 1910s.

This "ruralness," however, was increasingly more likely to be of the suburban variety. In the sample, the Boston schools attracted 20 percent of their population from the small towns and suburbs within twenty-five miles of Boston (see Table 5.3). Although the number of women born in the Maritimes remained high, the statistically significant shift over time was the increasing percentage of students who had been born in Boston

Table 5.3. *Birthplace of nursing students in the Boston training schools sample, by geographic location (in %)*

| Birthplace | Period entering training | | | |
	1878–99	1900–19	1920–39	All
Boston	8.8	5.2	7.7	6.7
Boston suburbs	13.7	20.0	25.2	20.3
New England	24.5	19.6	16.1	19.5
Rest of the U.S.	15.7	8.8	4.5	8.9
Maritimes	18.6	27.6	40.0	29.6
Rest of Canada	8.8	5.6	1.9	5.1
Rest of the world	9.8	13.2	4.5	9.9
N = 507				

Source: See Table 5.1.

suburbs. Thus, after 1900, over a quarter of the students had been born either in Boston or its suburbs. Ruralness, for nurses as for many other Americans, may have been increasingly a "state of mind."[15]

Birthplace data, however, reveal very little about a woman's actual life experience, migration patterns, or upbringing. A woman born on a Maine farm, whose family might then move to Boston, could be classified only as "rural-born." However, because application forms also asked for the prospective nursing student's current address, they give some sense of the migration patterns and the extent to which women were leaving rural and small-town areas *directly* for training.

Those who entered training did so about equally from communities that were rural/small town, medium-sized towns, and urban. This pattern did not change significantly between 1878 and 1939 (see Tables A.1 and A.2 in the Appendix). Although half the students were born in rural and small-town areas, only one-third were still in such communities when they applied to the schools. Almost half of the rural and small-town women had moved to either large urban areas or medium-sized towns *before* they applied to schools (see Table 5.4). The only important (although statistically not significant) shifts over time were the increasing suburbanization of urban-born women in the 1920s and 1930s, and the slightly greater tendency of the rural-born women of those application years (again pri-

Table 5.4. *Cross-tabulation of birthplace by address of nursing students in the Boston training schools sample, by size of community (in %)*

| | Address | | |
Birthplace	Rural/small town	Medium town	Urban
Rural/small town	52.0	18.9	28.7
Medium town	4.2	81.4	14.4
Urban	11.1	18.5	70.4
N = 507			

Source: See Table 5.1.

marily from the Maritimes) to still be rural when they applied to training schools (see Table A.3 and A.4 in the Appendix).

Much of this migration pattern thus entailed movement into the suburban ring surrounding Boston, and then into the training schools. The nursing schools' population, as with cities in general, came therefore from intermetropolitan migration. As did rural women elsewhere in the United States, the students moved in stages from rural areas to small towns or suburbs *before* they entered the large cities.[16]

To be meaningful, these figures should be compared with relevant segments of the American population. The Boston nursing students, in the years 1878–99, were living in rural communities in percentages just slightly above the rest of the Massachusetts population (26.5 vs. 21.7 percent), but were much less rural than the population for the entire Northeast (26.5 vs. 45.1 percent). Over time, however, as both Massachusetts and the Northeast became more urban, the percentage of rural women entering training was increasingly *higher* than the general population (see Table A.5 in the Appendix). The comparative figures, unfortunately, do not provide location information. Thus it is impossible to tell if these figures reflect farm living or suburbanization. But they do suggest that by the twentieth century, comparatively more nonurban women were drawn into training.

These figures are not surprising. As historian Richard Hofstadter noted, "The United States was born in the country and has moved to the city."[17] Nursing was just one way for an American woman to complete this move. But, as the nation as a whole became increasingly urbanized, women of "sound country stock," rather than their suburban or urban counterparts, continued to be lured by nursing's promise of a safe haven in an urban world.

Whether women entered training from rural, urban, or small-town homes, they did so at very particular points in their lives. When training was first introduced, a certain degree of maturity was expected from matriculating students. Women thus had to be in their early twenties to gain admission. Schools did not take those over 35, on the assumption that the training was too difficult for an older woman or she would be too set in her ways to be malleable. Thus in the Boston sample as a whole the average age of the entering students was 23.6. Less than 8 percent were over 30. These figures parallel those for white working women nationwide.

The rapid expansion in the number of nursing schools by the early 1900s and a shortage of applicants led to a decline in the age of admission. By 1912, Adelaide Nutting's survey found 55.2 percent of the schools were admitting women 20 or under, and 13.15 percent of these at age 18.[18] Similarly, in the Boston sample, the percentage of women in the 20–25 age group peaked in the 1910s. By the 1920s and 1930s women over 20 were much less visible as they were replaced by 17- and 18-year-olds, coming to training directly from school.

Nor were the educational requirements for training very strict, despite much continued effort among nursing educators to raise such standards. By 1910 in Massachusetts, almost two-thirds of the schools required some years of high school, but nearly a quarter expected their students to have only a common school education.[19] Boston City Hospital's entrance requirements included a writing and reading test, but other schools did not check their students' level of literacy. In the Boston sample, about 60 percent of the students had some high school education, but, where the number of years were listed ($N = 195$), only 55 percent of the students had more than two years (see Table A.6 in the Appendix). Even when a high school education became more common for women in the 1920s and 1930s, national nursing reports noted that nearly a quarter of all nurses had one year of high school or less.[20]

Familial obligation, or more typically, the lack of it, also helped to determine who entered training and when. Trained nursing was overwhelmingly a single woman's occupation. Unmarried women made up 96.7 percent of the Boston sample. Only eight widows, three married women, and one divorced woman appear. But since single working women often contributed part of their income to their natal families, those in training had to come from families that could afford to lose either the contribution of a daughter's wages or her help in the household. For daughters whose families needed their income or effort, nursing school was a more remote goal. "The most desirable pupils," the author of a popular article on nursing wrote in *Scribner's Magazine* in 1891, "are those who could be self-supporting outside the schools, and will not be a burden on their family while in them."[21] Many nursing students fit this criterion, but others scraped by. "We are poor," an anonymous nurse noted at a New England nursing meeting in 1907. "Two-thirds of us envied the women who had five dollars per month outside the hospital allowance, which we were supposed to use only for tools with which to do our work."[22]

Hospital and nursing superintendents also sought students not burdened by family demands for labor. Lucy Drown, the Boston City Hospital nursing superintendent, repeatedly told prospective students that the school could not take widows with small children or those with uncertain home arrangements. For the same reasons, although it was common for sisters to train at the same nursing school, hospital officials often discouraged them from coming together to avoid the possibility of losing two women to family responsibilities. Drown reminded her students they would be allowed to leave only when there was a serious illness at home. Any time lost had to be made up before graduation. Sick leave or personal leave did not exist.[23]

Nursing school applications asked the prospective student to report any domestic responsibilities that would keep her from fulfilling her obligations to the hospital. As might be expected, only one student in the sample answered that she had such demands. But in reality, next to their own illnesses, the major reason for women leaving training was to help at home. Elizabeth Denison, for example, never finished her training at Boston City because her sister's death in 1918 necessitated her return home. Olivia Schubert's brother went so far as to write damaging fictitious letters to Boston City because he so resented her leaving her "job" as his housekeeper to begin to train.[24] Thus, death, illness, or the needs of key family members all too often upset the delicate balance of the family economy and shifted a nursing student back into her domestic role.

Death, however, often freed a woman from the demands of the family and precipitated her application for training. Writing to Boston City in 1904, upon the death of her father, Anne L. McCormick stated:

> For years I have had the greatest desire to enter the hospital and make nursing my life vocation but knowing I was required at home could not do so before. However, I am perfectly free now and have my mother's sanction to prepare for training.[25]

Of the three hundred cases in the sample for which information on parents was given, in almost half (41 percent), one or both parents of the student had died.[26] Thus both the lack of parental objections and the need for wage labor made training a plausible alternative for many women. Often, only a family crisis made entrance into nursing, and eventually paid labor, possible.

When training was first introduced, it was social class and education that were to have distinguished the nurse from her untrained predecessor. The elite schools sought "refined and educated women, who have taken up the work not from necessity but choice." Thus, Bellevue Hospital in New York excluded women from what they called "the domestic servant class." Similarly, the founders of the Boston Training School at Massachusetts General sought "self-supporting women . . . of the comfortable classes for their new school."[27] At the elite training schools, the founders' intent was often carried out: At Johns Hopkins between 1889 and 1893, students were "a middle to upper-middle class group, drawn from the larger towns and cities rather than from rural areas." Similarly, the graduates of New York Hospital's training school between 1878 and 1920 were from "families which basically composed the span of the middle class and touched on the upper class."[28]

In contrast, the women who took their training at the three schools under study in Boston represented the middle and working classes. Using previous occupations as a very rough indicator of class background, their differences with those training in the elite programs becomes clearer.[29] Most of the women applying to the schools at Boston City, Somerville, and Long Island were not new to the paid labor force. Although a third (34.4 percent) reported themselves as "at home" doing "housekeeping" for their families at the time of their application, more than 95 percent also noted that they had previously worked for wages (see Table 5.5). In contrast, however, although nearly half (46.3 percent) of the elite New York Hospital's graduates also had worked for their families, they had never worked outside the home. The New York Hospital graduates who worked did so primarily as school teachers, untrained nurses, clerical workers, saleswomen, governesses, and companions.[30] Women in the Boston schools studied also held such positions, but in far lower numbers. Instead, the Boston women were much more likely to be waitresses, domestics, nursemaids, or any number of the diverse working-class women's occupations.

Comparisons among the Boston schools show some differences that reflect the status of the schools and changes over time in the occupational structure. Thus, as a large and somewhat prestigious school, in its early years Boston City Hospital's program attracted a large number of teachers (13.4 percent of its students). Somerville, in contrast, took many more young women coming to training directly from school and home. Somerville also drew more heavily from the lower white-collar occupations: 25 percent of its students had been either store clerks, saleswomen, office clerks, or stenographers; only 4.6 percent were former teachers. Long Island, as the smaller and more isolated program, more willingly

Table 5.5. *Leading previous occupations for nursing students in the Boston training schools sample compared to nursing students at New York Hospital*

Occupation	Boston sample		New York Hospital	
	Number	% [a]	Number	% [a]
Home	175	34.4	473	46.3
Teacher	48	9.4	149	14.6
Nurse	43	8.4	129	12.6
Housekeeper	41	8.1	6	0.6
Clerical worker	35	6.9	86	8.4
Saleswoman	23	4.5	30	2.9
Factory worker	19	3.8	6	0.6
Store clerk	18	3.5	0	0.0
Dressmaker	10	2.0	16	1.6
Other sewing	10	2.0	0	0.0
Bookkeeper	10	2.0	18	1.8

[a] The percentages do not total 100 because this is only a list of the leading occupations.

Source: See Table 5.1; Jane Mottus, *New York Nightingales: The Emergence of the Nursing Profession at Bellevue and New York Hospitals, 1850–1920* (Ann Arbor: University Microfilms Books, 1981), p. 230.

accepted women who had been nursing school dropouts, domestics, housekeepers, or untrained hospital nurses. Only 2 percent of Long Island's students had taught (see Table A.7 in the Appendix).

The criterion for selection suggests some of the limits to women's occupational mobility through nursing. To break the link between nursing and service, women who had been domestic servants were particularly discriminated against, especially in the better schools.[31] Home-based nurses were more welcome to train than those who had labored in hospitals. School officials believed hospital nurses were either too intractable or too unacceptable socially to be allowed to enter training. Only Long Island took both kinds of nurses in equal numbers. When Boston City's training school opened in 1879, fourteen of the first sixty-four students had previously been employed on the institution's nursing staff. Only six finished the course.[32]

Factory or mill workers were also discouraged from applying. Both

Boston City and Long Island took just under 6 percent of their students from such occupations, Somerville less than 1 percent. When a former shoe factory worker applied to Boston City, Lucy Drown commented, "If the environment of her work can be overlooked, I would recommend her acceptance." In contrast, the Waltham Training School expressly saw itself as taking women from the city's major factory, the Waltham Watch Company.[33] But in general, nursing school leaders sought a certain level of gentility in their students they thought factory work repressed.

Structural and racial changes in the work choices open to women also affected the previous experiences of nursing students over time. By the early twentieth century, as domestic service became increasingly a black woman's occupation, while nursing remained overwhelmingly white, fewer former domestics became nurses.[34] With the rapid growth of the clerical and sales work force, more and more nursing students, if they had worked at all, had been employed in such positions. Jean Latter, for example, had been a typist for three years when at age twenty she applied for admission to the training school at Somerville Hospital in 1922; her classmate Willa Rogers had been living at home in Nova Scotia, clerking in a local confectionery store.[35] The trend toward women leaving clerical work and sales for nursing was thus most noticeable in the first two decades of the twentieth century. By the 1920s and 1930s, over one-quarter of the women entering nursing had had such experience (see Table A.8 in the Appendix). However, as the demand for more students in the 1920s lowered the age requirement for nursing school entry to eighteen, an increasing percentage (41.9) of the students entering had never worked for wages.

A number of factors thus affected the supply of women who entered nursing. Changes in the choices open to women between the late nineteenth and early twentieth centuries meant the genteel former teachers so eagerly sought by nursing's founders often selected only the elite schools or sought other kinds of work. Former domestic servants, excluded from the "better" schools, still could enter nursing through the much more numerous smaller programs. The other most important change over time was the declining percentage of professionals, primarily former teachers, entering nursing training.

The lack of uniformity in entrance requirements, and the continued need for more students for the hospital's work force, prompted administrators to determine admission on the basis of physical stamina and health, rather than previous education or occupation. Furthermore, as the drudgery and difficulties of nursing became more widely known, many young women, less rural than their earlier counterparts, were both more reluctant to subject themselves to nursing's discipline and constraints and less fearful of the city's dangers. These "new women workers" of the early 1900s were unwilling to sacrifice freedom to gain the halo.[36] Often only recruits from more rural and protected backgrounds could be still lured in the 1920s and 1930s by the rhetoric of womanly service.

IN THE WORLD, NOT A PART OF IT

The difficulty of attracting "worthy candidates" became more visible in the twentieth century, but the problem emerged almost as soon as the nursing schools opened. In 1882, less than five years after the training school was started at New York Hospital, its principal admitted: "We are having difficulty getting into our school such women as approach the high standard of excellence which we aim at for our nurses."[37] By the turn of the century, with the growth in the number of schools, the nursing superintendents perceived their students not only as younger but less mature and lacking in discipline and home training. They were missing, one nursing superintendent bemoaned in 1920, "faith and spirituality."[38]

As the debate raged in hospital circles as to where the blame for this decline could be placed, nursing superintendent Mary Riddle at Newton Hospital in Massachusetts openly admitted that nursing's "failure to live up to promises is the reason for the dearth of young women."[39] Disenchanted nurses discouraged their sisters and friends from training. As a group of Boston nurses told a reporter in 1907, a woman would be better advised to take up teaching or stenography. "Nursing," they declared, "is not what it is 'cracked up' to be."[40]

Nursing school advocates maintained, however, that one of training's great virtues was that the schools provided a safe homelike haven for the young country woman in the urban environment. Their promise reflected the concern with the "drifting" of women to the urban world. For the young woman looking for work, the city was "a sort of Mecca for all in search of opportunity," sociologist Albert Wolfe commented in 1913, especially for those who "come from rocky farms and hill towns to escape the irksome drudgery and monotony of petty household duties." But a Sodom rather than a Mecca could await the naive and innocent, warned one of Wolfe's contemporaries, unless she had some money and "proper moral training."[41]

The nursing school, it was argued, could provide all this: income, good moral training, and, above all, protection from the sexual dangers of the city. The school, its advocates maintained, would be a way station into a safe and mature womanhood of service and virtue. A nursing superintendent in 1908 claimed the field "has opened up . . . rich opportunities of service to others, while *in* the world, not a part of it . . . because she [the nursing student] is shielded and her associates are those engaged in the same unselfish work." Nursing's noble goal, she concluded, was "to save

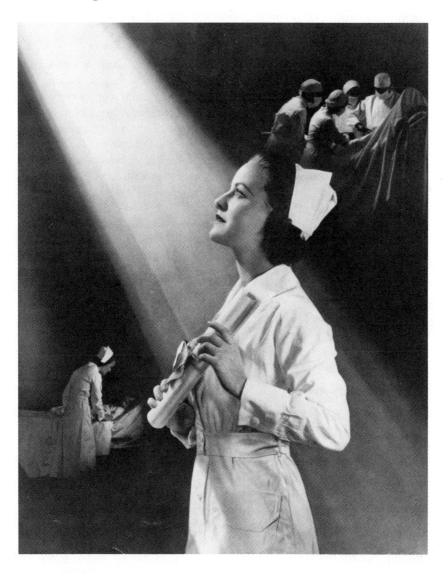

Popular books, posters, and advertising for nursing products emphasized the idealism and almost religious calling of the work. This picture was put out by Johnson & Johnson, circa 1930s–40s, as part of a calendar promotional campaign on nursing. The photograph was accompanied by this caption: "Forward, on the threshold of a noble career, the graduate nurse moves forward in a calling devoted to the service of humanity – Wherever she may serve, her uniform stands as a symbol of trained intelligence, her courage and loyalty inspire respect and confidence."
Source: Joan Brumberg Collection, Ithaca, New York

young girls from the perils that confront them in seeking other occupations." As if nothing more needed to be said, she concluded, "We are a family."[42]

Hospital and nursing superintendent Charlotte Aikens was far more candid when she admitted that the public saw nursing as making "the greatest demands but giv[ing] the least personal liberty of all the occupations open to women." But she argued, reiterating common cultural themes about the moral dangers confronting saleswomen, stenographers, and seamstresses, "The hospital nurse has at least the privilege of living in a 'protected boarding house.' " A nurse, after all, came to the hospital to live in a home. The bargain counter, Aikens contended, might be a pathway to a "brothel," the office the route to "low pay with the expectation of sexual factors for it," but nursing promised decent wages and moral protection.[43]

Aikens's argument was given currency in other cultural forms. The heroine of *End of the Road,* an anti–venereal disease, pro–sex-education film for women made in 1919, was a nurse. Spurning the sexual advances of a hometown boyfriend, Mary, of course, saved herself for true love and a marriage offer from an older and wiser hospital surgeon. In contrast, Vera, her high school classmate, contracted venereal disease from an unfeeling swain who picked her up at the department store counter where she worked. In the film's unsubtle message, nursing and purity, with the addition of informed education, were linked.[44]

Significantly, nursing school advocates stressed the familial environment of the hospital, the potential wages for nurses, and the opportunity to be of service, but not the actual *work* of nursing. Arguments that emphasized the sexual safety of nursing could ill afford to mention the obvious: that the work centered much of the time on the physical care of male strangers.[45] Nor could nursing's boosters afford to mention the drudgery that characterized the nurse's daily life.

Despite the continual emphasis on the virtues of training, by the 1910s there was a growing awareness among some nursing superintendents that the meager education, nagging supervision, hard work, narrow restrictions, and long hours were keeping women with more education and options out of the field.[46] In the hands of ill-trained and overworked nursing superintendents, the regimentation and labor, originally deemed necessary for the student's character development and moral uplift, were perceived only as petty tyranny. Yet as one nurse observed sadly, "There are unfortunately large numbers who continue to regard the training school as a reformatory, and the inmates as in need of discipline."[47]

What had begun as more of an institution to "finish" a young woman was rapidly becoming one to contain her. When there were few options for respectable women's work and large numbers of rural women coming to the cities, the restrictions in nursing training were accepted as necessity, in part to make work in the urban environment appear more acceptable. But by 1920, as a survey of the shortage in nursing students in New York City hospitals concluded, "Thousands of girls come to the cities yearly to enter business or art schools or college where there are no facilities for residence."[48] Many had already left the shelter of farms and small towns. The cloistered life the hospital promised was an anachronism.

By the late 1910s, nursing had fewer advantages to offer a young woman. The business world seemingly promised advancement, high salaries, and pleasant work while the hospital still saw "service to humanity" as its greatest drawing card. Yet, as a nursing superintendent commented, "The romantic glamorer [sic] of the profession has worn off. . . . Practical business training has knocked the sentimentalism out of the present day woman."[49]

It was also that the reality of nurse's training was more widely known. In the 1880s and 1890s popular women's magazines contained articles extolling the virtuousness and rewards of nursing, but by 1906 *Ladies' Home Journal* was publishing such articles as "Are Hospital Nurses Underfed?" A year later, a story on nursing in the *Boston Herald* ran under the lead "Romance Is Gone in Nursing the Sick."[50] By 1930, one popular writer summed up nursing's appeal.

Nursing is, in short, the one line of work left open to the uneducated girl which will not only raise her social status and pay her comparatively high wages but will provide her with a living while she is training and perhaps even a monthly allowance.[51]

The schools thus had to cast their nets even wider for students in order to keep their hospitals staffed. Even the larger schools, Adelaide Nutting argued in her 1912 report on nursing, were forced to admit and keep "pupils of pitifully low educational attainments and mental ability." In the smaller schools, she noted, the problem was even more difficult as women who had failed elsewhere were welcomed.[52] In 1918 the editors of *Trained Nurse and Hospital Review,* continuing the search for the virtuous, hardworking young farm woman, suggested that ads be placed in the farm journals as "these go into the best farm homes of the state and reach as a rule, just the kind of readers the school desires to interest."[53]

Ironically, as the women entering the schools became younger, less mature, or less willing to accept the rigors and the discipline, the necessity for the strictures of training seemed to increase. "The applicant of today," Nutting told a hospital convention audience in 1908, "needs a longer and more careful training to bring her up to standard of her predecessor in this work."[54] Nursing educators blamed the students' mothers, or even their grandmothers, for "failing in bringing forth daughters possessing stability, loyalty, strength of character and a dignity." As the number of "flapper nurses" (as they were labeled) increased, the mythical dignified country woman, willing to labor in the service of society and the hospital, was sorely missed.[55] To make up for the failures of upbringing, the nursing superintendents felt constrained to continue to emphasize discipline and conduct. But it was precisely these demands that often kept women with other options out of the nursing schools.

With admissions determined often by hospital needs rather than educational standards, the continued hard work, the restrictions of training, and a growing number of other work options for women, nursing became an occupation that could not attract an ideal and uniform band of genteel, educated women. By the 1910s, the daughter of respectable rural or small-town parents who had taught for a while might still enter training in one of the more elite and larger hospital schools. But at a nearby school, the daughter of a poorer, small-town family, who came directly from home or a clerical or sales job, with little educational advantage, might enter training at the same time. Both women, if they graduated, would be labeled trained nurses. It was this heterogeneity that characterized and therefore came to divide nursing. Nursing's promise of altruism and autonomy seemed to become less widely appealing as the field grew. And its leadership, raised on nineteenth-century cultural assumptions about womanhood, was increasingly out of touch with twentieth-century sensibilities.

6

Nursing as work: divisions in the occupation

The diversity that characterized nursing students and nursing training continued after the students received their diplomas and looked for work. In the nineteenth century, most students left the hospital behind after graduation. Unwanted by institutions staffed primarily by the untrained or student nurses, graduates were expected to find work, in competition with the untrained, in the private-duty market. A small number might secure an appointment as the superintendent of a training school or small hospital, or as the supervisor of an operating room or outpatient department.

By the turn of the century as hospitals grew in number and complexity, and public health became more organized, there was more demand for trained nurses in different institutional and public-health positions. But until the 1930s, although nurses might try out the various practice fields, the majority at any one point in time had to work in private duty if they wanted to nurse. Yet because of the heterogeneity in the nurses' social backgrounds, education, and training, large numbers of very differently prepared and educated women "crowded" into trained nursing practice and vied with untrained women for work. Within the nursing labor market, however, there was room for some horizontal job mobility and a good deal of geographic freedom.

While the labor market structured the demand and location of work for trained nurses, personal and institutional factors intertwined to shape their lives. Personal choices, age, marital status, and family demands obviously affected work patterns. In addition, the training school continued to label and direct a nurse's working life well after graduation. As with all working women, "choice" and "independence" were relative commodities.

INDEPENDENCE AND AMBIGUITY IN PRIVATE DUTY

Since hospital nursing was primarily reserved for either nursing students or untrained nurses until after World War I, graduation meant going into private duty and working in patients' homes. The medical student completing training went into private *practice;* the nursing student, however,

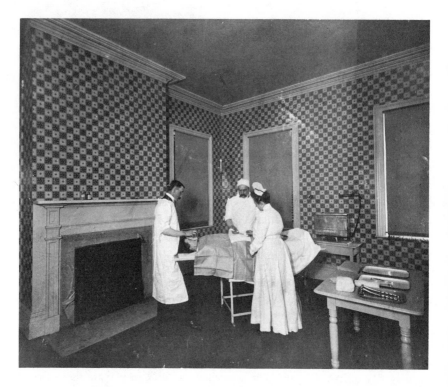

In the nineteenth and early twentieth centuries, nurses often assisted at surgery in a makeshift operating room in a patient's home. Pittsfield, Massachusetts, circa 1880–90. *Source:* Countway Library

went into private *duty*. Whereas physicians were expected to apply their skills in independent action, nurses, even without the control of the hospital and medical hierarchy, were still supposed to be submissive to higher authority and morally committed to their work. In private duty, a nurse was working for a *doctor's* patients. Although employed by a family, she was primarily dependent on physicians to define what she did and to help her get work.

Although devoted care to one private patient would seem to be the quintessential expression of a nurse's skill, nursing superintendents voiced grave concern about the dangers of private duty and worried that their students would find the work "exhausting." The exhaustion they feared was both physical and spiritual, a loss of sheer strength and moral fiber. It was frequently assumed that a nurse could only last ten years in private duty, her inevitable collapse owing as much to the danger of "moral laxity" as to the physical labor.[1] Warnings were issued about the danger of

nursing single men in hotels (no respectable woman should) or the tempt-
ing advances of a patient's unscrupulous husband (to be spurned at all
costs), along with admonitions to get enough rest. These warnings reflected less a fear of the vanquishing of the nurse's physical virginity than
fear for her spiritual virginity – the collapse of her moral purity, her gentleness, humanity, sympathy, and tact because of the long hours and strain.

The strain was not merely because of the inherent nature of the work.
The pressure to establish the necessity and role for trained nurses, the
ambiguity of their place in the household structure, and the psychic shift
from hospital to home-based work all created stress. In the 1880s and
1890s, the worth of the trained nurse remained to be proved to both
physicians and patients' families. Although much of what she did seemingly could be done, and was done, by untrained nurses, domestics, or
female relatives, she was somehow, through her personality, bearing, and
character, to present herself as a new and vital creation, necessary to
patient survival.[2] Many physicians were not convinced their patients
needed this kind of nurse, and they perceived hospital-trained nurses as a
threat.[3]

Trained nurses, even as their numbers swelled around the turn of the
century, never had a monopoly on the private-duty field. Many physicians
and families remained uncertain why the trained nurse's skills justified her
higher charges. In chronic and convalescent cases in particular, where a
companion-housekeeper was all that was needed, it was likely that a
family would hire an untrained nurse. If slightly more skill were required,
in some communities there were women called "trained attendants,"
graduates of short programs or "schools" run by voluntary associations
and the YWCAs. The income of the family or the nature of the patient's
illness often determined the kind of "nurse" hired.

The private-duty nurse was neither professional nor servant nor family
member, and her position in a household's structure was therefore uncertain. From the strict hierarchy of the hospital, the nurse was freed to find
her place in the vagaries of numerous household arrangements. Nursing
educator Isabel Hampton Robb succinctly captured the uncertainty when
she wrote that the private duty nurse was "neither for the drawing room
nor the kitchen."[4]

The difficulties were compounded by the contrast between the class of
hospital and home-based patients. In the hospital, the nurse, within clearer
lines of authority, served a patient population of primarily working-class
men and women. In the home, however, most nurses worked for families
whose social position was usually higher than their own. In a sample taken
of the families who hired nurses between 1880 and 1914 through a registry
for nurses at the Boston Medical Library, more than 50 percent of the
male family heads were either lawyers, owners of companies, or mer-

chants. The others were skilled or white-collar workers and professionals. Laborers, the unskilled, and the bulk of the working and lower middle class were conspicuously absent.[5]

The expense of private-duty nurses limited their wide usage. From the 1880s until the mid-1890s, graduates received $15 to $18 a week in Boston; by the late 1890s they were commanding $20 to $25. In New York, the rates were about $5 higher. By the early twentieth century, private nurses were averaging about $950 a year and by the late 1920s approximately $1,300.[6] Such an expense was beyond the grasp of the average wage earner.

Once in a patient's home, there were few guidelines to govern social relations for either nurses or families. Nurses, as a character in a nursing novel explained, were "always afraid of being asked to do too much. They're always afraid of being treated like ordinary servants."[7] Nurses were told during training that no work was beneath their dignity, but once in a patient's home a nurse had to draw the lines and decide for herself what were reasonable demands. If a nurse washed out a baby's clothes in one home because there was no laundress, should she be expected to do so in another home where such a worker was employed? Should a family be subject to a nurse's wrath because she was asked to eat at a second table or in the kitchen with the servants?

Clashes were inevitable between a family's expectation of servantlike behavior and the nurse's need to assert her standing above that of domestics and to establish her autonomy. Complaints from patients reflected the distance between expected and actual class-defined behavior and echoed those made of servants unfamiliar with the objects of a crowded bourgeois Victorian home. Nurses were thus faulted for being clumsy with precious objects, not knowing how to treat exotic pieces of furniture, and using expensive items carelessly. At a time of illness and stress, small mistakes in social conduct by the nurse became magnified and compounded by the fears of death and disease that pervaded a household. "The families want to know 'what are the rules,' " a Philadelphia physician inquired. Yet, as one nursing superintendent noted, "There are no definite rules to be observed."[8] A nurse's inability to judge correctly the unwritten rules could be costly. In 1892, a Philadelphia nurse reported:

If by any chance a nurse gains the ill will of her first few patients, her career is ended. She is not told anything of this, simply waits in her boarding house until her last dollar is gone, . . . in suspense . . . and wondering why a case don't come.[9]

The relationship of the nurse to the household's servants was often the most critical and difficult. This dilemma centered on where the nurse would take her meals. Nurses frequently insisted (to make sure they were treated as ladies, not servants) that they be served their meals in the dining room with the family, rather than in the kitchen with the servants. This demand was often resisted by families who saw the nurse as a servant and were uncomfortable with sharing their dinner conversations with a stranger from the working class. To lessen the conflict on this question, the Boston Medical Library Directory for Nurses, for example, asked both trained and untrained nurses on their application forms whether they would take their meals in the kitchen. In a sample from these records, only 40 percent of the trained nurses were willing to eat with the servants, as opposed to 74 percent of those without formal nurse's training. Of those unwilling to eat with the servants, 82 percent were trained nurses, and less than 20 percent were untrained nurses.

Managing relationships with the family's servants required tact as the nurse had to be understanding but distant, above but not superior. The June 1886 graduating nursing class at the Boston Training School for Nurses at Massachusetts General Hospital was told by a physician: "Never assume an air of superiority when dealing with the servants; but on the other hand, never be too familiar with them. At best they recognize your superior position unwillingly; therefore do all you can to conciliate them."[10] The countless stories of the overbearing, dictatorial nurse who left the household after an emotional uproar suggest that finding a path to conciliation was not always easy. In desperation, families turned to the more expensive private room in the hospital or called only for an "old-style" untrained nurse since in both cases the social relationships were rigidly defined.

The strain of the encounter between nurse and family was compounded by the work site. In the patient's home, the solitary nurse confronted a family social system. In the hospital, the patient was the lone individual, subject to a set of defined rules and a structured hierarchy. A private-duty nurse warned that hard work, with many patients, "under some circumstances [may] demand much less wear and tear on the nervous system than that consequent upon the supervision of her own solitary self while engaged in nursing one patient in the bosom of that patient's family."[11]

The nurse also had to learn to make do in the home without all the equipment and supplies that marked hospital care. The author of one of the manuals on "how to be a good private-duty nurse" recounted the story of an overzealous private-duty nurse who "thought she was distinguishing herself by extreme neatness, used to put thirty-five sheets in the wash in a week. She defeated her own end, for the laundress, naturally thought this a folly, and smoothed out those that looked clean, without washing them."[12]

The most obvious contrast between hospital and home-based care was the difference in structure. A system and schedule for performing duties was the sine qua non of the training schools. But as one private-duty nurse cautioned, "Indeed a too loyal adherence to one certain system may prove a huge stumbling block in the way of success."[13] The very work rhythms of the home and hospital differed. In private duty, a nurse's success depended on her ability to adjust to the needs and whims of the patient and family – not a premeasured schedule set to a timed performance. Private-duty nursing consisted of the performance of a series of tasks whose order was determined by the patient's illness and the needs of the family, much like a farmer's work depended on the weather. The patient and the family, not the work as in the hospital, had to be the center of the nurse's attentions. Thus differing personalities and flexibility, factors the training school tried to control, were of primary importance in the private-duty setting.

Private duty lacked supervision and control as well. Without the watchful eye of a head nurse or a superintendent, the nurse with poor techniques could "hide" in private duty for years. Only the market, rather than some kind of supervisory system, differentiated between the nurses, and because of the registry system (discussed later), patient choice often did not determine which nurse received the case. Furthermore, experience and skill were not generally rewarded. There was no real grading system and no differentiation in pay between those who had just graduated and those who had worked for years. In fact, patients often requested young and pretty nurses rather than older, more seasoned veterans. The only differentiation was made between the trained and the untrained nurse, yet this was a distinction the public barely understood.[14]

Private duty further tested the nurse's mettle as it was frequently exhausting and isolating work. Shifts of 12–24 hours were considered the norm until the 1920s, so that nurses were expected to be working from 84 to 168 hours a week. If the patients were convalescing or chronically ill, a nurse's tasks could be done at a leisurely pace. But because the nurse stayed in the patient's home or apartment, there was still a good deal of isolation from a "normal" life. An average case, for example from the Boston Medical Library Directory, lasted almost four weeks. When the nurse was not on a case, she had to be home or readily available to be called by phone or reached by messenger to take another. This left little time for outside interests, organized activities, or nursing politics. A nursing leader summarized the effects of the work on the nurse.

Its irregularity breaks down her health, its seclusions tend to narrow her interests. She cannot charge in accordance with any particular skill she had acquired; she is unethical if, after ten years of hard work, she charges any more than does the newest graduate in the field. Yet she must be all things to all people, she must remain human though she cannot live like most humans.[15]

Despite the uncertainty, nurses fashioned a variety of means for surviving and enjoying the work. In the traditional manner, the stories of patients who took their nurses to Europe on trips, married them, or left them large sums of money, however atypical, suggest that, as with servants and governesses, the "step up" in nursing was to marriage or life as a family retainer. But other nurses found more active ways to reshape the work and create alliances in the household. To repeat data presented earlier, 40 percent of trained nurses and 74 percent of untrained nurses were willing to eat in the kitchen. Nurses quickly learned, as the laundress story illustrates, that a resentful servant could make their lives miserable. Letters to the Boston Medical Library Directory rebuking nurses for being too friendly with servants and gossiping with them about the patient's illness and the household life suggest that congenial working relationships frequently developed. Other letters decried the nurses, especially on convalescent cases, who would leave the patient to go home, to go to the theater, or to visit friends or family. Some nurses had other businesses and conducted their other work while on a case. One nurse was disciplined for having another nurse call and lie for her by saying her aunt was ill. The nurse, when discovered, said she left the case because the patient was poor and the working conditions terrible. Other nurses slept on the job, abandoned patients, or refused cases.[16]

Most registries allowed nurses to state their case preferences. Comments such as "only surgical cases" or "no obstetrical cases" cover the application forms. Trained nurses, rather than their untrained counterparts, specialized more and were less willing to care for postpartum patients, presumably because such work almost always guaranteed they would be asked to do more household work. Untrained nurses, in contrast, willingly took the obstetrical work, may also have worked as midwives, and were much less likely to list a specialty.[17]

These attempts to control the work were perceived by the public and many nursing superintendents, however, as the shirking of duty. In a 1904 editorial entitled "The Path of Duty," for example, the *American Journal of Nursing* chastised nurses for refusing to take cases.

Such failure to meet our highest obligations, such violation of our common standards of right and duty, cannot be too sternly censured. The women who permit themselves to conduct their professional work in this manner are in this, at least, wrong through and through.[18]

Despite such attacks, however, the practice continued.

The biggest difficulty in private duty was the distribution system and the matching of patients to nurses looking for work. As private, individual workers, nurses found their cases through word of mouth, city directory listings, referrals from patients, physicians or druggists, and nursing registries. A nurse often had to make the rounds of physicians' offices to announce her availability and then go back to her home and wait to be called. Contacts made during training were often critical to a nurse launching her career. If the nurse ventured to a new city, finding work often took even more time.

By the depression of the mid-1890s, the difficulties of finding work were compounded as private duty became an overcrowded field in the major cities and on the West Coast.[19] The increasing supply of nurses, the continued competition with the untrained, and the expense of private duty (which limited the demand to the well-to-do) all contributed to the problem. The Boston Medical Library Directory, for example, supplied families with both untrained and trained nurses, although it allowed the latter to charge from five to ten dollars more a week. In an economic crisis, the graduates feared families would turn to their less costly competition. In Boston, however, the competition was more among the graduates themselves. Graduate nurses consistently received two or three times as much work as untrained nurses, and about 20 percent more than they should have, given equal distribution.[20]

Nurses waited for cases, visited and left their cards at physicians' offices, or registered at a number of different directories in hopes of calls. One nurse, upon resigning from the Boston Medical Library Directory in 1895, wrote, "If I had depended entirely on the Directory for a living of course I should have starved long ago."[21] Other nurses left the cities they were working in to find employment elsewhere. In 1914, a California nurse warned that even the West Coast was already becoming terribly overcrowded and suggested that East Coast nurses stay where they were.[22]

It is difficult to calculate how much work the typical nurse actually had. Trained nurses, on average, received only 3.2 cases a year from the Boston Medical Library Directory, the untrained nurses 2.3; this amounts to an average of thirteen and nine weeks' work a year, respectively. But this probably does not reflect the weeks of actual work since nurses could register with more than one directory or find cases on their own. A Cleveland nurse, for example, reported that in her eleven years of private duty (1895–1906), she worked thirty-three to thirty-five weeks each year. The only time she was employed fully was the fifteen months she spent on a "luxury" case as a companion, as well as a nurse, for one wealthy patient.[23]

Nursing was "seasonal" work, however, even in the best of years. There was a higher call for nurses in the midwinter months of January through March and a slowdown between May and July, caused perhaps as much by the exodus of the wealthy from the city during the summer as a difference in disease incidence. A comparison of twenty-five women's occupations in Massachusetts in 1890 shows nurses and midwives to be sixth in unemployment frequency.[24] Yet when a nurse worked, she earned more income on average than most other women workers in a given week. In 1910, a study of women workers' wages described anyone making over fifteen dollars a week as "prosperous."[25] Compared to women in clerical, sales, factory, waitressing, and kitchen work, nurses appeared to do "well."

Nurses found a variety of means for sustaining themselves through periods without a case. Some took other work or, if they could, returned home to the protection of their families. Others found institutional or public-health nursing jobs or branched into related health fields by selling surgical equipment or operating rest homes. Some simply lowered their expectations and waited for cases. Poignantly, the California nurse who warned of overcrowding, lamented: "The gradual fading away of resources, courage, hope – too often self respect – and sometimes suicide. The papers here suppress all that."[26]

As increasing numbers of middle- and upper-class patients began to use hospitals after World War I, private-duty nurses followed them into the institutions as "specials." Although it is impossible to date the actual change, by the late 1910s and early 1920s much of private-duty work was centered in the hospital's private rooms. Thus, although the private nurse might work in the hospital, she was employed by the patient, not the institution. Her work was still erratic and uncertain, her status continually ambiguous.

The irrationality of the hiring system complicated the employment situation. In an attempt to provide nurses (and to make a profit in their deployment), registries sponsored by medical societies and commercial agencies, as well as by hospitals and nursing alumnae groups, began to spring up. In any given city, any number of registries could exist with differing standards, fees, and available services. The registries usually established the wage rates, setting different standards for trained and untrained nurses. A "customary" wage was established for each group, although there was, at least in the Boston Medical Library Directory, a slightly greater variation in the fees asked for by the untrained nurses. Trained nurses were counseled, however, to keep a set rate.[27] However, it was not uncommon for a nurse to lower her rates when necessary, or, more often, to overcharge the patient on items such as carriage fares and laundry bills.

By the 1890s nurses' complaints about the lack of work through the registries had become part of an undercurrent of discontent. "Most graduates," a nurse reported, "do not feel they are fairly treated by the directory, but are afraid to complain for fear that it will be visited upon them."[28] In an attempt to equally distribute employment, when a nurse reported off a case, her name was supposed to be placed at the bottom of the rotation list. But, nurses charged, the registries played favorites, did not always follow this system, kept blacklists, and could not control whether a nurse received a "good" case that guaranteed employment for a length of time.[29] Private-duty work began to mean an endless waiting for calls.

Aware of the discontent over the registries, the extent to which both physicians' groups and commercial agencies were profiting from such services, and the necessity to control distribution, some nurses began to advocate the organization of nurse-controlled, centralized, and officially sponsored registries in each city. In Boston, for example, the Boston Medical Library Directory was closed as graduate nurses began to register with the nurses' officially sponsored Suffolk County Nurses' Directory. As one nurse commented, however, "It is not so much a share in the government of directories, as a share in the work given out by them that is asked by the majority of nurses. . . . Each one should have a share."[30]

There was no guarantee, however, that a nurse-controlled registry would mean any more work. In fact, nurses admitted that the commercial agencies often allowed the more experienced trained nurses to charge more, thus making such agencies more attractive for some than the official registries that set one rate.[31] The official agencies often enrolled only graduates from the "better schools," did not provide untrained nurses, and were thus less able than the commercial registries to meet varied community demands. Hospital and alumnae registries often provided only the institution's own graduates with positions as "specials" in the hospital. Thus the registries, at best, functioned only as nursing employment agencies or hiring halls for hospital specials, rather than as either community services or professional organizations. They were the continual focus of nursing discontent and concern.[32]

Despite the overcrowding, private-duty work continued to absorb the majority of nursing graduates because there was very little else they could do and remain in nursing. Some private-duty experience was considered essential for every nurse, but status in nursing quickly accrued to those in more "executive" positions within hospitals or public-health nursing agencies. Private-duty nursing, seen even within nursing as often no more than domestic service or a mother's work, bestowed little status. Furthermore, because there was no supervision, women with the weakest skills could stay in private duty. With the growth of hospital-based care in the early 1900s and the decrease in the debilitating sicknesses that required more long-term nursing care, the status of private-duty nursing continued to decline. By the late 1920s, nursing's Grading Committee could repeat the aphorism "Every nurse ought to do some private duty, but no good nurse ought to stay in the field more than a few years."[33] Aware of the overcrowding as early as the 1890s, Lavinia Dock counseled nurses to specialize "by branching into auxiliary lines of work not strictly nursing, yet which can be better done by one having the training of nurses." Her suggestions, however, entailed specializing *outside* of private-duty work itself.[34] Lucy Drown, the superintendent of nurses at Boston City Hospital, was even more blunt in her advice. Sharing her concern in 1899 over the lack of work with the physician in charge of the Boston Medical Library Directory, she wrote:

[There is] . . . less survival of the fittest [in nursing] than in some other walks of life. My advice to these young women would be that if they cannot make a place for themselves as nurses, to go back to the work they left when they came into the hospitals, and maintain themselves as teachers, stenographers, dressmakers, etc.[35]

In fact, however, most stayed in nursing.

THE LIMITS OF OTHER OPPORTUNITIES

An institutional position as either a superintendent of a training school or administrator of a small hospital beckoned some nurses. Although on paper an "executive" position, the superintendency of a nursing school could mean a prestigious position in a large urban hospital or more commonly, a more lowly job, often akin to staff nursing, in a small, twenty-to fifty-bed, hospital.

The training school a nurse attended frequently determined the kind of institutional position she was offered. In 1898, one administrator calculated that 60 percent of the nursing superintendents in 327 different schools in the country trained at only 24 schools.[36] Those working in the better schools tended to be either the schools' own graduates or graduates of a comparable program. Such women moved from superintendency to superintendency, but rarely back into private duty.[37] As Nightingale had envisioned, women from the elite training schools served as "nursing missionaries," starting and organizing schools in the American hinterland beyond the major East Coast cities. It was thus common for a nurse to graduate from Bellevue, Massachusetts General, or Johns Hopkins directly into a superintendency in another institution.

"Mature age," *Trained Nurse and Hospital Review* suggested, was necessary for a nursing superintendent.[38] But the expansion in the number of schools undermined this requirement. The Grading Committee survey found in 1928 that nearly 13 percent of the superintendents of nurses and over 15 percent of the nurses who were both hospital and nursing superintendents were out of nursing school five years or less. The estimated average age of the superintendents was only twenty-six. Maturity and special training may have characterized women from the leading schools. But the Grading Committee found that half of the superintendents of nurses, and more than half of the nurses who were hospital administrators, had never taken any special training. Further, 40 percent of the administrators, 25 percent of the nursing superintendents, and 33 percent of the women who served in both positions, had three years or less of high school.[39]

Wages also varied. In the 1880s and 1890s superintendents' salaries ranged from $900 to $2,000 a year with maintenance. At a small hospital, *Trained Nurse and Hospital Review* noted in 1916, a nursing superintendent might expect to be paid $600–$1,200 with maintenance and to be on twenty-four-hour call. At a large hospital, her pay might increase to a range of $1,000–$2,000 a year, and her hours to twelve a day, six and one-half days a week. By the late 1920s, the Grading Committee survey found that wages varied with both locale and hospital size. Administrators in small hospitals were receiving from $1,500 to $2,000 and those in larger hospitals, $2,000–$2,500. All these salaries included maintenance since it was assumed necessary for an administrator to live within the hospital's walls. A nurse who became a hospital administrator might expect a wage approximately $500 more than that of the nursing superintendent.[40]

There was very little stability in such positions. Three-quarters of the 1,440 superintendents surveyed by the Grading Committee had stayed in their current positions five years or less. Minnie Goodnow, for example, was the superintendent in nine different training schools over a forty-year period, often staying less than a year in each position.[41] Unfortunately, the Grading Committee survey did not inquire what else the superintendents did. The school and qualitative evidence suggests, however, that certain women, once in the superintendency circles, moved as did Goodnow from school to school. Others might be superintendents one year and private-duty nurses the next. Thus the unevenness, lack of education, and experience of those in superintendent positions in nursing were common.[42]

It was also possible for a nurse to be hired as the head administrator of a small hospital, even one without a training school. In 1909, *Trained Nurse and Hospital Review* editorialized that half the members of the American Hospital Association were nurses; similarly in 1920, Adelaide Nutting estimated that nurses were the administrators in half the country's hospitals.[43] C.J. Parnell, the medical superintendent at University Hospital in Ann Arbor, explained in 1920 that hospital administration frequently attracted physicians who were "medical derelicts" whereas "the reasons for the almost universal employment of trained nurses as hospital executives has been simply that a higher quality of intelligence could be purchased for the money than could be secured in the service of men in the positions."[44] It was assumed that nurses would administer smaller institutions while male doctors and other trained men would head the larger ones.[45]

This nursing presence in the administration of the hospitals was further documented by a 1927 American Medical Association survey. Nurses administered 20 percent, or 1,506, of all hospitals in the country, but were much more likely to run "nongovernmental charitable hospitals of less than 100 beds."[46] By 1933, nurses ran 2,542, or 41 percent, of all U.S. hospitals, but again predominated in the smaller charitable and church-affiliated institutions. Nurses that year were the administrators in 77 percent of the hospitals under 100 beds.[47] This pattern was to hold until the period of great hospital expansion and financing after World War II. In 1949, when hospital and nursing superintendent Charlotte Aikens died, one eulogist recognized this nursing role and the change by beginning with the comment that with Aikens's death, "an epoch in welfare history – the period of the woman hospital administrator" had closed.[48]

A trained nurse could also take an institutional position as a head nurse, assistant superintendent, or operating room supervisor, but rarely as a staff nurse. The day-to-day nursing on the hospital floors was still reserved either for students or untrained women. So common was this pattern that Charlotte Aikens in a three-part series in *Trained Nurse* never once mentioned staff nursing. Similarly, an article on vocational opportunities run by the journal six years later did not list staff nursing among the thirty-eight different jobs open to nurses![49] Even the Grading Committee study in the late 1920s did not differentiate between head nurses, supervisors, and staff nurses in its "institutional" nursing category.

There were, of course, some graduates working as staff nurses in some hospitals in the country. In general, these hospitals were either the larger public institutions or specialty hospitals that had difficulty attracting untrained nurses and could not sustain training schools. An early twentieth-century hospital administrator counseled that "women who 'wouldn't do' as private nurses" would do in keeping "order and nurs[ing] the patients in a large public hospital."[50] Many of the graduates from Boston's Long Island Hospital, for example, had to work in chronic, almshouse, and infectious-disease institutions in the Boston area because they were denied access to the private-duty market.[51]

Low pay and chronic overwork plagued the staff nurse and limited the number of graduates willing to take up the work. Dr. Kleinert told the medical staff at the New England Hospital in 1890 that it was impossible to get graduate nurses for general work "because they know from sad experience that they will be asked to do much more than is ever expected of them elsewhere." Kleinert reported that the hospital kept a ratio of four graduate nurses to forty-four patients in the maternity wards. She argued to the hospital's staff that at least "half a dozen" had to be hired at a time and a less "penurious" policy of payment had to be instituted.[52] Staff nursing, while it promised the graduate nurse steady work and maintenance, did not equal what she could make on her own as a good private-duty nurse. Staff nursing also required the nurse to live in the hospital and to put up with its rules and control.

The unwillingness of trained nurses to take such positions was not limited to the small hospitals. "How can we retain the efficient graduate in our service?" Boston City Hospital's nursing superintendent Emma Nichols wrote to the head of the training school committee in 1911. Eight nurses had left one of the hospital's departments in a short time, she reported, "the cause being financial reasons. In every case the nurses have felt they could better themselves." Nine years later her successor would be writing a similar letter to the hospital superintendent with the same complaint.[53]

By the late 1920s, the Grading Committee survey found nurses disliked the strain and responsibility of this work, without commensurate authority and the uneven hours, more than they did the low pay.[54] By this time, staff nurses were averaging ninety-six dollars a month with maintenance, a wage probably greater than they could make on the average in private duty. When discussing the positive aspects of such work, however, nurses mentioned their ability to keep up with the latest techniques, the stimulation of working with students, and the steadiness of employment.[55] But the independence they had hoped for as students seemed to vanish in the sterile atmosphere of the hospital.

Hospitals were reluctant to hire graduates for two main reasons: They were harder to control and relatively expensive. The administrator of New York Hospital complained in 1906 that the difficulty with graduates was that they were "wage earners" and demanded such special concessions from the hospital as two hours' absence a day for recreation or recuperation. He noted that the hospital did not feel it owed even its own students this privilege.[56] Graduates brought different techniques to a hospital from their own training, refused to accept the authority of the hospital administrators, and had the freedom to leave whenever they felt oppressed by work. Superintendents also worried about what the graduates would tell their students. As one administrator noted:

We have had so much trouble with graduates coming in and causing some uprising in our training school. Our place is so small and the girls are so closely in contact with each other. They talk shop talk and things they pulled while in training, or how different their school was to what they have to put up with.[57]

Graduate nurses sometimes were hired as supervisors, anesthetists, or head or operating-room nurses. The nursing superintendent at Boston City Hospital in 1928 requested an increase in the graduate nursing staff of the hospital. Her list of requirements for the main department of the hospital, though it detailed the need for 114 graduates, listed none for general or staff duty. Instead, they were to be supervisors, head nurses, operating-room, and outpatient department nurses.[58] By 1916 such positions carried more prestige than staff nursing and a higher wage of between $40 and $100 a month with maintenance.[59]

Public-health nursing was the third and smallest major area of employment for trained nurses. Public-health, or visiting or district nursing, as it was originally labeled, grew out of the visiting of the poor by philanthropic and religious organizations in a number of cities. For example, a graduate of Bellevue's first class was hired by the Women's Branch of the New York City Mission and Tract Society in 1877 to serve as a "missionary nurse" among the poor to bring, the society reported, "unspeakable comfort to many who have no one to minister to them."[60] Seven years later the Women's Education Association in Boston, in conjunction with the Boston Dispensary, developed a nursing service that was to bring "instruction in the principles of hygiene and simple nursing care" to the poor. By 1886 it had become an independent charity entitled the "Instructive District Nursing Association," with its own board and ten nurses assigned to different districts in the city. A similar autonomous association was formed in Philadelphia the same year. This kind of nursing grew slowly, however, because it required an endowed charity large enough to support the nurse's entire salary (since the service primarily was provided free of charge to the poor). Public-health nursing leader Mary Gardner estimated that there were only 300 public-health nurses in the country in 1900.[61]

After 1900, with increased immigration and government concern with health, both voluntary and government-supported public-health agencies began to grow. This kind of nursing, a "student of social problems" was quoted as saying, "is the safest and most practical means of bridging the gulf which lies between the classes and the masses."[62] By 1912 there were an estimated 3,000 public-health nurses; by 1938 the number had climbed to 19,390 nurses in 5,091 agencies, working for "department stores, industries, insurance companies, boards of health and education, hospitals, settlement houses, milk committees, baby saving funds, playgrounds, and hotels, as well as visiting nurse associations."[63]

Debate continued about exactly what the public-health nurse was supposed to do when she brought her "unspeakable comfort" to the poor. In some cases, she was an instructor, bringing the message of prevention and hygiene to the masses, or a practitioner, providing direct patient care, or sometimes both.[64]

Despite much disagreement over their duties, most public-health nurses queried by the Grading Committee gave very positive reports about their jobs.[65] Furthermore, by the 1910s, wages were slightly better than in hospital work, averaging $80 to $125 a month for supervisors and $50 to

$85 for staff nurses. But such wages did not include maintenance; thus a nurse's real income in public health was considerably lower than in institutional work.[66]

Public health allowed for the most independent judgment and autonomy of all the nursing practice fields. As in private duty, the public-health nurse had to use the force of her personality to obtain patient compliance, her own ability to improvise procedures, and her own judgment as to what kind of care should be provided. Unlike hospital or private duty, there was no head nurse to check with or even a doctor to easily advise on treatment patterns. "The success of district nursing depends," the superintendent of the Visiting Nurse Association of Chicago wrote in 1901, "more than in hospital and private practice, upon the character of the nurse; and the character of the nurse depends much more upon the nature of her training and the continuance of those helps, physical and moral, which that training has supplied to her."[67]

Success also entailed providing the predominantly lower- and working-class patients with lessons in proper middle-class health behavior. Thus the demeanor and teaching skills of the nurse were considered more important in public health than in hospital work. Public-health agencies tried to be quite selective in choosing their staffs. Agencies reported they almost always had an excess of applicants for positions yet experienced difficulty in finding nurses with the proper skills. "Lack of theoretical course work in public health" and inadequate "academic background" were given as reasons for 54 percent of rejections.[68] Ironically, at a time when public-health medicine was increasingly seen as the backwater of the medical profession, public-health nurses, because their practice involved autonomy from medical and hospital control and the provision of cross-class care and education, were perceived as the elite in nursing. At the same time, public health remained the smallest of nursing's practice fields.[69]

Thus when trained nursing was first introduced, private-duty work absorbed most of the graduates, while a small number found positions in public health and hospitals. In the nineteenth century, estimates of the numbers in private duty ranged from 55 percent to 80 percent of all graduates.[70] By the turn of the century, increasing specialization and the growth of public-health, school, industrial, and hospital nursing somewhat increased the options for graduates. By 1927, the Grading Committee concluded that the usual estimate that 70 percent of the profession were in private duty and 12 percent in public health was not accurate. According to their calculations, by then 57 percent of graduate nurses were in private duty, 14 percent in public health, and the remaining 29 percent in institutional work.[71]

Nursing thus provided its practitioners with a number of job possibilities. Addie E. Kelton, an 1887 graduate of the Waltham Training School, for example, spent most of her entire working life in private duty, alternating this with the responsibility of caring for her parents and teaching massage. Charlotte Conor, who graduated fifteen years later, was more adventuresome. She spent several years in private duty in Waltham and a year as a head night nurse at a state sanatorium in Rutland, Massachusetts. She subsequently became the superintendent for several years of a small hospital in upstate New York. Somewhat restless, she resigned in 1916 and headed west. She became a homesteader in Montana, an accomplished handweaver, and a private nurse in a small mining town located, she wrote, "practically on the summit of the Rocky Mountains." During World War I, she enlisted through the Red Cross and spent the war at the Presidio in San Francisco. When mustered out, she stayed in California and resumed private-duty work. By the mid-1930s, she was considering moving to Silver City, Nevada, with a friend to "stake her own claim" in gold-mining country.

In contrast, Agnes Ryan, a 1901 graduate of Waltham, married a physician within three years of graduation and retired from active nursing. Grace Stuart, however, worked for ten years as a district private-duty nurse, head, and tuberculosis nurse, and superintendent in Massachusetts, New York, and Connecticut before her marriage, also to a physician.[72] Nursing could thus lead to very different work patterns, job statuses, and perceptions of the problems, advantages, and disadvantages of the work.

PROFESSIONAL LIFE TABLES AND CHOICES

Personal inclinations and skill, as well as luck and opportunity, shaped a nurse's work patterns. But age, marital status, family demands, training school, and year of graduation also determined work histories. In general, nursing was characterized by a good deal of horizontal mobility among the practice fields and jobs, but very little upward mobility.

Age, for example, affected the nurse's career opportunities. Unlike the "professed nurse," whose skill was supposed to come with age, the "professional nurse" was expected to be young. The physician's journal *American Medicine* editorialized in 1912 that nursing required "the young and vigorous, who can bend to the strains and not break."[73] Both physicians and families seemed to expect that a young, often pretty, nurse would effect a better cure. Requests for private-duty nurses in one New York hospital registry, for example, were overwhelmingly for nurses in their twenties.[74] The average age of nurses registered between 1880 and 1914 with the Boston Medical Library Directory for Nurses was 28.81, with a mode of 25. In contrast, untrained nurses in this directory were on average 35.97, with a mode of 40.

As compared to all female workers in the national statistics, between

1910 and 1940, fewer nurses were represented in the age groups below 19 and over 45. In 1940 when the number of older women (defined as over 44) in the work force climbed to 22 percent, trained nurses in this age bracket accounted for only 16.5 percent of all working nurses. In contrast, 54 percent of all untrained nurses and midwives were in the "older" category.[75]

For most white nurses, as with other white female workers, marriage meant dropping out of the paid labor force. But a very large percentage of nurses who trained between 1873 and 1940, as with women in other professions, never married.[76] Although there were slight differences among the nursing schools and over time, the proportion of nurses who never married, again as in other professions, was consistently higher than the percentage of single women in the population of women as a whole.[77]

Beginning in the 1920s, however, increasing percentages of married nurses, as with other married women, remained in, or reentered the nursing work force. By the mid-1920s, it was becoming quite clear that marriage did not mean the complete termination of a nurse's active working life. By then one in five working nurses was a married woman.[78] During the Depression, work for married nurses, as for other women, was often a necessity.[79]

Class differences mediated the effects of marriage on the nurse's work experience. For working-class nurses, marriage meant either the abandonment of paid labor for household and child-rearing responsibilities, or, when necessary, a return to employment. Women whose husbands' positions provided them the opportunity for volunteer labor had the option of serving on public-health nursing and hospital boards or performing other health-related charitable work.[80]

The Grading Committee attempted to create a "professional life table" for nurses from the records of 73,271 graduates of 423 different training schools.[81] As in other women's work, nursing had a high "professional mortality" rate in the early years after graduation, followed by a long plateau and another large drop-off when nurses reached the ages of 55–65.

The records of the alumnae of the Waltham Massachusetts Training School confirm this pattern, suggest its dynamic, and introduce a small exception. Within five years of graduation from Waltham, a large number of nurses "dropped out," overwhelmingly for marriage rather than some other career choice. About half of the Waltham nurses who married did so a few years after graduation. However, another half who married worked for over ten years before marriage. Clara M. Cann, for example, was in private-duty, visiting, and tuberculosis nursing in Cambridge, Massachusetts, and Seattle, Washington. She did not marry and "retire" from nursing until thirteen years after graduation. Helen Geary, from the class of 1911, worked in hospitals from Waltham to South Carolina as an operating-room supervisor, assistant matron, and superintendent before her marriage seventeen years after graduation.[82]

Family demands that interrupted a nurse's career impinged on single nurses as well. Jessie F. Le Bosquet received her diploma from Waltham in 1908. She worked as a private-duty nurse for seven years until her mother became ill. Because of this illness, the notes on her in the *Waltham History* state, "She had to take shorter and shorter cases until in 1926 her mother became seriously ill and she stayed home, taking care of her until her death in 1930. She has never resumed work but keeps house for her sister, with whom she lives." Of the 24,389 nurses queried in the Grading Committee's study, 50 percent of those in private duty, 45 percent in public health, and 37 percent in institutional nursing responded they had performed such familial duties.[83] Families demanded such labors from their "spinster" members as they had for generations. Given the trained nurse's obvious expertise, however, such demands were perhaps even more inevitable for her than for other single women.

The training school experience clearly shaped, and in some cases determined, a nurse's work patterns. As Nancy Tomes has suggested in her study of the Pennsylvania Hospital nursing school, there were two "tracks" within most nursing schools: Those labeled as having more "executive ability" were encouraged to go on into superintendency or to become head nurses, and the remainder were expected to go into private duty.[84] Differences existed among schools as well. Comparing the graduates from the Massachusetts General and Boston City hospitals for the years 1857–1909, those from the more elite MGH program were nearly twice as likely to find positions as either superintendents, supervisors, or head nurses in other hospitals and training schools. The differences between the schools are even clearer when the figures are recalculated by subtracting the number of nurses who married, died, or retired. Only slightly over half (54.3 percent) of the Massachusetts General graduates were in noninstitutional positions, whereas 86.9 percent of the Boston City nurses were working in either private duty or public health.[85]

This pattern did not change over time as is illustrated by a comparison of the graduates of the Waltham Training School with those from the more elite programs at Johns Hopkins in Baltimore and Presbyterian Hospital in New York for the years 1887–1942. Waltham graduates were more than twice as likely to enter private duty, and institutional positions went predominantly to nurses from the more elite schools (see Table 6.1).

By the turn of the century, as the health field was growing, nurses had many more options as to where to work. "It is a striking fact," the Grading Committee concluded in 1928, "that nurses shift from one field to another with great frequency."[86] As the committee's statistics indicate, 74 percent of those in institutional work had done private duty, whereas

Table 6.1. *Comparison of the practice fields of the active nursing graduates of Johns Hopkins Hospital, Presbyterian Hospital, and the Waltham Training School, 1887–1942*

Nursing school	Private duty	Institutional	Public health	Missionary	Other[a]
		Practice fields			
Johns Hopkins 1889–1939	263	398	186	16	111
(N = 974)	27.0%	40.9%	19.1%	1.6%	11.4%
Presbyterian 1892–1942	143	245	113	0.0	135
(N = 636)	22.5%	38.5%	17.8%	0.0	21.2%
Waltham 1887–1936	401	158	110	3	33
(N = 705)	57%	22.4%	15.6%	0.3%	4.7%

Note: The numbers were calculated by subtracting all the nurses listed as either married, housewives, retired, or deceased in order to make the figures comparable.

[a]Other work in nursing and other occupations.

Sources: Elsie Lawler, "The School of Nursing – Fifty Years in Retrospect," *Johns Hopkins Hospital Alumnae* 38 (July 1939): 124–25; Eleanor Lee, *History of the School of Nursing of the Presbyterian Hospital 1892–1942* (New York: Putnam, 1942), p. 278; Annette Fiske, compiler, *A History of the Graduates of the Waltham Training School* (Waltham: Waltham Graduate Nurses' Association, 1937).

43 percent of those in private duty had previously been staff nurses (see Table 6.2).

The history of the Waltham graduates confirms this pattern of movement. Just under one-third (32.7) of all of the Waltham graduates did only private duty nursing, about half for a few years, and the rest for their entire careers (see Table 6.3). But the other two-thirds either went into another practice field or combined private duty with other kinds of work. As more work options developed after 1910, the percentage doing only private duty dropped from 36.7 to 29.9. After 1910, Waltham graduates, as did other nurses, more regularly found jobs as staff or head nurses within hospitals, although clearly not so readily as did graduates of the major programs. Further, the increasing specialization within health care was obvious after 1910 as nurses became laboratory and X-ray technicians, social workers, and physiotherapists. Waltham nurses who dropped out from practice often found other ways to stay in the health-care field by opening their own rest homes and small hospitals. Others took up com-

Table 6.2. *Nurses now in private-duty, public-health, and institutional work who have at some time done each specified type of work, 1928 (in %)*

Work done at some time	Current employment		
	Private duty	Public health	Institutional
Private Duty	100	88	74
Nursing a relative free of charge	50	45	37
Hospital nursing staff	43	47	80
Hospital floor duty	41	33	37
Hourly nursing	17	15	7
Visiting nursing	14	62	11
Other public health	9	59	11
Physician's office	9	9	8
Industrial	7	20	5
Sanatorium staff	8	9	9
Anesthetist	6	7	14
Nursing school teacher	5	13	23
Resident in school, orphanage, etc.	4	5	5
Dentist's office	2	2	1
Demonstrator of drugs, appliances, etc.	1	0	0
Other	6	13	11

Source: Committee on the Grading of Nursing Schools, *Nurses, Patients and Pocketbooks* (1928; reprint, New York: Garland, 1984), Table 55, p. 257.

pletely different forms of work that allowed a certain degree of independence: running poultry farms, selling real estate, opening a tearoom, teaching, or entering the antique business.

Nursing provided women with both job and geographic mobility, if they wanted it. Ada Mayo Steward graduated from Waltham in 1893 and became the first industrial nurse in the United States when she went to work for the Vermont Marble Company in Proctor, Vermont, in 1895. She became superintendent of the company's hospital. She later was a surgical nurse in Texas, assistant superintendent of hospitals in Vermont and upstate New York, and practiced and taught massage and private duty from Washington to Florida. In 1918, when she was probably in her later

Table 6.3. *Comparison of the practice fields of the graduates of the Waltham Training School for Nurses from the classes 1877–1910 and 1911–1936*

Practice field	1887–1910		1911–1936		1887–1936	
Private duty (total)	178	62.1%	223	53.3%	401	57.0%
Private duty only	105	36.7	125	29.9	230	32.7
Private duty & staff	10	3.5	36	8.6	46	6.5
Private duty & public health	26	9.1	21	5.0	47	6.7
Private duty & superintendent	21	7.3	3	0.7	24	3.4
Private duty & head nurse	13	4.5	37	8.9	50	7.1
Private duty & registrar for directory	3	1.0	1	0.2	4	0.6
Institutional (total)	55	19.2	103	24.6	158	22.5
Staff nurse	2	0.7	39	9.3	41	5.8
Head nurse, supervisor or instructor	22	7.9	51	12.2	73	10.4
Matron or superintendent	31	10.8	13	3.1	44	6.3
Public health (total)	42	14.5	68	16.3	110	15.6
Public health only	16	5.6	38	9.1	54	7.7
Public health & superintendent	7	2.4	3	0.7	10	1.4
School nurse	9	3.1	15	3.6	24	3.4
Industrial nurse	7	2.4	8	1.9	15	2.1
Public health & head nurse	3	1.0	4	1.0	7	1.0
Other nursing or health work (total)	11	3.8	24	5.7	35	5.0
Doctor	1	0.3	1	0.2	2	0.3
Missionary	2	0.7	0	0.0	2	0.3
Misc. other work	8	2.8	23	5.5	31	4.4
	(N = 286)		(N = 418)		(N = 704)	

Note: Nurses were assigned to the categories to which they made their primary work commitment. The last class graduated from Waltham in 1936.

Source: Figures computed from descriptive work histories in Annette Fiske, compiler, *A History of the Graduates of the Waltham Training School for Nurses* (Waltham: Waltham Graduate Nurses' Association, 1937).

forties or early fifties, she married a retired businessman in Vermont. In contrast, Elizabeth Manning spent twenty-five years in one family's employ. Others worked a few years before marriage. Jessie Pease did some private duty for a year in 1916 before her marriage to a dentist and her retirement from nursing. Eva L. Merrifield did private duty and hospital specializing for three years before her marriage.[87]

In sum, nurses were primarily young single women whose work patterns reflected the demands made by marriage, family, economic necessity, and the labor market. In general, those from the more elite training schools were more likely to obtain responsible positions in public-health and institutional work, whereas the majority from the less elite programs worked as private-duty or staff nurses. Although geographic mobility was common, most job moves were to parallel, rather than higher, positions. Those who left nursing usually did so either for marriage or for work in a health-related field. But those who stayed in the profession moved a great deal between jobs, cases, practice fields, and locales.

A DIVIDED HOME

As an occupation, trained nursing had an ambiguous and uncertain status. Although wage labor, it was seen as akin to a woman's devotional acts on behalf of her family. As women's work in a field dominated by male physicians, it was subordinate labor. As woman's labor, it demanded self-sacrifice and self-abnegation. As an occupational group, it was divided into numerous different practice fields and locales.

As work, however, nursing could provide a woman with a skill to practice for a lifetime or until marriage, and an opportunity for adventure and geographic mobility. For a few, there was the chance to move up the ladder of successive superintendent positions and gain a modicum of authority, however circumscribed. For the majority who moved from case to case, or spent their lives with one family, nursing could bring comfort, freedom, a sense of independence, and self-worth. But by the 1890s, for most nurses, this independence also meant difficult, isolating, financially insecure work in an overcrowded field. Joy was frequently replaced by bitterness, change merely one of locale or institution, rather than responsibility.

Nursing was thus shaped by its position as subordinate service work for women in the health-care hierarchy and by the divisions in the class backgrounds, education, training, and work experiences of its practitioners. This position, and subsequent divisions, shaped the politics of nursing reform.

PART III

The "re-forming" of nursing

7

Professionalization and its discontents

The problems in nursing elicited the beginnings of an organized response by the late 1880s. The necessity for a national organization of trained nurses was discussed in the pages of *Trained Nurse and Hospital Review* by 1889, and, the same year, the first alumnae association was formed at Bellevue Hospital in New York. By the early 1890s, a small group of nursing superintendents from several of the larger, more prestigious, schools began to seek professional recognition and power for nursing. In organizing professional nursing associations, they sought, through voluntary and legislative means, to limit the numbers in nursing and to standardize and raise its educational requirements.[1]

The professionalizing effort placed the superintendent leadership of the nursing associations in a series of dilemmas. They had to exalt the womanly character and service ethic of nursing while insisting on the right to act in their own self-interest, yet not be "unladylike." They had to demand higher wages commensurate with their skills and position, but not appear "commercial." Denouncing the exploitation of nursing students as workers, they had to forge political alliances with hospital physicians and administrators who perpetrated this system of training. While lauding character and sacrifice, they had to measure it with educational criteria in order to formulate registration laws and set admission standards. In doing so, they attacked the background, training, and ideology of the majority of working nurses. Such a series of contradictions were impossible to reconcile.[2]

Their professionalizing efforts were also fraught with conflicts peculiar to nursing. Physicians and hospital administrators, fearful of the competition from nurses or the loss of the nursing student work force, and unwilling to let a group of women determine their own destiny, fought their efforts. The public, barely convinced of the necessity for training in the womanly art of nursing, did not rally to their demands for professional status and autonomy. And, as nursing organizations focused on state registration laws and educational reforms in the schools, they became isolated from the majority of working nurses, whose concerns were different.

Both ideology and social position splintered nursing as an occupational group undergoing the pressures of a professionalization effort. "Traditionalists," as historian Barbara Melosh labels them, working mainly in private duty, continued to emphasize character and spirituality as the essential core of nursing.[3] Other nurses, often in private duty but less sentimental in outlook, could be called "worker-nurses" because of their focus on direct, work-related reforms that linked an altruistic spirit to an autonomous occupational outlook. "Rationalizers," nurses mainly in hospital-management positions, tried to find ways to control the growing division of labor in nursing without focusing on the special position of the trained nurse. All these groups contended with the "professionalizers" in the nursing associations to define nursing's future.

Nursing thus serves as a special example of the particular interplay of gender and class in shaping any occupational group's professionalizing attempts.[4] The sex-segregated labor market "crowded" working- and middle-class women into the same field, yet tracked them into differing occupational opportunities and visions. Nursing's increasing internal stratification and its place in the health-care hierarchy stymied efforts to achieve professional autonomy.[5] The cultural and religious emphasis on womanly sacrifice and self-abnegation continued to have meaning for many nurses, but it could not serve as the basis for professional reform in an increasingly secularized world. Trade-unionist demands provided neither the language nor the strategy for improvements in the context of the powerful ideological force of service, character, individual independence, and extremely scattered work sites. Organized nursing thus found itself, unlike the physicians whose model for professionalizing it attempted to follow, unable to garner the power it sought to standardize and control the nursing field.[6]

THE BEGINNINGS OF PROFESSIONAL REFORM

Occupational loyalty, the basic consciousness necessary to begin a professionalizing and standardizing effort, proved difficult to elicit within nursing. The first efforts in the forms of alumnae associations of the various training schools were often, at first, as much to provide some kind of mutual benefit society for graduates as to organize nurses for collective action. Such organizations, however, helped to create what one nursing educator called a "clan spirit."[7] Fidelity to the "home hospital," deeply engrained during training, thwarted efforts to develop broader occupational loyalty, particularly toward graduates of the smaller, less prestigious, training schools.

Nevertheless in 1889, the same year the first alumnae association was being planned, a nurse wrote to the editor of *Trained Nurse* proposing a national organization to be called the "American Nurses' Association" and suggesting that it seek state registration for nurses. Supported by positive letter responses, the journal's editor proposed first the formation of state associations and helped to encourage such a group in New York. In February 1890, *Trained Nurse* printed a constitution for a national organization as suggested by several nurses. But subsequent issues dropped the question because of opposition from the elite schools.[8]

In 1893, Isabel Hampton, the politically astute nursing superintendent at Johns Hopkins Hospital, organized a meeting on nursing as part of the special section on hospitals at the International Congress of Charities, Correction, and Philanthropy in Chicago at the Columbian Exposition. Through the prestige of her position, skillful planning, and carefully cultivated connections with other nursing superintendents in major training schools, Hampton was able to set up a forum in which the problem caused by a lack of standards and the need for a national organization of nurses could be openly discussed.[9]

Strategically, Hampton argued the necessity of organizing a society of superintendents before creation of a national organization of nurses based on alumnae associations. Immediately after the meeting, eighteen nurses met to found the American Society of Superintendents of Training Schools in the United States and Canada, the association that later was to become less cumbersomely known as the National League of Nursing Education (NLNE). Six months later, forty-four superintendents attended a convention of the society in New York and approved a constitution and bylaws. High standards for admission were set that excluded superintendents of small hospitals or specialty institution schools, and issues of educational standards, ethics, registries, and organization were debated.[10]

Following Hampton's strategy, plans were laid for a national organization of alumnae associations. At meetings in September 1896 and February 1897, the Society of Superintendents created the Nurses' Associated Alumnae (NAA) of the United States and Canada. Isabel Hampton Robb (she had married Dr. Hunter Robb in 1894) was elected the group's first president. The problems of nursing recruitment in the Spanish-American War, a code of ethics, and the organization of funds for an official journal (to be called the *American Journal of Nursing*) took up the early meetings.[11]

As an association of alumnae groups concerned primarily with raising nursing educational standards, and dominated from the beginning by the superintendents of the larger training schools, the NAA reserved entry for the alumnae associations of schools that gave two full years of training in general hospitals of 100 beds or more. It consciously did not attempt to be a broadly based, inclusive nursing organization. Associations were to pay dues and send delegates to annual meetings. Despite the geographic mobility of nurses and the growth of state associations and nurses' clubs, there was no direct individual membership and no membership for other nursing organizations. The question of the basis for membership was repeatedly debated during the NAA's first fourteen years. In 1911, entry requirements were eased somewhat and the organization's name changed to the American Nurses' Association (ANA). Alumnae associations, however, retained the responsibility for determining individual membership.[12]

As with other professional associations, the ANA and the NLNE never became broadly based, as only a minority of nurses and superintendents ever joined, or indeed were expected to join.[13] Furthermore, the organizations' leaders differed widely in training and outlook from their membership and from trained nurses in general. Of ninety women identified as the key leaders in nursing between 1873 and 1945, nearly 50 percent (forty-four) trained in only six major large nursing schools located in teaching hospitals: Johns Hopkins, Bellevue, New York, Boston City, Massachusetts General, and Connecticut Training School-Yale/New Haven; nearly one-third had trained at Bellevue or Hopkins. Most spent their entire careers as superintendents, university-based educators, officials in state and national nursing organizations, or directors of major public-health agencies. Private-duty nursing was seen, at best, as a good "foundation" acquired early in their careers, not as desirable lifetime work. In addition, middle-class background and high school and college education differentiated the nursing leadership from their occupational colleagues.[14]

Efforts to gain control over who was allowed to enter training, manifested in a debate over the payment of allowances to students in training, were the focus of early endeavors in professionalization. Such allowances, in reality small monthly wages, helped attract women to training and justified the use of students as the hospitals' workers. As early as 1889 in an article in *Trained Nurse,* Mrs. Seth Low, the lay president of the Brooklyn Training School for Nurses, objected to the payments because she felt such remuneration interested women who only wanted the salary. She did not oppose what she called "worthy poor" candidates and suggested that scholarships be set aside for such women. But her article elicited a round of angry letters from graduate nurses that reflected a continuing argument in nursing. They attacked her "aristocratic views" and defended payments as reasonable compensation for the harshness of training.[15]

A year later the debate resurfaced in the *New York Medical Journal* where New York Hospital superintendent George Ludlam defended such payments, comparing them to the money given to cadets in military academies. Such allowances, he contended, helped nursing to attract women from families of "refinement" who were caught in financial reverses. Such a group, he concluded, was a "very large and constantly rising class."[16]

At the first meeting of the Society of Superintendents in 1894, educators Lavinia Dock and Isabel Hampton decried the payments. But other nursing superintendents supported them, noting that the repetitiveness and difficulty of nursing made such remuneration reasonable since only self-supporting women who needed the money and the work would actually apply.[17] The allowances were also seen as "payoffs" for the exploitation. As *Trained Nurse* editorialized in 1902:

Would nurses who were paying a good round sum for education be willing to abide by the rigid rules now in force, or would they, when they considered they had provocation, and things were not to their liking, pack up their belongings and go home. . . . The question then arises, if nurses are in position to *demand*, will they submit . . . ?[18]

Thus the debate over payments raised the questions of both the exploitation in training and the class background and motivation of potential students.

Some of the leading schools, under pressure from their nursing superintendents, introduced the nonpayment system, but the overwhelming majority did not. The experiences at New York Hospital underscored the difficulties. When Annie Goodrich became superintendent of nurses there in 1902, she insisted on several reforms to upgrade the program, including ending the allowances. Instead, the school supplied students with uniforms, caps, and books. By 1907, however, when Goodrich left New York Hospital for the superintendency at Bellevue, her replacement requested a return to the monthly payments. She argued that "cultured women" would not enter training unless there was financial necessity requiring the allowance. The hospital returned to the payments.[19] An anonymous nurse, writing to the *American Journal of Nursing* in 1902, clearly stated the key underlying issue:

By all means, let there be hospitals in which for their own good reasons no remuneration be given, but let us have no more of that twaddle of "raising the standard" by such means.

Rather, let the standard be raised by character, by refinement and intelligence, and by natural qualifications, than by a question of mere money.[20]

When the elimination of payments did not work as a strategy to raise entry standards, the American nursing leaders, as had the British, turned to state registration.[21] To achieve such legislation state by state, the NAA urged the formation of state affiliates, expressly to push for these laws.[22] As efforts to control entry into the field centered on a legislative strategy, a measurable quality – educational attainment – had to become the nursing standard. "It is easier to maintain a criterion from an educational standpoint than from the moral and social aspect," a nurse pointed out.[23] Thus proper character for nursing became redefined, in part, as requiring a reasonable educational background and rigorous theoretical and scientific training.[24]

Although partially aware of the limitations of registration, nursing leaders believed, as did other Progressives, that legislation would transform their field by placing the power of the state behind their efforts. Their views were similar to those of the early leaders of women's suffrage. As historian Ellen DuBois has argued, suffrage advocates regarded their goal not as a narrow institutional reform but as promising, through bringing women into the public sphere, "a total transformation of their lives."[25] Similarly, nursing, although structurally outside the private domestic sphere, was still ideologically within its parameters. State legitimation of high standards, set by nurses, would free nursing, it was hoped, from this ideological constriction. The struggle for women's suffrage brought before the public the question of a woman's role and patriarchal control; the parallel struggle for nursing registration publicly raised the question of the nurse's role and physician and hospital control.[26]

When the issue of control moved out of the sickroom and hospital corridors into the legislative arena, the battle over nursing became more visible and vituperative. The difficulties varied considerably among the states and depended, in part, on the political skills and alliances nurses were able to build, the structure of the nursing education system, and the peculiarities of the political process and administrative machinery for licensure. Opposition in many states came more from the doctors affiliated with small, specialty, or mental hospitals, which stood to lose their work forces as a result of legally enforced standards, than from physicians in private practice, in large hospitals, or the state medical societies.[27] Nurses often found themselves in tenuous alliances with officials from larger hospitals who were willing and able to accept certain standards. These collaborations were necessary because women could not yet vote in most states and could not sit on state-mandated examining boards. But such alliances could easily dissolve into hostilities when nurses attempted to act independently.[28]

The laws differed from state to state and changed over time, but most were permissive rather than mandatory and did not cover "all who nursed for hire." They differentiated nurses more by education than by practice; only those wanting to be labeled as "registered nurses" needed to sit for the examinations and/or graduate from approved nursing schools. The laws thus tried to mandate educational requirements within the training schools, rather than define the scope of nursing practice.[29]

Qualifications for taking the state examinations and control over the examining boards focused the real question: legal acknowledgment of nursing's right to determine its own occupational future. Few physicians were willing to concede to nursing, through state mandate, what they were unwilling to give up in practice. As one physician bluntly questioned, "Is it but justice to assert that the nurse's fitness is to be decided in the sick chamber, and who is the judge of her fitness but the attending physician?"[30] In addition, physicians repeatedly argued that the "market," not legislation, could determine the good nurse. Furthermore, such Progressive Era epithets as "nursing bosses" and the "nursing trust" were hurled at registration organizers, while others derided them for being "trade unionists."[31]

Opposition also was voiced by nurses who had graduated from the smaller schools. Even with "grandmother clauses" in most of the legislation, they stood to have their status and standing lowered when strong registration laws passed. In many states they aligned themselves against the state nursing associations during the legislative battles, forcing continued compromises in the state association bills.[32]

Even when registration was passed, the administration of the laws and the nursing boards proved to be as weak as most of the laws themselves. In her case study of the administration of the New York law, Nancy Tomes found that when the first law passed, only nineteen of the state's ninety-eight incorporated schools met the guidelines.[33] This law, and many others in different states, forced training schools to add affiliations or expand their programs to meet requirements. The necessity for state reciprocity extended the power of the laws in the major states beyond their borders.[34] But because such registration was not mandatory, many schools chose instead to forgo it rather than change their training programs.[35]

In other states, the lack of money, clerical help, time, or inspectors meant that nursing boards had to "pass" schools they never visited.[36] The boards were further hampered by their own composition as political appointments weakened efforts to gain uniformity. In 1922, when the Board of Directors of the ANA went on record calling for high school graduation as a minimal requirement for entry into training, one nursing leader reminded them that most state nursing-board members, who would have to enforce such a requirement, were not themselves high school graduates.[37]

The focus on registration pushed the nursing associations into seemingly contradictory positions that undermined the possibility for improvements through other legislative means. In California, the state nursing association joined the hospitals in 1913 to fight a bill to include student nurses in laws that restricted the hours of women's labor.[38] Many California hospitals fought the legislation because it would have increased the number of students needed and limited their use of students in private duty. The California State Nurses Association *joined* the opposition to the bill because it did not want nursing classed as a trade and nurses as workers. As the association argued, "Real nursing, self-sacrificing service, cannot be timed by the clock. It never has been, and it never will be."[39]

The state association's concurrent lobbying for a registration act played a role in its opposition, as it searched, in activist Anna C. Jamme's words, for a more "dignified manner" to combat the long hours.[40] The legislation was passed, however, and withstood repeal efforts by the hospital and nursing associations.

The California state association's stand was not shared by many working nurses, however. As one nurse wrote in some confusion and naïveté:

The attitudes of those in charge of training schools is what puzzles graduate nurses. Why they did not at once start their eight-hour system – a system that ought to have been established in all training schools ere now – without exhibiting such bitter antagonism towards the law, is a matter for surprise.[41]

Paternalism, on the part of hospitals and physicians, and the link between nursing and mothering could also be justified, ironically, in the name of professionalism. This particular twist surfaced in legislative attempts in Illinois in 1917, as in California, to regulate nurses' hours. Chicago hospital executives formed an association expressly to gain the exemption of hospitals from an hours' bill. In a circular presenting the arguments for their position, the hospital association willingly classed nursing as a profession, albeit a womanly one, to justify exclusion from the law. Nursing stands, they asserted, "in the same relation to the sick of the world as the medical profession. The work of nurses can no more be regulated by a hard-and-fast law than the work of doctors or mothers." Denying there was any exploitation of the student they declared:

Nurses in training are part of the hospital family, and are cared for as a father cares for his children. The money given them is only given as pin-money to take care of books, carfare, etc., not as wages. Their whole so-called working time is devoted to the study and practice of nursing.[42]

Such arguments proved effective. By 1920, only California included nurses, and then only students, in its laws determining women's hours.[43] Thus nurses did not achieve much of the legal protection accorded *either* professionals or other women workers.

The professional nursing associations' focus on registration and educational reforms often brought them into conflict with their own constituencies and physicians, and into precarious alliances with the larger hospitals and their associations. Although legislation slowly upgraded standards in the schools, it did not achieve the goal of legitimating the professional nursing associations' right to regulate nursing or facilitate the creation of a united occupation.

HOSTILITY AND INDIFFERENCE IN THE PUBLIC REALM

By 1900 trained nursing *was* becoming more accepted as a necessary part of the medical world. But acceptance of nursing's importance did not translate into cultural and political willingness to support nursing in its professional efforts. The public remained indifferent and physicians and hospital administrators, hostile.

There was still a good deal of ignorance and uncertainty about the trained nurse. Families who sent their daughters into training might come away with some understanding of the work, whereas those who hired nurses frequently saw them as "semimenials" and were unlikely to support any effort to change their conditions.[44] Sentimentality toward the woman working to support herself through devotion to others could quickly be replaced by hostility when a family, in the midst of crisis, had difficulty finding a nurse, paying her charges, or putting up with her demands. A reform-minded upper- or middle-class woman might be sympathetic toward, and even support, the claims of an immigrant woman making shirtwaists in a tenement firetrap, but have much less concern for a nurse who charged twenty-five dollars a week, refused certain tasks, and left her home in an uproar after a fight with the servants.

In the hospitals, the student status of the nurses, and the institutions' claims of paternal and maternal authority over their charges, kept public inquiry into the working and wage conditions of nurses at a minimum. With two exceptions, there were no major investigations into conditions for nurses within hospitals outside those done by nurses themselves during the Progressive Era. Yet during these years almost every other kind of women's employment was subject to careful scrutiny and social investigation. Even the Women's Bureau, which began issuing reports on the conditions for women workers in 1918, did not examine nursing until 1943.[45] Ironically, the assertion of nursing's professional status by nursing leaders protected it from such investigations. As a consequence, nurses had a difficult time making the public understand their work and the need for reform.

Nursing had been supported, of course, by women active in charity efforts. But as the schools developed into hospital departments, such women were relegated to advisory positions on women's boards and frequently were viewed as interfering busybodies.[46] In addition, as Nancy Tomes has argued, nurses' claims to special authority and professional status forced them to separate themselves from the women who wanted to do the work for patriotic reasons during World War I. Such divisions made political alliances difficult, although they surfaced periodically during legislative battles as nurses sought the support of federations of women's clubs.[47] Such alliances appeared to have existed primarily on an ongoing basis in the public-health nursing agencies and associations, in part because this nursing field depended on the charitable contributions of such women for its very survival.

The kinds of feminist support networks so important for women entering medicine, however, did not appear to exist in nursing once other professions and careers became more acceptable for women of the middle class.[48] The very lack of autonomy of nursing work and its link to traditional women's labor both seem to have kept nursing from capturing the imagination and interest of feminists concerned with expanding roles for women. A few visible wealthy benefactors such as Frances Payne Bolton in Cleveland and Helen Hartley Jenkins in New York did support nursing. But the outpouring of funds, raised so successfully by women's colleges, eluded nursing. In turn, with the notable exceptions of Lillian Wald, Lavinia Dock, and Adelaide Nutting, most nursing leaders shied away from organized feminist and suffrage activity. Although nurses did march in suffrage parades, public links to the women's rights organizations were not forged.[49]

Much physician opposition to the upgrading and control of nursing standards by nurses also underlay and influenced public lack of sympathy. An exchange between Dr. A. W. Catlin and graduate nurses in the pages of the *Brooklyn Eagle* during the depression of the 1890s is a classic example of the ideological expression of these struggles.[50] Catlin voiced concern with the high fees of private-duty nurses and the inability of the average wage earner to pay such prices at the height of a severe depression and amid growing physician concern with overcrowding in medicine. His solution to the problem, unique because of its outrageousness, nevertheless contained the major continuing elements of the physician's answer to what was to be labeled the "nursing question."

Catlin called for the endowment of a "home" for private-duty nurses. In such a "home," the nurses would be selected and trained by physicians and, "if the doctor so decides," would lower their fees substantially below the current standard in Brooklyn – to nothing, if necessary. Catlin reasoned that such charity would be possible because the nurses' living expenses would be covered in the endowed home, and presumably because only women willing to be so devoted would enter this kind of training.

Other physicians were not so blatant in calling for what amounted to a stable of "kept nurses," but Catlin's idea that a physician should control a nurse's training, income, and even her living arrangements was not so unusual. His suggestion for a home in many ways typified what physicians wanted nurses to be: compliant and ever-present daughterlike creatures, never quite ready to live on their own, forever dependent on a father's largess and his conception of their world. His proposal of a supported home also played into contemporary feminist reform efforts to improve conditions for women workers by providing them with cheaper and more controlled living situations.

Catlin's proposals sparked an outcry from Brooklyn nurses.[51] One nurse suggested the concerned doctor spend more time employing graduate nurses than trying to find cheaper substitutes. "What *right* has Dr. Catlin to set our prices?" an irate nurse queried. Another chastised him for trying to oppress "a woman who is only trying to earn a decent living." Perhaps, another nurse ventured to inquire, there could be as much loyalty toward nurses expressed by doctors as nurses were expected to give in reverse. An enterprising nurse accepted the terms of Catlin's suggestions and asked:

How about building a home for cheap doctors? I am sure the trained nurses will be willing to teach them free of charge. What a beautiful memorial that would be for future generations – a HOME where anyone could go and get a doctor for 50c. Trained nurses could easily charge $30 a week.

Neither home was built.

Medical and hospital journals continued to reflect the attitude, clearly stated in a 1928 Michigan State Medical Society report on nursing, that "nurses are helpers and agents of physicians; not co-workers or colleagues."[52] Indeed, the very definition of doctor appeared to depend on nursing's remaining both a woman's occupation and subordinate to medicine.[53] There were, of course, numbers of physicians who supported professionalizing efforts in nursing. But, in general, as JoAnn Ashley and others have forcefully argued, "Physicians spent a great deal of time attempting to convince both women in nursing and the public in general that nursing was subordinate to medicine and should remain so for the public good."[54]

THE WORKER-NURSE

Nursing might have been able to overcome physician hostility if it had been united itself. But the leadership's professionalizing ideology and strategy were perceived by many working nurses, particularly those in private duty, as either irrelevant or in opposition to their definition of nursing and its problems. Unashamed of the necessity to work, they saw nothing wrong in their focus on such "mundane" issues as wages and conditions. They resented bitterly those who impugned their motives and attacked their seeming "commercialism." They refused to accept the judgment that only those with pure, noneconomic motives could be true nurses. The sentimentality that infused the assumptions of why women would enter such service work was either abandoned or never held by these women.

A nurse who signed herself "Candor" clearly articulated this position in 1888. She rejected the heavenly image of the nurse for a more earthly form. In a letter to *Trained Nurse* she declared:

Where there is one nurse with a missionary spirit . . . there are forty-nine others who are obliged to make the humiliating confession: "I am a nurse because I must earn a living for myself and those dependent on me, because my nursing is well-paid, honorable, and to me interesting."

. . . Of course this spirit of self-immolation is very beautiful and lovely, but is it practical? Is it the motive power which had induced the army of sensible, practical women to take up this work? . . . Let us be honest, even at the sacrifice of sentiment. Let us not hesitate to do a good deed when opportunity offers, but let us not try to make people believe we are angels and that to do good is the chief object in our lives, with a small remuneration thrown in, to which we scarcely give a thought.[55]

These opinions, repeated in numerous other letters and statements, and associations of primarily private-duty nurses, could be called the "worker-nurse's position." It entailed a pragmatic conception of women's motives for entering nursing, a concern with conditions and wages, and pride in the practical skills and independence of nursing labor.[56] Such a position frequently brought the women who held it in conflict with those who were articulating a more "professional" vision of nursing. An *American Journal of Nursing* editorial in 1904, for example, warned that women who shared "Candor's" perspective on nursing were bringing to nursing "traditions – traditions foreign to the whole spirit of nursing as we understand it." But such a spirit had long been part of the motivation of women entering nursing, as the letters of application attested.[57] At stake in the argument was who defined that spirit.

The need for work as a valid and honorable motive for entering nursing was a perception shared by many women. At the same time, nurses who held these views were increasingly forced into a defensive position to ward off the label of commercialism. Such nurses also resented the notion that women had to have different motives from those of men to justify their working. Commenting at a 1903 Boston meeting on the charge that women entered training because of a desire "to earn big money," a nurse declared that need, and a lack of experience, often necessitated such seeming obsession with wages. With a view of work that reflected the experience of native-born, middle-class white women, she declared:

Everyone expects a man to earn his living and respects him for doing so. With women it is different. We have not been at it very long, not more than two generations; and it is not unnatural that the thoughts of others perhaps our own, should dwell upon the matter rather disproportionately.[58]

The question of independence and the necessity for decent wages was raised clearly in the debate that centered on a proposal for a nurse's pension fund. In 1892, the English hospital leader, Henry C. Burdett, the editor of *The Hospital,* founder of the Royal National Pension Fund of England, and a staunch foe of registration for nurses, proposed an American National Pension Fund for nurses, physicians, and other "hospital workers." It was part insurance scheme and part charity (Burdett persuaded J. Pierpont Morgan and W. O. Mills each to contribute $50,000 to the fund). Burdett even suggested that grateful patients could send contributions in the name of specific nurses, rather than offer them gratuities.[59]

The plan did not come to fruition, but three years later it was revived by physicians attached to the Nurses' Directory of Philadelphia. Neither plan, however, was organized or controlled by nurses. The idea was denounced by a number of nursing leaders, who contended that the plan would "pauperize" and degrade independent nurses. "Nurses with the true spirit of American independence," one nursing leader wrote, "and the requisite amount of self respect, will not tolerate the idea." Lavinia Dock added that nurses' wages might be lowered once it was known such a "benevolent" fund existed.[60]

The worker-nurses' response to the failed scheme was more divided. Such assistance, one Bellevue graduate thought, was patronizing. Given nurses' low wages, she contended, what they needed was "justice." An Irish-born nurse agreed, adding she and her American colleagues did not believe nurses should be the "objects of charity." But other nurses saw it not as charity but as payment for self-sacrificing work. Asserting their own independence, they focused on the scheme's necessity for premium payments rather than the charity. Another nurse stated that she was willing to share her "pension fund" with other health workers and did not see the necessity for a fund only for nurses.[61] These nurses did not equate independence with a refusal to think collectively about an insurance program, even one with elements of charity. When Burdett's scheme failed, they turned to their alumnae associations and nurses' clubs for such assistance.

Worker-nurses accepted the reasonableness of demanding decent wages *and* expressed the desire to be of service to those in need. As one nurse noted, "A nurse is willing to work; she would be glad to help the sick and suffering, but she must also help herself."[62] Nursing's Grading Committee survey in the 1920s revealed that many nurses did a month's charity work a year.[63] Many nurses, of course, rejected this kind of work and refused to take such cases. But the desire to be of service to those poorer than themselves was not limited to nurses who could easily afford such sentiments.

"Candor's" "army of sensible, practical women" expressed pride in their own skills and abilities to overcome the difficulties encountered in their work. The pages of the nursing journals were filled with examples of their ingenuity in devising equipment, modifying hospital techniques, and coping with the uncertainty of private duty.

Yet a frequently voiced sense that many nurses were both technically and behaviorally ill equipped for the work underlay the bravado. One nurse, signing herself "One of Them," frankly admitted her training in a small obstetrical hospital left her feeling like a "fraud"; she counseled others to train in large institutions where more experience could be gained.[64] Others, more defensive about their training, responded angrily to the attack that their meager educations in small hospitals should deny them entry into the ranks of trained nurses. Explaining why nurses often did not attend meetings of the local nursing associations, *Trained Nurse* editorialized in 1911 that they were "ashamed and humiliated of being from a small school, one that might be seen as disgracing the profession."[65]

These nurses deeply resented the charge that they lacked gentility, tact, and knowledge because of their social backgrounds and training. Those who readily admitted to their humble origins chafed at the suggestions that their newly learned behaviors were deficient. Others, who claimed a place in the middle class by birthright, similarly resented the attacks on their motives for entering training. They shared the assumption that a nurse had to have character, a certain amount of gentility, and a middle-class demeanor to accomplish her tasks.

The question of character, and whether it could be a measure of a nurse's worth, underlay the tensions between worker-nurses and the leadership. When the state associations sought to use educational requirements and the size of training schools to determine a nurse's right to sit for state registration examinations, many nurses saw hard-won skills and status being maligned. One nurse rather defensively attacked the drive for registration in New York State. She argued that such efforts would not be "fair play" or an accurate determination of a good nurse. In her opinion:

The nurse who possesses tact, whose manners are those of an innately refined woman, who dresses quietly, yet well, the nurse who can turn a pillow deftly and please her patient will always be far more successful than, it may be, her sister who perchance has a dozen ologies [*sic*] on her tongue and a license to practice issued upon recommendation of the State Board of Examiners.[66]

Further, she noted, the reality of the lives and training of most private-duty nurses made them fearful of such exams. "Are you prepared to pass this examination?" she inquired rhetorically. "Can you spare time from your duties to study for it?" The concern of those eager for registration and higher standards focused on entry requirements and nursing education, whereas nurses already in the field were occupied with the conditions they faced at work.

These viewpoints and resentments shaped the struggles that emerged between organizations led primarily by private-duty nurses and those controlled by prominent nursing superintendents. As Susan Armeny has demonstrated in her study of such organizations and disputes, many of the groups created by private-duty nurses, however ephemeral, were inclusive rather than exclusive in their membership, concentrating more on mutual benefit and lenient registration laws than educational reform.[67] Issues of membership and leadership in nursing organizations underlay many of the disputes among groups. Celia R. Heller, the chief organizer and defender of a late nineteenth-century New York nurses' group called the Nurses' Protective Association (NPA), counseled other nurses: "The unity of the graduate should be our first thought. Do not ask a nurse if she graduated from a large or small school. If she is a good nurse and respectable, she is your equal."[68]

The NPA, organized in New York in 1897 to gain a state law on nursing practice, proposed legislation that would have given licensure to nurses who graduated from small hospitals or took short courses. It was attacked at meetings by Lavinia Dock and in writing by the nursing superintendents of seventeen New York training schools. The attack centered, as Armeny has suggested, on the low standards for licensure proposed by the NPA, the inclusiveness of the membership, and the right of graduate nurses to determine their political goals without nursing superintendent leadership.[69]

When the dispute spilled over into the pages of *Trained Nurse,* elitism within nursing came under fire. The ire of the nursing readership of the journal was raised when a letter from the group of nursing superintendents was published warning nurses against the NPA and questioning its representativeness, since it had not elected delegates from alumnae associations and had neither nursing school superintendents, heads of hospitals, nor any non–New York City nurse in its membership. Angrily, one nurse wrote: "I do see something very objectionable in women who certainly can have no jurisdiction over nurses after graduation, using such means to interfere with nurses who are trying to help themselves."[70] Five Illinois graduates who joined the letter-writing debate were insulted by the superintendents' position and questioned the implication that nurses could not make judgments for themselves. "Women with pride and self-respect," they concluded, "will not submit to being governed by and dictated to by those who have no authority beyond the training school. . . . They are not capable of judging of the needs of the graduate in private practice."[71] Another nurse, taking the time-honored worker's position of questioning the ability of those in authority to do her job, queried, "How many of these superintendents have in fact engaged in private practice?"[72]

Such sentiments touched on the resentment against nursing superintendents built up during training and rekindled after graduation. It reflected a traditional working woman's anger against infantilization. Supporting this viewpoint, a *Trained Nurse* editorial in 1900 argued:

Nurses are rapidly becoming weary of having full-fledged projects thrust upon them without being allowed to assist at the birth, and of being told like little children, "We know what is best for you. Take what is set before you and ask no questions."[73]

Efforts by the more elite nursing associations to reach out to worker-nurses also proved relatively unsuccessful. In 1915, a county division of the Massachusetts State Nurses' Association called for a statewide organization of private-duty nurses. Although the plan was to establish an autonomous organization separate from the state association, membership recruitment consisted in asking nursing superintendents for names of nurses who were already state association members. A small Private Duty Nurses' League, with thirty charter members, was founded.[74]

The league met three times a year at the same time as the Massachusetts State Nurses' Association to hear papers on a variety of topics of interest to those in this practice field. The war, the time constraints of private-duty work, or perhaps the very professionally oriented nature of the organization kept the league from ever reaching large numbers. By 1919, the league was three years old but had a membership of only eighty-one, and yet, a survey revealed, it was the only "thoroughly well organized private duty nurses' league" in the country! By 1920 the league had fewer members after four years than at its initial meeting and was folded back into the state association.[75]

The physical and emotional constraints of private duty meant that the institutional support and time necessary to form viable separate sustained organizations did not exist. The very existence of nursing organizations, organized by hospital alumnae associations, directed by superintendents, and led by women who had the time and financial security to do the work of sustaining the organizations, made it even more unlikely that an organized opposition could find a base. As *Trained Nurse* editorialized, anyone who organized against the leadership's goals found herself "regarded with suspicion and branded as one 'opposed to progress' and 'without high ideals.' "[76]

At best, groups of nurses were able, in Armeny's words, to "resist professionalization" by thwarting the registration and educational reforms of the leadership, but not to offer a feasible alternative strategy to improve nursing. A different understanding of nursing could provide support at the workplace; anger and resentment, however, could not coalesce into a political force.[77]

TRADITIONALISTS AND RATIONALIZERS

Efforts to provide such support did appear outside the more elite nursing organizations. It was mainly articulated by individual nurses and widely circulated through *Trained Nurse*. But neither the journal, nor those who wrote for it, developed a politically adept leadership whose strategic and tactical plans served as the focus for an alternative organizational force within nursing. The publication's editors and writers attacked the professionalization efforts of the leadership, but emphasized individualism rather than organization. As early as 1889, seven years before the Nurses' Associated Alumnae was formed, the editors of this magazine had called for a broadly based organization of nurses, and attempted to help begin its formation.[78] By the 1910s and 1920s, however, the journal's editors retreated to even questioning the necessity for organization, arguing, not unexpectedly, that character rather than organization mattered in nursing.

These editorials and articles continued to be supportive of private-duty nurses and those trained in the smaller institutions. But rather than articulate a working-class vision of trade unionism, the journal equated professionalism with unionism.[79] Further, a *Trained Nurse* editorial in 1919, during the growing anti-left political climate, proudly declared, "We have not published articles on socialism, anarchy, woman suffrage and other subjects which are out of place in a nursing magazine."[80] Nor would they advocate any actions aimed at questioning the authority of physicians or the necessity of accepting doctors as nursing's "friends."

While defending, at best, the needs of nurses that evolved out of their narrow economic and occupational position, *Trained Nurse* did not defend needs that stemmed from their social class or gender. "Feminism, socialism, and anarchy" were all linked and defined "out of place" in a nursing journal and nursing. The editors' condemnations of the occasional nursing strikes and organization efforts were even more vituperative than those appearing in the *American Journal of Nursing,* the official journal of the ANA.[81] The term "trade union" was used as an epithet against the ANA, rather than as a suggestion for nurses seeking another organizational form.

Their editorials condemned the efforts of nursing leaders who were variously labeled "bosses" and "merely politicians," and attacked their elitism and "dictatorial spirit." Appealing to "our American forefathers," *Trained Nurse*'s editors argued that opposition to the centralizing tendencies of the nursing leadership stood for "individual liberty." Refutation of professional reform was thus based on a doctrine of individualism and a belief in the necessity of nursing's submission to physician authority and patient needs.

Strategically, the journal's editors and writers opposed not registration per se but the kinds of exclusive registration laws being proposed by the state nursing associations.[82] Their opposition to the registration laws thus grew out of their attacks on the nursing leadership's efforts to upgrade educational requirements and form selective nursing organizations. Demands for educational criteria in nursing, particularly through the use of the cudgel of state registration laws, smacked of "class legislation," it was editorialized. Instead, editorial after editorial argued, "in the selection of the nurse the supreme test should be *character* . . . not titles or degrees, not educational attainment, but a high grade of character." Examples of high school graduates in training who lied in their nursing notes about procedures and medications were detailed. "No amount of education," it was concluded, "could possibly make up for the lack of character."[83] Nursing was, it was argued, hard and responsible labor that required women willing to suffer in silence for the sake of patient care and hospital stability.[84]

These viewpoints were reiterated by two frequent contributors to *Trained Nurse,* Annette Fiske and Charlotte Aikens. Both consistently supported the worker-nurses in their writings and proposed solutions to nursing's dilemmas, which only served, however, to reinforce nursing's ideological and economic binds.

Fiske, by class background and education, was an unusual candidate for nursing training and appeared even more unlikely, once trained, to have challenged the professionalizing views of the leadership. She was born in 1873 in Cambridge, Massachusetts, the daughter of Amos K. Fiske, a Harvard graduate and the financial editor of the *New York Journal of Commerce.* She was sent to private school, as behooved a respectable upper-middle-class Episcopalian girl of her age, and then on to Radcliffe in 1890. She received an A.B. in 1894 with a magna cum laude with Final Honors in Classics and was elected to Phi Beta Kappa. She stayed on at Radcliffe for three more years and took a master's degree in the same field.[85]

Like other women of her generation and class who desired an escape from the stifling life of the family or genteel women's work, Fiske sought more purposeful labor by entering training four years after completing her master's degree. Perhaps the esoteric and scholarly nature of her chosen field of study did not meet some deeper need. In an article on nursing for *Radcliffe Magazine* in 1914 she closed with these personal comments: "For myself, I never really lived till I went to the Waltham Training School for Nurses. . . . There may be nothing spectacular in [the nurse's] work but in a quiet sort of way she has the opportunity opened before her of doing more than most for the welfare of mankind."[86]

From the time of her graduation from Waltham till her death at age seventy-nine in 1953, Annette Fiske devoted her nursing career to the private-duty ideal and the Waltham School. She was a private nurse for a number of years, interspersed with work as an assistant principal and nursing instructor in other training schools, as well as public-health nurse in milk stations. An instructor at the Waltham Training School beginning in 1918, she stayed until the last class entered in 1932, while spending thirty years editing the school's *News Letter* and writing its history. She was active in the short-lived Massachusetts Private Duty League (serving as its recording secretary) and later in the Massachusetts Nurses' Association. She became a trustee of Waltham Hospital, secretary of the Waltham

Graduate Nurses' Association, and author of two small science books for nurses as well as innumerable articles for *Trained Nurse* and *Hygeia*.[87]

Fiske's articles on nursing ranged from practical suggestions for private-duty nurses to discussions on ethics and professionalization. She consistently upheld the view of a nursing "traditionalist" that a good nurse was defined by her innate character and devotion to service. "Here, as everywhere else and more than anywhere else," she wrote to her Radcliffe classmates, "personality counts and it is the woman of refinement and tact who succeeds – if she has the true love of service."[88] Even more directly, in another article she declared, "Yet *service* is the nurse's only excuse for existing, and if her training does not make her pre-eminently of service to others, it is a failure."[89] Only through strict training and instilling of the "spirit of service" did she believe the "self-sacrifice and devotion" necessary in nursing could be developed. She willingly admitted there were problems in nursing, but she blamed the training schools and the nursing leadership, not individual nurses, for them.[90]

By the 1920s, Fiske had come to agree with the leadership that nursing was a profession but, she queried rhetorically, the issue was "where to place the emphasis."[91] Answering her own question, she pointed to women's greater manual dexterity and spirituality. She attacked the leadership's efforts to measure a nurse by her educational attainment, arguing "it is the ideal side rather than the learned side that distinguished the profession from the trade, for knowledge of some kind is needed in every calling."[92] While she lamented the loss of self-sacrifice and character in the women entering training, she did not believe raising the educational standards was a substitute for greater discipline and emphasis on service in the training schools.

As had the first generation of training advocates, Fiske believed in a discipline that enriched the nurse's spirit and deepened her commitment to service. She strenuously objected to a discipline that taught routinization and ritualized devotion to methods. Thus she believed private duty was the most important field of nursing because it required the nurse to be her most humane, caring, and innovative. If devoid of spirit, she declared, "Nursing degenerates into a commonplace, utilitarian occupation that any one could follow, that calls for no special ability, no refinement of character, no unusual endowments. . . . Is the word [nurse] going to degenerate till it means only a superior kind of machine?"[93] Emphasize "devotion and self-sacrifice," she promised, and "the profession will win all the love and respect and admiration that anyone could wish it to enjoy."[94]

Fiske supported worker-nurses and attacked the elitism of the leadership, but in a voice that by the 1910s and 1920s was out of tune with the structural and ideological changes in nursing. The celebration of devotion voiced by Fiske and the *Trained Nurse* might confer dignity, but it did not speak to the needs of private-duty nurses who faced longer and longer waits between cases and a professional leadership that increasingly viewed them as a threat and an anachronism.

Nor did the emphasis on individual effort provide nurses with a strategy to build an organization either to improve conditions or counter the leadership's efforts. By its very nature, Fiske's belief denied the necessity for organization. Her Calvinist insistence on the need for personal conversion to a life of service was increasingly out of place in the growing secularization of American culture in the 1920s. Although comforting, such an ideology could not, and did not, provide the basis for a political grouping in any real opposition to the professional associations.

In contrast, Charlotte Aikens, a trained nurse and hospital superintendent, attacked the strategies and goals of the nursing leadership by articulating the "rationalizer" position closer to that of other hospital administrators. A Canadian-born and college-educated woman, she trained for nursing at a large Ontario city hospital in the 1890s and then immediately came to New York to take a course in ward administration. Her education led her to the hospital superintendency at several American institutions. Aikens was best known, however, for her numerous articles and editorials in *Trained Nurse* and the *National Hospital Record*. She also wrote or edited six books on hospital management, nursing administration, education, and ethics. An active leader and vice-president of the American Hospital Association, she most clearly tried to suggest strategies for improving and standardizing nursing that did not clash with the needs of the hospitals.[95]

In many ways, Aikens's views were similar to those of Fiske and other nurses who wrote in *Trained Nurse* emphasizing character rather than educational requirements. But unlike Fiske, Aikens sought to find a way to improve nursing by raising its standards through the use of the organized power of the hospital association. Furthermore, unlike the nursing leadership in the professional associations, she sought to raise standards *and* provide hospitals with a cheap nursing work force.

Aikens proposed an alternative strategy: the grading and classification of *all* who nursed for hire, whether trained or untrained. Through her position of leadership within the American Hospital Association (AHA), she either led or was the moving force behind a series of the association's reports on nursing issued between 1908 and 1916.[96] Through these reports, she advocated a clear classification and division of labor among nursing workers that recognized what she labeled the "natural division among nurses."[97] The reports suggested various schemes for training nurses either in large hospitals or in smaller institutions affiliated with other institutions for training purposes, while allowing unaffiliated small hospitals to train "attendants." These plans thus were an effort to provide a cheap labor force for the small hospitals, keep nursing education within the larger hospitals, and still improve nursing standards.

The nursing leadership, however, perceived this strategy as a threat. Aikens's proposals, the writer of her obituary recalled, were "like setting off a stick of dynamite." Critics emphasized the difficulty of enforcement inherent in any grading scheme once the variously trained "nurses" or "attendants" began to look for work. Fearful of any system of grading that allowed for more than one level of *hospital*-trained nursing worker, a nursing educator argued against Aikens's view by asserting "the grading of nurses to be impractical because they cannot be kept in grades."[98]

After several reports were issued, representatives of nursing associations met with an AHA committee in 1916 and a new report was subsequently written. In the compromise, classification of different grades of hospital-trained nursing workers was replaced by a weak recognition that there were differences between those with and without hospital training.[99] Those lacking hospital training were no longer to be allowed to call themselves nurses.

Aikens's strategy, the classification and grading of the already existing nursing work force, was ideologically defeated. The professional nursing leadership made clear that its concerns were primarily upgrading and protecting trained nursing, not helping to create a system acknowledging and classifying all who nursed for hire.[100] In the context of the unregulated nursing marketplace, and the hospitals' continued demand for cheap labor, the leadership's opposition was justified. Aikens's plans, if they had been enforced either voluntarily or through legislation, might have further diluted the meaning of training.

The failure to devise a system to regulate the work force within nursing, however, was a defeat as well for the worker-nurses. It left them with no viable way to control the continued chaos in the labor market. At best, they could only hope that the educational reforms and registration efforts promulgated by the professional associations would eventually bring about change without undermining their status. Yet for the worker-nurses, fearful about not finding enough decent work, and tired of being labeled "unprofessional" or "commercial" for voicing such concerns, the professionalizing effort of the leadership offered little solace. But Fiske's position, which demanded more individual self-sacrifice, and Aikens's strategy, which required more standardization, neither spoke to their needs nor generated any real alternate solutions.

CONTESTED TERRAINS

By the early 1890s a small group of nurses, with nursing superintendents in the lead, began the difficult struggle to standardize the nursing field by professionalizing trained nursing. While trying to obtain state legitimation for their claim to professional status, the nursing associations had to try to set educational criteria by which to upgrade the meaning of training. They had to do so, however, in the face of public indifference and increasing physician and hospital administrator hostility to their efforts. As their goal became professional recognition and power, they also fought to disassociate nursing from legislation beginning to protect other women workers and to thwart the attempt to devise a system to regulate all who nursed for hire.

By focusing on educational reform and exclusive registration laws, the professional nursing associations also found it impossible to generate much support within the ranks of working nurses. The professional leadership, in order to exclude "badly trained" or "unprofessional" nurses, saw such women, and the small institutions where most of them trained, as nursing's gravest threat. The concerns of such nurses – for improved working conditions, income, and recognition for their skills – were perceived as antithetical to the professionalizing effort.

In turn, for the majority of working nurses, the goals of the state and national nursing associations seemed either hostile or irrelevant to their own pressing needs. A professionalizing strategy, emphasizing upgrading of standards for the training schools and their curricula, threatened the already shaky status and economic situation of many practicing nurses. Using nursing's commitment to the importance of character and devotion to service, many worker-nurses and traditionalists thus tried to counter the professionalizing efforts by arguing that competency in nursing should be judged by such qualitative standards. Their adherence to nursing skill measured in womanly virtue was less a conservative and reactionary stance than a belief, transcending class and educational background, in the nurse's individual character and workplace skills. Such a belief grounded altruism in supposedly natural, rather than educational, soil.

Worker-nurses often declared there was no inherent contradiction between duty to patients and concern for adequate wages and work. But the ideology of sacrifice, coupled with the isolation of their work and the continued criticism from the nursing leadership, militated against a sustained oppositional organization. Nurses might "resist professionalization" and criticize it, but could not yet feasibly organize against it. Their rejection of it left them in a political void, however. Calls for greater devotion to service or acceptance of a graded nursing work force did not solve their problems. A different way of reconciling the dilemmas within nursing had to be found.

8

Nursing efficiency as the link between service and science

Despite slight improvements in nursing education, by the early twentieth century the old barriers continued to thwart reform.[1] The leadership's educational concerns and professional goals were rejected, or ignored, by the majority of working nurses who remained unorganized and increasingly under- or unemployed. A paid and specialized hospital nursing work force could not be created when students were still perceived as the best, and cheapest, nursing personnel. Nursing could not gain professional control while the hospitals' needs still governed entry into training and the nursing education process. Educational improvements were continually fought by physicians who wanted the nurse to be merely a kindly woman and a practically trained subordinate. And the necessity to professionalize nursing education was not understood by the public as long as the difference between the trained and untrained nurse was uncertain.

When the professionalizing strategy of seeking voluntary educational improvements and mandatory registration laws barely seemed to be staving off disaster, many nursing leaders began to search for another language and set of practices that could transform nursing's nineteenth-century service ethic into more rationalized twentieth-century terms. Not unexpectedly, the Progressive Era's "mania" for efficiency seemed to them an appropriate forum within which to redefine nursing's content and meaning. Such an effort, it was hoped, would elevate the practice and status of nursing.

Efficiency in this era had both a moral and a managerial definition. It signified a hardworking, disciplined, unemotional person, willing to break with traditions to become an effective "expert." As promulgated by "scientific managers," efficiency required the systematic breakdown, analysis, and timing of the steps in a work process; the search for standards and the "best way" to perform each task; the separation of mental from manual labor; and ultimately, managerial control over the planning and execution of work.[2]

Accepting these ideas of capitalist rationality was not perceived as antithetical to nursing's historical commitment to service and duty. Efficiency was to be the link between service and science, the bridge over which nursing traveled to be accepted as a profession. The traditional emphasis on the "one right way" of doing work was to be replaced by a "scientific" search for, in the words of management engineers, the "one best way." The efficiency and order that trained nursing produced through its military, religious, and familial models of hierarchy and discipline were, therefore, to be given a new veneer more in keeping with the cultural and economic world of the new century. Nursing, as were other professions, was thus subscribing to a "morality of efficiency" to validate its claims for autonomy and power.[3]

Nurses also struggled with efficiency as a way to assimilate new meanings of science into their ideology, behavior, and practices.[4] Aware that changes in medical and hospital practice had serious ramifications for nursing, they were often divided and ambivalent about the transformations they were reacting to, and advocating. Physicians, too, found the changes demanded by medicine's new relationship to science difficult to assess. However, nursing's clinical position, its identification with caring and service, and its divided place in the health-care hierarchy, made its embrace of science quite different from that of medicine.

The pressures to come to terms with new ideas of rationality and science also came from the institutions within which nursing was embedded. By the 1910s, hospitals had grown in number, size, complexity, and importance to the structure of medical- and nursing-care delivery. A redefinition of the hospital's purpose, a reordering of its division of labor, and a rethinking of its management methods were necessary. The "once charitable enterprise" became what it had not been before: a medical and nursing institution that sold care as a commodity.[5] It was within this context that the effort was made to use the ideas and methods of efficiency and scientific management to legitimate, upgrade, and standardize nursing.

BORROWING A VOLUME FROM INDUSTRY

Surveying the rapid increase since 1873 in the number of hospitals, a Chicago surgeon entitled his lead article for the journal *Modern Hospital*'s first issue in 1913, "Hospital Growth Marks Dawn of New Era."[6] Numbers alone, however, did not reveal the changes in the hospital world. Shifts in urban demographics and living patterns, changes in philanthropic funding, municipal reform, and economic crisis all reshaped the nature and place of the hospital. The "therapeutic revolution" of the late nineteenth century was also beginning to be a part of the transformation of hospital care.[7] The acceptance of antiseptic and then aseptic techniques, the deployment of X-ray machines, and the establishment of clinical laboratories all made possible the use of the hospital for more acute medical and surgical care, although the differences between discovery and diffusion made for slow and uneven changes among institutions. However much leading physicians proclaimed the wonder and safety of their new procedures, or hospital administrators declared the comfort of their institutions, until well into the 1920s, surgery in the kitchen and births in the bedroom remained common. Nevertheless, by the second decade of the twentieth century, the hospital was becoming a multiclass institution and the linchpin in American health-care delivery.

This "new entity," as a *Modern Hospital* editor labeled it, was increasingly expensive to create and run.[8] Surgery, hospital trustees soon found out, required vast expenditures for operating rooms, equipment, and supplies. Discussion of the crisis caused by the cost of rubber gloves, oxygen, and gauze filled the pages of economy-minded hospital journals and annual reports. Despite such concerns, the trustees' beneficence and the community's social standing were frequently still measured by the gleam of the chrome on new surgical equipment and the marble flooring on an imposing hospital pavilion. Pressures to economize had to be balanced against recalculations of such conflicting measures.[9] Under these circumstances, hospitals increasingly saw their patients as sources of income rather than objects of charity, even when such changes caused great uncertainty.

This uncertainty created an "identity" crisis for hospitals as institutions. Debate raged over whether the hospital was to be seen as a charity, a hotel, a medical factory, or a workshop. Above all, it centered on whether the hospital's management had to act as if it were a business. Speeches, articles, and editorials declared the necessity for "sound business principles" in the hospital world. The business rhetoric, however, was often defensive or propagandist in tone, as if its proponents were trying to reassure themselves as much as convince others. Many hospital officials remained uncertain as to how much business policies were compatible with either the older charity impulse or the new scientific demands.

By the 1910s, a compromise language had evolved, typical of the Progressive Era, that melded the conceptions of charity, business, and science. The hospital was to be administered as if it were a *public trust*. In this way the moral duty of the institution to become a business was clothed with both the nineteenth-century understanding of charity and the twentieth-century promise of science.[10]

As a public trust, it was agreed the hospital should provide "efficient" care.[11] But it was easier to genuflect verbally before the Progressive Era's altar of efficiency than to determine what adherence to its doctrines meant in practice. As the author of a 1913 New York City study into hospital management concluded, "The investigation . . . deals with a field having no established standards . . . by which to judge the efficiency of hospital practice."[12]

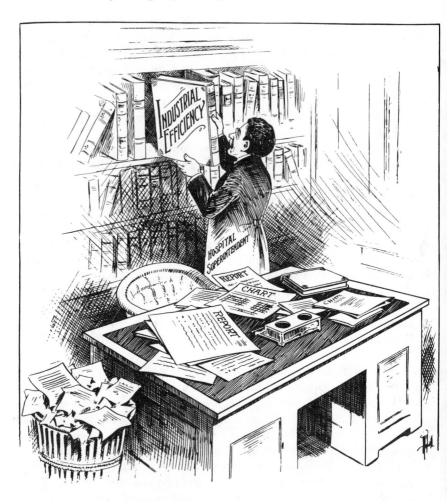

Hospital superintendents in the early 1920s were increasingly encouraged to "modernize" their institutions by "borrowing a volume from industry." *Source: Hospital Management* 10 (November 1920)

For some in the hospital, the meaning of efficiency could be taken directly from the business realm and measured in its coin.[13] Rather vaguely, efficiency and economy were linked. As a *Hospital Management* cartoon suggested, hospital administrators were counseled to "borrow the volume" of industrial efficiency from industry. A hospital administrator warned: "No superintendent who wants to keep up with the times will overlook the factory, store, or office which must apply modern methods to survive."[14]

FACTORY PRODUCTION SHEET

Motors...............253
Transmissions.....342
Chasses...............301
Finished cars......271
Shipments...........263
On hand.................24
Unfilled orders....212

HOSPITAL PRODUCTION SHEET

Discharged............?
Diagnoses..............?
Infections..............?
Consultations........?
Deaths...................?
Autopsies..............?
Causes of Death.....?

TRUSTEE   SUPERINTENDENT   DOCTOR

The hospital administrators' growing concern with efficiency and industrial models was tempered by their uncertainty over what counted as hospital production. *Source: Hospital Management* 9 (April 1920)

How to apply the lessons from industry's borrowed volume was not readily apparent. As yet another *Hospital Management* cartoonist noted, hospitals, unlike factories, did not keep accurate records of what they "produced." In the industrial realm, the criteria of profitability and growth offered some concrete measures of the value of various management schemes. But in the hospital, as one administrator noted, the "dollar yardstick" alone could not be used to measure the institution's worth.[15] Physicians, a hospital surgeon warned, were willing to see the hospitals spend "millions and billions of dollars . . . without any reference to what this expenditure will do toward real efficiency."[16]

There was disagreement not only over what the "yardstick" had to measure but also over who would apply it. In industry, efficiency or scientific management plans usually empowered a new layer of management experts. For physicians, just beginning to solidify their ideological and political power in the hospitals, the suggestion that an authority and a measure outside their professional control would be used was anathema. They were not willing to accept what one superintendent characterized as a "business system" instead of their own "faith system." Nor did many believe, as one surgeon declared, that it was possible to "standardize an art."[17] Physicians, who were just obtaining "master craftsmen" status in the hospital-workshops, were not about to allow themselves to be managed by others in a "health factory." Even these physicians who tried to institute patient outcome as the criterion for efficiency, however, found their fellow doctors unwilling to be measured.[18]

There were some attempts to apply scientific management techniques to both surgical procedures and hospital management. Frank Gilbreth, one of the leading figures in the scientific management movement and its most public spokesman, became intrigued with the idea of the application of motion study to the hospital and to surgery in particular. Interested at one time in becoming a surgeon himself, Gilbreth filmed a number of operations in hopes of studying the doctors' motions and improving on the efficiency of their techniques.[19] At meetings of both the American Medical and Hospital Associations in 1914, he elaborated on his suggestions for the application of scientific management to the hospital.[20]

Aware of physician resistance to his ideas, and even hospital management reluctance to use his measures, Gilbreth nevertheless ended his speeches with a call to restructure the hospital. He received polite applause for his speeches and found them printed in medical and hospital journals. But editorials discounted his approach. His suggestions, which would have meant the real acceptance of the hospital as a capitalist industry and physicians as workers within it, were too radical and too threatening.

These debates over scientific management were part of the larger struggles within the medical community to come to terms with the institutional and professional consequences of the new meanings and promise of science. Thus, at the same time as the growing concern with scientific management, a small group of elite surgeons within the professional American College of Surgeons recognized the necessity for a physician-controlled set of standards for the hospitals. Aware of the unchecked growth of hospitals that were more like hotels than medical facilities, and of the number of physicians who were labeling themselves "surgeons" without special training or skills, the leaders of the college sought to control surgery by setting standards for the hospitals.[21]

They knew that without improvements, the public would question both the hospitals' and surgery's commitment to science and service. "The god of science," surgeon and *Modern Hospital* editor John Hornsby admitted, "[is] walking with feet of clay."[22] To return the god to a place of honor, Hornsby and the college's surgeons declared, would take the effort of physicians and surgeons dedicating their institutions to science. With the support of the American Hospital and Catholic Hospital Associations, as well as the American Medical Association, and funding from the Carnegie Corporation, the college promulgated *minimal* hospital standards based on structural assessments. Even with such standards – the keeping of case records, the setting up of a clinical lab, prohibition against fee splitting, and requirements for a staff organization – only 89 of 678 one-hundred-bed institutions surveyed in 1919 were able to pass, and the records of the survey were destroyed. The college's standards, which were raised over time, became the measures against which hospitals were judged. While serving as the basis for improvements, these standards guaranteed physician control over the hospitals and staved off the efforts to establish management control over individual physicians' work.

Efficiency committees were established in a number of institutions for short periods of time but were usually abandoned when physicians expressed either lack of interest or hostility.[23] The applicability of scientific management and efficiency to the work of physicians would lie buried for at least another generation, while the doctors cemented their power in the hospitals.

This was not true, however, for others in the institutions. The prescient comments of a Boston physician reflected a growing consciousness. Upon hearing her hospital's efficiency committee report, she remarked that "she could not help thinking that hospital efficiency really depended more on the nurses – who were on hand all the time – than on the doctors."[24]

THE APPEAL OF EFFICIENCY

Many nursing leaders shared this physician's belief, as concern with efficiency began to be widely discussed. The very ambiguity of the terms "efficiency" and "scientific management" gave the concepts their wide appeal. While a hospital administrator might define efficiency as obtaining more work from his or her nursing student staff, a nursing leader could use the same language to demand more science in the nursing curriculum or the hiring of aides to do the hospital scut work.

Underlying this growing belief in efficiency was the effort by some nursing educators to transform the content of nursing by adding more basic science to its training and more objective study of nursing's methods and practices. Aware of deep-seated cultural, medical, and nursing assumptions that assigned "natural" male and female characteristics to the doctor and nurse, they sought a way to modify this genderization. They shared the conviction, presented by Columbia University zoology professor Henry Fairfield Osborn at the 1907 graduation of the Presbyterian Hospital School of Nursing, that "science without sentiment" failed its moral purpose.[25] Cognizant of the demands medicine was increasingly putting on nursing, nursing educators argued that skilled nursing required more than "mere deftness in precise manipulations and the scattered fragments of scientific knowledge." More scientific training in "observation and judgment" was, they declared, essential to good nursing.[26]

In linking "science and sentiment," nursing professionalizers also had to restate the traditional nursing concerns for patient care and hospital efficiency. Caring, unlike curing, was more tied to institutional arrangements. Nurses could easily state that they had always been concerned with efficiency in both patient care and hospital administration. It was precisely a concern with detail, systematizing, and proper organization that trained nursing had brought to the hospitals.[27]

Nurses were not simply reiterating the need for the old nursing commitment to getting the work done through traditional methods and blind discipline. Aware of both the financial stresses and demands for medical care being put on hospitals, they argued that only nursing, if upgraded, could clearly find the *best way* to be efficient economically and scientifically. Efficiency schemes, the leading nursing educators suggested, could be used both to improve patient care and to free nursing from drudgery.[28]

The methods of efficiency engineers appealed to nursing leaders. Moral exhortations and legislative arguments had not convinced hospital officials and physicians of the need to upgrade nursing. The more "scientific" and "objective" evidence drawn from time studies seemed a better means of proof.

The impetus behind this interest in the "tools" of the managment engineers is illustrated by a story Annie Goodrich, the distinguished nursing educator and leader, related to her biographer. One day, while in training in 1891, Goodrich was assigned an overwhelming work load. The hospital superintendent abruptly criticized her for not doing what Goodrich clearly thought was impossible. Incensed by his demands and rudeness, Goodrich considered leaving nursing. Instead, she made a time study of the work to show the superintendent "how long it really took to do what he expected." She concluded that a student would need seventeen hours to finish what she had been told to do in eleven. Taking her figures to the hospital superintendent, Goodrich reported that given the time and the demands, he was teaching his nurses either to be "deceitful" or "to do poor work." The superintendent was apparently unmoved either by her remonstrances or her research. But Goodrich, along with other nursing leaders, remained convinced that such "scientific" evidence was necessary to prove the case for change in the organization of a nursing service.[29]

This interest in scientific management was reinforced through the nursing leaders' contacts with efficiency experts. In 1912, fully two years before his appearances at the American Hospital and Medical Associations' meetings, Frank Gilbreth presented his arguments to a national nursing convention.[30] He argued sagely that "the entire hospital system must be systematized – and will be in time – but, if you desire it, why should not the *nurses* lead the way?" Always the excellent ideological salesman, Gilbreth promised that scientific management would mean greater cooperation, eliminate waste and drudgery, raise standards, and even increase happiness in the hospitals. In response to Gilbreth's paper there were no condemnatory editorials in the nursing journals as there would be two years later in a hospital management magazine.[31] Instead, Annie Goodrich proposed that a nursing committee on scientific management be established. Gilbreth and his wife, Lillian, a management expert in her own right, frequently consulted with nurses. When a nursing educator came to their Providence, Rhode Island, home for a meeting, they set up beds in their living room to demonstrate their methods. After Frank's death in 1924, Lillian Gilbreth continued to work for various nursing groups for the next thirty years.[32]

The home economics movement also provided a context in which nursing leaders could see the applicability of efficiency schemes to nursing. Through her position within the Division of Nursing Education at Teachers College, Columbia University, Adelaide Nutting became friends with Melvil Dewey and his wife, two of the leading organizers of the Lake Placid Conferences on Home Economics. These summer conferences brought together various reformers concerned with the creation of greater efficiency in the household, the applicability of scientific management techniques to housework, and the development of the new field of home economics.[33] Nutting attended regularly and gave papers on institutional management.

These advocates of household efficiency sought, in the words of one of the participants at the 1902 conference, "to bring the home into harmony with industrial conditions and scientific ideals that prevail today in the larger world outside."[34] The concern of these household reformers was the ever-disintegrating middle-class home and the void the loss of productive work had left in women's domestic lives. They argued that the scientific management of housework would transform the drudgery and mindless quality of housework into mental stimulation, freeing the housewife to improve her standards and perhaps herself. This application of "science" to the household was miraculously to bring the household out of its isolation, yet preserve it as a female domain.[35]

The promise that such techniques could end drudgery, raise standards, and still enshrine a woman in her own sphere had obvious appeal to nursing. Ellen Swallow Richards, the movement's leading figure and theoretician, recognized the parallels between nursing and her own work. She cited the introduction of trained nursing and the trained woman superintendent as examples of "the first successes in modern housekeeping."[36] It is no wonder that a nursing educator like Nutting would find a congenial home among such reformers.

It was not just women in nursing and domestic-science reform who were captivated by the promise efficiency held. The very flexibility and numerous interpretations of the efficiency schemes, the societal acclaim given to "science," and the seeming elevation of women into experts in their domains were vague, yet specific enough, to appeal to differing groups of women reformers searching for legitimation and status for women's work. No other set of principles or proposals at the time could hope to answer so many diverse needs.

The application of scientific management to women's work also appeared to bring women out from under the seemingly arbitrary and traditional paternalistic control over their lives exercised by fathers, husbands, physicians, and bosses. For many women, such possibilities were almost revolutionary. Sue Ainslie Clark and Edith Wyatt, for example, expressed this hope in their study on women's work for the New York Consumers' League in 1911. Despite some anxiety over scientific management, they concluded:

The whole tendency of Scientific Management towards truth about industry, toward justice, toward a clean personal record of work, established without fear or favor, had inspired something really new and revolutionary in the minds of both the managers and women workers when the system had been inaugurated.[37]

Similarly, many nursing leaders thought that scientific management could be used as part of such a bourgeois revolution in the hospital to free nurses from the shackles of physician and administrator control.

Nursing leaders saw concern with the improved management of the hospital nursing service and the upgrading of nursing education as compatible. Annie Goodrich readily conceded at a meeting on hospital efficiency in 1916 that it was *not* "an easy problem to work out, how the nursing staff shall be pupils in the school and at the same time do actual work in the hospitals."[38] Goodrich, along with the other nursing leaders, was only just beginning to realize that the logic of their professionalizing strategy for nursing depended, in part, on the separation of nursing education from the hospital's nursing service.[39] But because work in the hospital was still inextricably linked to nursing students, the hospital's nursing service and the training school's educational program had to be considered, and improved, together. Nursing standardization, the leaders realized, was necessarily connected to hospital standardization.[40]

FORMS OF RATIONALIZATION

The rhetoric of concern with scientific management and efficiency took several different forms. Nursing's voices were first heard in the loud debates over hospital construction. The increasing cost of urban land and building to accommodate the needs of private-pay patients necessitated an architectural revolution in hospital design. Long, self-contained wards were replaced by private rooms and "skyscraper" hospitals. New conceptions in hospital construction also developed in response to the replacement of sanitarian beliefs by germ theory, engineering advances in metal frameworks, and the shifting architectural emphasis on functional design.[41] Hospitals began to be planned around the centralization and specialization of functions. Individual wards with their own supplies, diet kitchens, and drug rooms were replaced with centralized units, pneumatic tube exchanges, and dumbwaiter services.[42]

Florence Nightingale had been an important hospital "architect" who linked the physical structure of the institutions to the nature of the nurse's work. Her name was given to the dominant ward plan in England, and her ideas influenced the building of scores of hospitals worldwide, including the Johns Hopkins Hospital in Baltimore.[43] Carrying on in this tradition, many nursing superintendents argued to nurses and administrators alike that it was nursing's "moral obligation" and "right of experience" to be intimately involved in hospital construction and alterations.[44]

Influenced by Lillian Gilbreth's studies on industrial psychology and fatigue in housework, the nursing concern focused on the wasted energy, enforced drudgery, and subsequent fatigue that poorly planned hospitals foisted on nurses.[45] Emphasizing proper "structure" rather than "ornate appearances," a nursing superintendent stated in her talk on scientific management, would make it possible to "conserve the time, health, strength and nerve force of those who are engaged in this most interesting, absorbing and splendid work."[46] Reflecting a growing belief that drudgery need not be inherent in nursing, Charlotte Aikens argued that the "ease and comfort" of nurses should not be considered "among the seven deadly sins."[47]

Hospital architects, administrators, and physicians who helped to design the new modern hospitals were much more focused on how space could be designed to economize, reorganize, and manage the nursing service. Two influential planners pointed out that more inexpensive help could be hired if centralized linen, supply, and drug rooms were built so that the nurses could spend more time at the bedside.[48] Another physician tied pedometers to a group of nurses to record their mileage, weighed their heavy wooden patient trays, and measured the distances they traveled to bring screens and bedpans to patients in large wards. But he used the subsequent evidence of overwork to argue that physicians had to play a larger role in reforming the training schools' curricula and in keeping nurses more focused on "intimate practical and humanitarian aims."[49] The study of the physical structure of the hospital's impact on the nurse's work did not always lead to agreement that the nurse's comfort, or right to determine her own work pace, was an important consideration in hospital efficiency.

As had Annie Goodrich in her student days, many nursing leaders hoped time and motion studies would provide a quantitative and qualitative measure of nursing work. Aware that no real studies or standards existed, nursing leaders in New York began to work with hospital investigators in 1913 to develop an ideal ratio of nurses to beds. Such a measure served as a rough guide for the number of necessary personnel but did not take into account the actual content of the nurse's work.[50] In 1921, Elizabeth Greener, superintendent of nurses at Mt. Sinai Hospital in New York, undertook what is regarded as the first time study of nursing.[51] This study, and similar ones in the 1920s, tried to determine the number and kind of nursing personnel needed for particular divisions in the hospitals. In a preliminary way, these studies began to document the disparity between the number of nursing procedures called for in the hospital and the number actually being performed.[52] Many were used to build a reasonable nursing *load* and to determine weaknesses in the nursing teaching and service structure.[53] Thirty years after Annie Goodrich made her own time study, the chronic overworking and understaffing of the nursing service were being measured.

This concern with task analysis and development of a proper division of the nursing load led to the development of the "functional" or "efficiency" method of nursing.[54] A series of nursing tasks was identified and then apportioned to a particular nurse or student. Under this method, a nursing educator noted:

> . . . the patient is not the unit or centre of thought. But the *work to be done* is classified into, beds to be made, baths to be given, temperatures to be taken, treatments to be given, diets to be prepared and served, medications to be given, charting to be done, dressings to be done, etc. *The thing to be done* is the unit and centre of thought and endeavor.[55]

Task analysis, nursing leaders soon realized, made sense if the procedures studied themselves were deemed "efficient" or "effective."[56] At

Teachers College in New York, nursing educator Isabel Stewart sought to have students use comparative studies to evaluate different methods of instrument sterilization, hand scrubbing, and colonic irrigation.[57] Science and scientific management for a nursing educator like Stewart were thus ways of examining a series of problems; her focus was more on method than clinical investigation.[58]

Whether it was attempting to change the construction of the hospital, measure and reapportion the nursing tasks, or study the effectiveness of nursing procedures, in the most general sense, nursing leaders were trying to move from nursing's adherence to each school's "one right way" to the scientific management concept of finding and standardizing to the "one best way." But nursing leaders were also really attempting to redefine the content of nursing and to shed the tasks that associated nursing with dirty work and lowly domestic service. Carefully hedging her argument, for example, Minnie Goodnow agreed that "probationers and young nurses" should know how to dust, clean rooms, and make beds, but they should not be required to do so incessantly. "A nurse should not be above her job," she concluded, "but there is no reason why she should spend her time in monotonous repetition of things which a servant can do as well, thereby missing *real training* in nursing."[59] Similarly, a perceptive management expert told an international gathering in 1927 that forcing nurses to scrub floors must be done for the sake of discipline since it could hardly "be justified by analysis of the professional requirements."[60]

Scientific management's tools and concepts could thus promise to end the drudgery for nurses and to recognize, on the grounds of efficiency, the need to add more science and theory to nursing education. Ironically, by using the very methods that made industrial work more mechanical, nursing hoped to free itself, in nursing leader Lavinia Dock's always appropriate words, from "martinet discipline, routinism, and institutionalism."[61] Thus, the nurse-author of a text on hospital economics assured her readers that "scientific management of tasks improves the spirit of workers."[62] The introduction of standardization techniques, time and motion studies, and more theory in nursing education was, it was hoped, to make it possible to restore dignity to nursing, rekindle its ideals, and upgrade its status.

AN UNCERTAIN PROMISE

Behind the hopes, the calls for job analysis, and the beginnings of a research program, however, were the twinges of uncertainty, the questioning of a promise too broadly made. Even those who most advocated the advantages of scientific management left themselves open to the question of whether all these new techniques were going to make nursing into something that contradicted, rather than complemented, its greatest ideals. Acutely aware of this problem, a nursing educator insisted that the use of process charts in the hospitals was "not intended to make workers mechanically minded, but to make them think and feel that they are doing their work in the most efficient way."[63] But if nurses had to be *made* to think and feel this way, what was really happening on the hospital floor?

As nursing tried to shed the limitations of its military and religious past, it became ensnared by the constraints of a businesslike future. Once again, in the search for a basis for professional reform, nursing leaders found themselves attacked for destroying the very moral fiber and spirit of nursing. Their embrace of the new efficiency modes allowed critics of professionalization to use the charge, made repeatedly by other critics of expanding capitalist orders, that the process led to the "mechanization" of the human soul.[64]

Meta Pennock, an editor of *Trained Nurse,* in a talk on nursing ethics in 1924, appropriately enough before an organization called the American Evangelical Hospital Association, thus evoked a rather romanticized portrait of the craftsmanship of the trained nursing order. The new functional methods, she argued, affected nursing the way factory work changed the work of artisans, by taking "the heart out of nursing." Such methods, she declared, left the nurse without an individual identity and sense of responsibility.[65]

Critic Annette Fiske similarly charged in the wake of postwar jingoism that these new nursing standards were merely "German efficiency . . . something heartless and brutal."[66] Such criticisms and structural constraints weakened nursing leaders' abilities to either introduce new efficiency models or to use efficiency as a unifying ideology in nursing.

Uncertainty over the basis for defining good nursing also undermined the press for more science and scientific management. In an interesting, self-critical report released in 1906, the Training School at Massachusetts General Hospital admitted its students were strong in theory but lacked knowledge of "how to make the patients comfortable." The alumnae queried reported that their training paid "too much [attention] to the case" and "too little regard . . . to the patient." A physician concurred, noting that while the "science of nursing is well taught, the real spirit is not." Such training, another MGH doctor concluded, meant the school was turning out women who learned "too much of the practice of medicine and too little of the practice of nursing."[67]

It was the continual conflict, however, between the nursing service and nursing education that undermined the somewhat naive efforts of nursing leaders to use scientific management to upgrade nursing. Stewart and others began to realize that any activity analysis of nursing functions had to be based first on more qualitative understandings of what constituted "good nursing." In 1943, looking back on the wave of enthusiasm for efficiency of which she was very much a part, Stewart roundly criticized the attempt to approach the hospital and nursing as an "industrial plant" since it left the student with "little real knowledge of any case as a whole."[68] Yet as nursing leaders clearly recognized, the similarities between a hospital and an industrial plant came down to, as a number of them phrased it, "the necessity of getting the work done."

Nor could support be garnered among most nursing superintendents. They were still administrators of nursing services first before they were educators. Success in their hospital was measured by how smoothly and economically the nursing service was run, and not by how well the students were educated in nursing theory. Such administrators often felt in more congenial and useful company in the American Hospital Association meetings than at the Society of Superintendents sessions. As a nursing leader bluntly stated, "The nursing profession, to a strikingly large extent, shares the business viewpoint of the hospital boards and executives."[69]

Hospital officials were aware, however, that the public image of training had to be improved if enough students were to be attracted to nursing. A great effort was made, as part of the vast expansion in hospital construction in the 1910s and 1920s, to improve the living quarters of students. New nurses' "homes" were built with larger bedrooms and recreation areas.[70] In the 1920s, a visiting European hospital administrator quipped, upon seeing a New York hospital's nursing students' residence, that he hoped when he died he would be reincarnated as an American nurse.[71] As a human-relations emphasis in industry became more common, hospital administrators appealed to nurses in the language of "joint efficiency" and "mutual cooperation," rather than military and charitable duties.[72] But the work load continued to become both heavier and more complex, while administrators remained reluctant to commit hospital resources to the educational program.[73]

Furthermore, hopes that more science could be added to the curriculum, or scientific methods used to evaluate procedures, were not fulfilled. As Isabel Stewart honestly lamented in 1929, "The scientific content of nursing is little more than a thin veneer covering a larger body of traditional material and practice gained largely through experience."[74]

THE REALITY OF EFFICIENCY

By the early twentieth century, the hospital was becoming a more essential part of the medical- and nursing-care system. Increases in acutely ill patients, greater complexity in surgical and medical care, and expansion in the numbers of paying patients all increased the demands placed on the hospital's nursing service. The task of caring for patients became more specialized, and a functional division of tasks had to be instituted in order to "get the work done." The demands of work often overcame the concern with quality. While an Isabel Stewart might worry about the best way to insert an intravenous needle, in most hospitals, nursing and hospital administrators were concerned with how quickly student nurses could perform the task. But once the methods and tools of the efficiency experts were introduced they could be used, not to upgrade nursing, but to subdivide and increase the work. Once again, as in the nineteenth century, the benefit from a seemingly positive structural nursing reform accrued primarily to the hospitals.

Many nursing leaders had also hoped that efficiency would be the key to the realm of the seemingly "objective" practices and expert status increasingly accorded science.[75] Efficiency looked as if it would allow nursing to redefine, and almost secularize, its ethic of order and caring. It promised to "degender" nursing by taking it out of the secondary sphere of women's labor by placing it in a more neutered and seemingly powerful arena. It was not that nurses expected to emulate medical practice, or the physicians' reliance on science per se. Rather, they saw science as a gender-free zone that could transform the content of their work and the status of their field. As zoologist Osborn had implored, they wanted to link "sentiment and science."

As long as the hospital's nursing service and the nursing school's educational program were linked, neither registration laws, nor voluntary educational standards, nor efficiency schemes could upgrade the nursing situation. However, if graduate nurses, rather than students, could become the hospital's nursing work force, while other workers took on the drudgery and "menial" tasks inherent in the work, several problems seemingly could be solved: the overproduction of students could be stemmed, employment found for the graduates, and a subsidiary role created for the untrained or quickly trained nurse. To do so, nursing still had to gain acceptance for the necessity for professionalization by raising the barriers to entry, severing nursing education from the hospital's nursing service, and differentiating the trained from the untrained nurse. Yet again nursing leaders searched for other tactics to bring about the changes they desired.

9

The limits of "collaborative relationships"

Despite all the efforts put into the professionalizing strategy, by the second and third decades of the twentieth century a growing crisis in nursing became noticeable. Licensure laws had made a difference in some states in pressing for small improvements in many schools.[1] But numbers overwhelmed these changes. Between 1910 and 1927, hospitals grew by 56.3 percent and the available beds by 102.6 percent, whereas the number of student nurses jumped 138.2 percent. Trained nurses seemed to be everywhere. In 1900, for every 100,000 people in the United States there were 173 physicians and only 16 nurses; a mere twenty years later the number of doctors had dropped by 21 percent to 137 and the number of nurses had climbed by 781 percent to 141. Ten years later, in 1930, trained nurses overwhelmed their untrained counterparts by over 40,000.[2]

Although periodic outcries about "overtraining" and a nursing scarcity were still raised, the overproduction of nurses, low standards, and a heterogeneous work force continued to characterize the field. By the early twentieth century, both overpopulation and the changing and increasingly complex demands in nursing exacerbated an already difficult situation.

In the aftermath of physicians' successful efforts at professional reform through creation of a unified profession, surveys of conditions in medical schools, and support from elite foundations, nursing leaders embarked on a similar quest. In the 1920s and 1930s, nursing entered a period of increasing self-assessment and what nursing editor and historian Mary Roberts characterized as nursing's "collaborative relationship" with physicians, hospitals, and the foundations concerned with the broad rationalization of the health-care system.[3]

As physicians had for medicine, nursing leaders sought to document the reasons for nursing's ills, to define professional nursing, and to gain from the foundations ideological and financial support for their goals. They hoped to create a unified, well-educated work force by severing nursing education from hospitals' nursing service demands. They wanted to develop collegiate programs for an elite, close the weaker hospital schools, and define poorly trained nurses out of the profession. They tried to protect the title of nurse but could not find a way to cope with, or control, the untrained or partially trained subsidiary nursing workers.

The continuing demand for nursing personnel always threatened, however, the improvements that could be achieved. Furthermore, the uneasy nature of such collaborative relations drove the nursing leadership more narrowly into elite educational reform and heightened their contempt, rather than their understanding and concern, for those already working. As the worldwide Depression of the 1930s deepened the problems in an already depressed industry, the need for a solution to nursing's long-standing difficulties took on new urgency.

WORLD WAR I AND THE NURSING "MADNESS"

By the eve of the First World War, the idea that high-quality nursing care depended on more than a nurse with practical skills, a kind heart, a well-developed sense of duty to the patient, and deference to the physician was just beginning to gain wider acceptance. When the United States entered the war on April 6, 1917, the demand for nurses in both civilian and military hospitals almost shattered that fragile understanding. Clara Noyes, director of Red Cross nursing, wrote to Adelaide Nutting two days after war was declared:

Tell Anne of Albany [Annie Goodrich] that if I were not convinced before, I should be now that the most vital thing in the life of our profession is the protection of the use of the word *nurse*. Everyone seems to have gone mad. I talk until I am hoarse, dictating letters to doctors and women who want to be Red Cross nurses in a few minutes.[4]

The military's willingness to use a supplementary voluntary aide system to meet the nursing need and the desire of thousands of patriotic women to "nurse" created the "madness" Noyes feared. Nursing leaders quickly recognized the situation as a serious threat to nursing standards.

The lines on policy were quickly drawn. On the side of increasing the supply of nurses through the use of "aids" (as they were called) stood Red Cross nursing, represented by Jane Delano, in alliance with Dr. S. S. Goldwater, the influential superintendent of New York's Mt. Sinai Hospital and chairman of the Committee on Hospitals of the General Medical Board of the Committee of National Defense. On the side of meeting the demand through the ranks of trained nurses stood an array of powerful nursing leaders on several governmental committees, led by Adelaide Nutting's Committee on Nursing of the General Medical Board.

The issues were fought out in the press, in nursing circles, and in numerous governmental meetings. They came to a head at a debate before a joint meeting of the nursing associations in May 1918. At that time, Delano and Goldwater argued that the "nursing crisis," as Goldwater labeled it, had to be met by the use of voluntary aides. The nursing aides Goldwater sought to mobilize were not working-class women but the very educated "leisure class" women whom the nursing leadership had long hoped to attract to its own ranks.[5] These women, Goldwater promised, "when the war is over, . . . will melt away into private life, strengthened and chastened by their experience, leaving the nursing field in the hands of the professional nurses."[6]

Annie Goodrich, representing the nursing leadership's position, forcefully argued that the need could be met through the establishment of an Army School of Nursing, stepped-up enrollments in civilian training schools, and a special training program for college-educated women. At the heart of her claim was the fervor of nearly half a century of the struggle to have nursing defined as skilled work needing more than womanly sympathy to achieve results. Goodrich was clearly fearful, as well, of losing from nursing the very women Goldwater hoped would fade back into private life. After the debate and discussion, the nursing associations went on record as endorsing the Army Nursing School scheme.[7]

The scheme was rejected, however, by the Army General Staff. It took the considerable political talents of Nutting and her supporters, among them the influential upper-class nursing sympathizer, Frances Payne Bolton of Ohio, to reverse this decision. In August 1918, the debate was reopened at a meeting of the General Medical Board. The eloquence and marshaled statistical evidence of the nurses, their promise of trained nurses' greater discipline and efficiency, and the divided opinions of the physicians on the board staved off the aide onslaught. The Army school was authorized. The armistice three months later, however, seemingly ended the military aspects of the aide question.[8]

Far from settled when the European fighting ended was the question of how civilian nursing care was to be provided. The flu pandemic, which began to sweep the world two months before the war's end, posed even more of a threat to nursing's position. The pandemic, which caused more deaths than the military battles, raised the question in personal and vivid terms of whether the nation had enough nurses. As mortality figures rose and the need for nurses multiplied, the Red Cross, in the face of increasing military nurses' deaths from the flu, revived the plan for military nursing aides less than a month before the end of the war; the American Hospital Association called for the training of "hospital helpers" for civilian care.[9]

During the pandemic some nurses, trained and untrained alike, took advantage of the public's fear and desperation to demand higher wages. Once again, it was charged, trained nurses were merely concerned with their own incomes and available only to the rich. "It is perhaps inevitable," Isabel Stewart wrote with some degree of resignation in 1920, "that

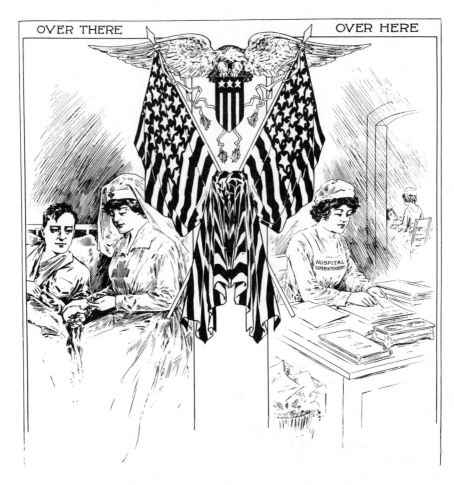

During World War I, hospital managers emphasized patriotism and nursing's importance at home and in the war. This magazine illustration portrays a nurse's many possible roles: in the Red Cross at the war front, in the hospital superintendent's office, and at the patient's bedside. The caption read: "Both are serving the nation." *Source: Hospital Management* 5 (June 1918)

the difficulty of securing nurses during the last year or two should have revived again the old agitation about the 'over-training' of nurses and the clamor for a cheap worker of the old servant-nurse type." Yet she concluded more hopefully than was warranted, "Scarcity may be a blessing . . . if it only shows up clearly the very shortsighted, unbusiness-like and ungenerous policy which most hospital officials have consistently employed toward their schools."[10]

The seeming scarcity of nurses during the war and pandemic years brought nursing more damnation than blessings, however. In a widely circulated interview on the "nursing problem" published in the popular journal *Pictorial Review* in 1921, Dr. Charles Mayo, of Minnesota's Mayo Clinic, revived a hackneyed and romanticized solution: the training of "100,000 country girls as sub-nurses." Mayo did not mean nursing aides but rather a lowering of the nursing educational requirements and length of training to reach out to the "girl" born to nurse. Mayo's scheme confirmed the worst fears of the nursing leadership that any plan to create more than one kind of nurse was, at bottom, an attempt to undermine trained nursing's standards and professionalizing efforts.[11]

Nursing leaders carefully developed, and then had published in *Pictorial Review*, two responses to Mayo's "solution."[12] It was deemed politically safer, however, to discuss the need for high standards in nursing rather than the necessity for training another kind of nursing worker. The leadership's refusal to confront the issue of another grade of nurse was made clear in the correspondence between Adelaide Nutting and Richard Olding Beard, a Minnesota medical school physician and supporter of collegiate education for nursing. Beard had been chosen by the nursing leaders to write one of the responses to Mayo. As a draft of his article circulated, Nutting tried to convince him to take out the paragraph that called for the training of nursing assistants. Well aware that there was a need for such workers, she still argued:

I do not think we can keep these women, if they are semi-trained, in the class of trained attendants. I believe we must find some mechanism or method of organization by means of which the well-trained nurse can serve all classes in the community at a price they can fairly pay.

Nutting's "instinct for social justice," as she labeled it, also made her fear the creation of a two-class nursing system based on ability to pay rather than need. Beard, while disagreeing with her on practical and strategic grounds, acquiesced and struck out the offending section.[13]

The nursing leaders continued to oppose acknowledging or accepting more than one track of "trained" nurses. Arguments over whether the trained attendant could be controlled and kept from "passing" as a nurse, or whether she would only provide "cheap" nursing for the poor, continued to dominate nursing and hospital discussions. Nurses appeared more willing to accept the *untrained* attendant, relegated to household chores in a patient's home or in the hospital, than the *trained* attendant who would be doing more "nursing" tasks. But the hospitals, when unable to attract enough nursing students, began to offer short "training" programs for "hospital helpers."

In public-health work, the health commissioners in both New York and Chicago tried to develop programs in which "competent bright women" could be quickly trained as health workers to care for chronically ill and convalescent patients. Chicago's health commissioner, Dr. John Dill Robertson, established the Chicago Training School for Home and Public Health Nursing, which offered a two-month program and claimed to have produced 4,321 "nurses" in its first year.[14] As Clara Noyes had feared, even without a war, it was exceedingly difficult to protect the use of the word "nurse."

"THE GREAT HOPE"

In the early 1920s new hope was raised that order could be brought out of the chaos. The first major national study on nursing was being prepared by social investigator Josephine Goldmark under the aegis and funding of the Rockefeller Foundation. Originally commissioned by the foundation in 1918 as a study of public-health nursing, the study quickly broadened into an examination of the entire problem of nursing education and distribution.[15] The Rockefeller Foundation was itself not directly concerned with the upgrading of nursing. Focused on improvements in medicine and public health, the foundation's officials saw nursing merely as an "ancillary service."[16] But these officials also understood that the changes they wanted to make were often hampered by poorly trained and unskilled nurses. Aware that the foundation's commitment to nursing was somewhat half-hearted, the nursing leaders still felt it was an opening wedge.

If Abraham Flexner's report on medical education was written from the perspective of the Johns Hopkins Medical School, the Goldmark Report, as the study was popularly called, was shaped by the views of nursing educators at Columbia's Teachers College.[17] The nursing leadership hoped it would be for nursing what the Flexner Report had been for medicine: the legitimation of their professional goals by an outside "objective authority" and the basis for requesting foundation funding. Ever since the publication of the Flexner Report in 1910, Adelaide Nutting had been trying to interest the Carnegie Foundation in a similar investigation of nursing. In Nutting's view, this was *the* opportunity to legitimate the nursing leadership's goal of separating nursing education from the nursing service in the hospital. Hope that the old struggles would be, in Nutting's words, a "stage of history" reflected the leadership's expectations.[18]

The report's final conclusions did indeed back up many of the leadership's complaints about the exploitation of students and supported their demand for improvements.[19] It pointed to the need for nurses with post-graduate course work in the public-health field; similar additional training for educators, supervisors, and superintendents; the maintenance of high educational standards, including more basic science courses; a properly funded training school with a graded curriculum of twenty-eight months; and the endowment of a university-based school of nursing to train the profession's future leadership. Further, in a fairly controversial section, it called for the replacement of student nurses by graduates in hospitals and the training of "hospital helpers" in the execution of routine duties of a "non-educational character."

As might be expected, the report had a very divided reception. The views of Winford Smith, a member of the report committee and superintendent of the Johns Hopkins Hospital, reflected the institutional difficulties any implementation faced. Commenting in a letter to Goldmark on a preliminary version of the report's conclusions, he rhetorically noted that the nursing system which was proposed would not "be of practical application to the average general hospital." Furthermore, it would require a training school "upon the same basis as that of the medical school." Whereas medical schools were increasing their "practical" training, he noted, nursing appeared to be heading in the opposite direction of more theoretical education. Such a curriculum he thought unwise and unnecessary.

Nursing standards had to be raised, he agreed, but not by sacrificing the hospital's needs. Smith feared advocating a nursing education system he called "far in advance of the thought of the hospital authorities." (On her copy of Smith's letter, which Goldmark presumably sent her, Nutting mockingly added "oh, oh" in the margins.)[20] But Smith's position reflected the kind of support, at best, the Goldmark Report was to get in hospital administration and physician circles. Although the report legitimated, as the nursing leaders had hoped, most of their views and goals for nursing reform, the political consensus needed for implementation was much more elusive.

The report was also criticized by many nurses, particularly by those who feared any plan that supported the training of another grade of nurse. Rather diplomatically, the report called for the "definition and licensure of a subsidiary grade of nursing service," and for a trained subsidiary nurse for patients with mild and chronic illnesses or in convalescence to work, under physicians and "possibly" under nursing direction, in "certain phases of hospital and visiting nursing." Goldmark wrote Nutting that such a conclusion was necessary. She asserted that any discussion after the report's publication had to take up the subsidiary worker issue. Warning Nutting, she wrote: "If nurses do not take the matter into their hands, those hostile to them will."[21]

Although sympathetic to nursing's fears of subsidiary workers, Goldmark had spent too much of her own career concerned with the "inefficient" use of women workers to give in on this issue. "For different grades of need," she argued, "different grades of service should be provided."[22] Aware of the danger of abuse of the subsidiary workers, she nevertheless thought in terms of efficiency and the necessity for swift, decisive action on nursing's part.

Nursing remained divided on this issue. Mary Beard, the director of the Providence Visiting Nurse Association, and other leaders in public-health nursing were willing to discuss the use of a trained attendant to give bedside care in public health *under* the direction of a better-trained nurse. The editors of the *American Journal of Nursing* even admitted that "nothing is gained by turning our back and then assuming that what we do not see does not exist."[23] But many in nursing, both in private duty and in administrative positions, opposed the acceptance of another trained nursing worker. They hoped untrained workers would become a thing of the past and feared any form of training or licensure of trained assistants. Thus, Richard Olding Beard claimed that trained subsidiary workers were not economical for either hospitals or patients. With the debate with Mayo so recent a memory, he declared: "The mere fact that a certain section of the medical profession wants, or thinks it wants, a less highly trained nurse, is not enough."[24]

The issue of subsidiary nursing workers remained unsettled. There was a slow shifting of nursing opinion toward reluctant acceptance of the necessity for training and supervising attendant nurses. But the general fear of such workers receiving some training and then "passing" as nurses, coupled with the growing unemployment and oversupply of graduate nurses, blunted nurses' willingness to deal seriously with this issue.

Legitimation of professional goals, without the funds or political power to implement them, became nursing's Pyrrhic victory. In medicine, the support of the Rockefeller and Carnegie foundations turned the recommendations of the Flexner Report into the reality of full-time instruction, new laboratories, and endowed medical schools.[25] After the publication of the Goldmark Report, the Rockefeller Foundation did support a bachelor's degree program in nursing at Yale, fund some other collegiate programs, and provide fellowships for research in nursing, mainly in public health.[26] But at Yale, nursing's supposedly showcase collegiate program, it became obvious that the foundation funding was almost penurious compared to the millions of dollars that poured into the medical school and other Yale institutes. Furthermore, it was abundantly clear that the funds were limited by both foundation and Yale University officials.[27] The creation of a few underfunded collegiate programs did little to improve conditions in the vast majority of training schools, to stem the continued overproduction of nurses, or to settle the question of training subsidiary-level workers.

Unlike the Flexner Report, the Goldmark study, while suggesting mod-

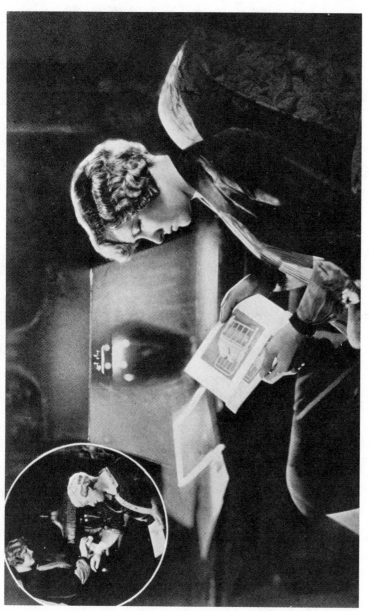

In the twentieth century, correspondence schools promised young women the "rewards of a nursing career . . . through home study." Prospective students were reassured, "The competent nurse gains many friends," and "Study and begin practice in your own home." Chicago School of Nursing, *Splendid Opportunities in Nursing* (Chicago: Chicago School of Nursing, 1935, p. 13). *Source:* Joan Brumberg Collection, Ithaca, New York els and standards for reform, did not survey and classify training schools. Goldmark's report, in contrast to Flexner's, had neither applauded the best programs nor sought to discredit the worst ones by name. It was the Flexnerian model of survey and classification that still beguiled the nursing leaders and kindled their hopes for real reform. Flexner, however, had studied only 133 medical schools; by the early 1920s, there were nearly 2,000 schools of nursing.

FAILURE OF THE GRADING SOLUTION

By 1922, preliminary responses to Goldmark's recommendations were making it clear that the report would provide neither a classification scheme for nursing schools nor a mechanism for surveying and grading them. The National League of Nursing Education's Committee on Grading, which had been waiting to assess the Goldmark Report's impact, began to mobilize the political and financial resources to undertake the herculean effort of such a survey. They moved with some urgency since the American Medical Association (AMA), increasingly chary of nursing's own upgrading efforts, was beginning to organize its own nursing curriculum committees.

The league, in conjunction with the other national nursing organizations, moved quickly to organize an "independent" joint study with foundations and representatives from all the major nursing, hospital, public-health, and medical associations. There appeared to be a consensus, except within the AMA, that the time for such a study had finally come. The AMA, after putting the grading proposal off and transferring it from various committees, was less than pleased about a joint, non-AMA-controlled project. As Isabel Stewart wrote candidly to Richard Olding Beard: "I fancy their idea of the Lion and the Lamb lying down together is for the Lamb to be *inside* – but I don't think the League is quite so submissive and lamb-like as they may think. However, we are hoping for the best."[28] The AMA finally agreed to tentative participation by William Darrach, the dean emeritus of Columbia University's College of Physicians and Surgeons, and by Winford Smith, the director of Johns Hopkins Hospital and veteran of the Goldmark Report Committee.[29]

Representatives from other major health organizations were chosen and, in 1926, the group, named the Committee on the Grading of Nursing Schools, adopted a five-year program (later extended to eight years). They raised nearly $300,000 for their expenses, mainly from the organized nursing associations and the individual contributions of nurses, with smaller amounts from the Rockefeller Foundation and nursing's benefactor, Frances Payne Bolton.[30]

The Grading Committee's objectives were nothing less than to survey comprehensively nursing's ills and to propose the necessary mechanisms for change. A study of the supply and demand for nursing services, a job analysis of nursing work, and the grading of nursing schools were all set as projects. Determined to prove quantitatively and seemingly objectively the problems nursing faced, the committee sought a director skilled in both statistical compilation and its graphic display. May Ayers Burgess, a Ph.D. statistician with experience in health surveys and a technocrat without the political and feminist orientation of Josephine Goldmark, was selected as the director of studies.[31]

The hopes for reform that the Goldmark Report had raised, but did not implement, were transferred to the Grading Committee's study.[32] Some nurses perceived the work as nursing's equivalent to the hospital-standardization efforts of the American College of Surgeons. As early as 1925, the always irascible (and somewhat misogynist) hospital administrator S. S. Goldwater warned that hospital standardization was "a program outlined and applied by practical men; whereas [the Grading Committee] is a program that will eventually be the glorified work of a group of idealistic women."[33] These "idealistic women," however, saw the Grading Committee as the "practical" culmination of the nursing reform movement: a combination of the Flexnerian and standardization approaches applied to nursing. Standards had to be set to force smaller schools to close or upgrade as a way to keep poorly trained women out of nursing. The argument had to be made boldly and statistically that overproduction of graduates was the root of nursing's difficulties and that nursing education and a hospital's nursing service had to be separated.

As in the Flexnerian and standardization efforts, nursing leaders were implicitly trying to narrow the gateway into their field. Anne Strong, the director of the School of Public Health Nursing at Simmons College in Boston, in a long private letter to Isabel Stewart, stated the need to exclude certain women from nursing.[34] Giving up on nursing's nineteenth-century promise to mold the good-hearted country woman's character and skills, she bluntly stated:

I do wish we could be honest. Immature girls with less than full high school education and the limited or poor background that goes with such lack of educational opportunity do not seem to me to fulfill any definition of a professional worker, in spite of the really noble qualities that nursing ultimately develops in a small proportion of them.

Musing about what to do about the situation, Strong suggested a division between nursing schools and separate titles for the different graduates. Those from the "inferior" schools, she suggested,

would really have only a good attendants' course, which is all they are able now to profit by and carry away and use. And the doctors would have their bedside nurses they are always crying for. And then we could concentrate upon the other schools which should train really professional workers.

There would be objections to this, she noted, because of its undemocratic nature and its "closing of the door of opportunity" to women with "inferior training." But she argued that such women were already locked out by their lack of education. "The trouble with us," she concluded, is that

we constantly cling to our stock dishonesty that in this democratic country everyone is just as good as everyone else, and probably a little better. I wonder how long we can best serve nursing by failure to admit facts.

Facts were precisely what the Grading Committee produced. An extensive statistical survey of the field was undertaken, utilizing census reports and questionnaires. Every findable nursing registry and public-health agency, subscribers to the *Journal of the American Medical Association* in ten states and every member of the AMA, a sample of these physicians' patients, a ten-state selection of nurses, hospital superintendents, and nursing superintendents were surveyed. Two different extensive grading questionnaires were sent to all nursing schools in the country.

The first finding, published in 1928 as *Nurses, Patients and Pocketbooks,* was a long, devastating book presenting the facts of the situation. The oversupply of nurses and their increasing unemployment were carefully documented. The undersupply of nurses able to provide skilled and complex care at reasonable costs was also noted. The consequences of this situation of surplus and unmet needs for nursing, physicians, hospitals, and the general public were discussed.

The committee appeared shocked by its own findings. Writing to Teachers College nursing professor Elizabeth Burgess, the committee's director, May Ayers Burgess (no relation), stated that the profession "faced . . . a bald set of facts which are rather dreadful to think about." Her dreadful facts were indeed the basis for what she called a "crisis" facing nursing.

At the present time one out of every 590 people in the United States is an active graduate nurse.

There are 2296 schools of nursing in the United States. The number seems to be increasing.

This year nearly 20,000 new graduates are entering the profession. . . .

The average professional life of the nurse is a little more than seventeen years.

Of the 20,000 new graduates this year, nearly half are women who have never finished high school. Their academic education is less than that required for stenographers, typists, or file clerks in high grade business offices or for saleswomen in the better department stores.

These undereducated young women are coming not only from the small hospitals, but from the larger ones as well.

Dissatisfaction and unrest are particularly noticeable in what might be called the non-professional nursing ranks. The expressions of this unrest are not always fortunate.

Out of every ten active graduate nurses in the United States, three belong to the American Nurses' Association, seven do not. Control of the nursing profession now rests in the hands of a small minority body.[35]

The facts, so explicitly stated, did make the problem painfully obvious. Six years later in its final report, the Grading Committee recommended the expected: reduction in the number of schools; higher entrance requirements; separation of nursing education and nursing service in hospitals; aid to hospitals to assist in the funding of nursing services; and public funding of nursing education.[36]

The facts, even more clearly stated and backed up by evidence than in the Goldmark Report, did not, of course, immediately translate into action or funds. Sympathetic reviews of *Nurses, Patients and Pocketbooks* added to the call for restricting the number of schools, raising standards, and introducing graduate nursing in hospitals. The AMA's response was predictable and rather sanctimonious in light of its own professionalizing efforts. The *Medical World* reviewer thought the book sounded "more like the yell of the nurse who does not want any more nurses graduated in order to lessen competition"; and the AMA's *Journal* decried the implication that nursing needed college-trained women in the field.[37]

As might be expected, hospital administrators, to a large extent, were unsympathetic to the reform effort. They still denied that the hospitals were profiting from student labor or that the hospitals had "kidnapped" nursing, as one nursing leader had charged. In a revealing choice of words, the president of the American Hospital Association (AHA) responded that the hospitals had instead "sired" nursing, adding, "Do you not all agree, that nursing is the one and only legitimate daughter of hospitals? The history of nursing makes plain that without hospitals there could hardly be graduate nursing as a profession." The obvious reverse truth, that without nursing there could hardly have been hospitals, was not mentioned. Finally, the president noted, referring to the old platitudes, that nursing training was good preparation for womanhood. The hospitals, by training large numbers of women, even if they never practiced, were therefore providing a valuable service.[38]

The Grading Committee was aware that gaining support for its recommendations would be difficult. Particularly cognizant of the burden the findings placed on nursing superintendents, May Ayers Burgess sympathetically noted: "It is so difficult for many people to realize that a criticism of existing conditions is not necessarily a criticism of the person who is caught in those conditions."[39] The criticisms of nursing superintendents and their schools were made very directly and seemingly personally, how-

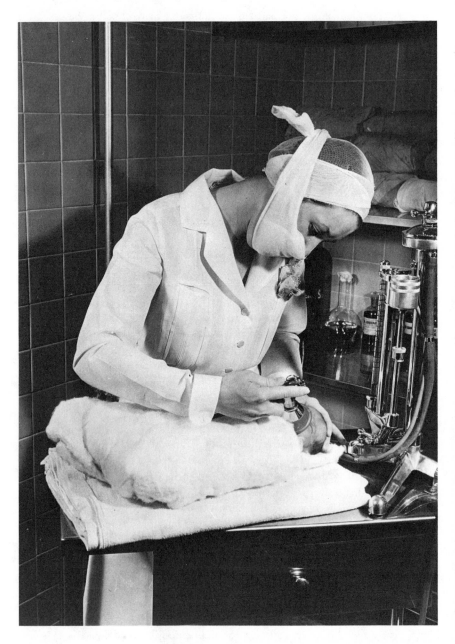

By the 1930s, nurses were working with increasingly complicated equipment. Here a nurse resuscitates a newborn with a Kreiselman machine. Boston Lying-In Hospital, delivery floor, 1939. Photographer, Hansel Mieth. *Source:* Countway Library

ever, through the committee's grading forms. The grading was based on a school's responses on a number of items on a long list compared to replies from other schools.

An outside authority rating a school in red ink did not always engender goodwill for the Grading Committee or for nursing reform. At a meeting in 1930, one Grading Committee member reported that a nursing superintendent told her, " 'When I saw that Miss Goostray [Stella Goostray, Children's Hospital nursing superintendent and consultant to the Grading Committee] did not like what we were doing, I just said "Bunk," ' and threw the book into the drawer.' " Another said they looked too good and didn't show it to her board.[40] Similarly, despite the recommendation of separating nursing education and the hospital nursing service, a 1927 Grading Committee survey of 500 superintendents found that 76 percent emphatically preferred a student nursing service.[41]

Grading Committee members reported that even when nursing and hospital superintendents were sympathetic to the findings, they had difficulty getting their boards to either read or keep an open mind on the reports. One committee member stated that her board and hospital administrator returned the report unopened "partly because they are scared by the number of graphs and the bulk of the material." More important, a physician member of the Grading Committee noted that there was little public understanding of the demand for nursing reform. He related a meeting on nursing with the education regents in New York State: "They say 'why don't you nurses do what the doctors tell you to do?' That is their conception or comprehension of the nursing situation."[42]

In some cases, nursing superintendents were able to use the grading reports and the broader findings of the committee to force changes. A typical letter from a nurse-hospital superintendent to the committee read:

Our class work has increased, the educational requirements have advanced; the entrance age of students has been advancing, and since 1929 we have engaged graduate floor duty nurses, head nurses in charge of the floors. We have also engaged a general floor supervisor.[43]

Nearly 81 percent of the nursing schools responded to a second grading in 1932, and, in 75 percent of the items on the questionnaires, the records of the schools were better than in 1929. But both the number of students and the average number in each school had still *increased* in the intervening years. Improvements on such a low base were clearly just a beginning.[44]

The most serious problem with the Grading Committee's work was its failure to prepare either a public "white list" of the best programs or a "black list" of the worst schools. The question of classification and publication of lists was debated throughout the history of the committee. At a meeting in November 1931, the decision was made not to publicize the grading results or to devise a publicly available grading scheme. The decision was justified on a number of grounds: the difficulty of obtaining up-to-date, fair data on the over 2,000 schools without personal visits; the arbitrary nature of such classification programs; the lack of clear consensus on what constituted good standards; general committee doubts as to whether they were the appropriate body to establish accreditation standards; and whether they could withstand the criticism such a process would entail.[45]

In the end the Grading Committee was swayed, not by the physicians or hospital administrators, but by the conservative arguments of its educator members, Henry Suzzallo, president of the Carnegie Foundation for the Advancement of Teaching, and Samuel P. Capen, the chancellor of the University of Buffalo. These men argued that the injustice to borderline schools and the danger that classification would freeze schools at certain levels were too grave to warrant anything more than a public educational campaign. Only Elizabeth Burgess, the NLNE representative, dissented from this crucial vote; Edward Fitzgerald, dean of the graduate school at Marquette University, abstained.[46]

The committee also had to decide if it was going to promulgate standards at all. In an informal letter to Adelaide Nutting, May Ayers Burgess stated the committee's dilemma: either set very minimal standards to obtain cooperation from the American Hospital Association, the American Medical Association, and the American College of Surgeons, or set up standards that would almost certainly generate their "active opposition." Aware that Nutting would oppose low standards as the price for cooperation, Burgess pledged herself to fight for higher standards. But an angry Nutting penciled in her comments that she did not fear "active opposition" since nursing had "never had cooperation" when it came to improvements.[47]

Committee members, however, were not that forthright or brave. Standards were set, but at a relatively moderate level. Committee members clearly worried that any minimal standard would prevent, rather than encourage, improvements. As the registration laws had shown, a standard in name only would have been worse, they thought, than the committee's inaction. May Ayers Burgess even speculated that if the standards advocated in the Goldmark Report had been used as a guide in 1926, "not five percent of the nursing schools could be on an accredited list."[48]

The nurses on the committee clearly had other solutions in mind. By 1932 the Grading Committee was placing its hopes in the power of the economic pressures of the Depression and their own publicity to force the weaker schools to close. Nor could the NLNE, given the Depression and the outlays to support the work of the grading committee, pay for a major accreditation effort even if it had wanted to.

Furthermore, it was becoming obvious that the nursing leadership was already informally thinking about forming an association of "a group of schools of sufficiently high standards" to do some of the grading themselves. By 1932, the Association of Collegiate Schools of Nursing was established. It went on to set standards and accrediting procedures for university-based schools of nursing, abandoning until nearly ten years later the effort to have the NLNE accredit all schools of nursing.[49]

The entire thrust of the committee's work could be summarized in the title of one of May Ayers Burgess's speeches, "Why Not Improved Training for Fewer Nurses?"[50] Although the committee did not develop a mechanism for grading, its ideological impact should not be underestimated. It provided, for those willing to use it, concrete evidence of overproduction and exploitation. As a joint, heavily funded project, it legitimated nursing's push for reform. In no small way, it prepared the way for the acceptance of graduate staff nursing in the hospital. It also focused much of the political effort on establishing collegiate programs for an elite.

The Grading Committee project also made explicit the class concern underlying reform efforts. May Ayers Burgess consistently made this quite clear. When she spoke about "overproduction," she coupled it to the problem of "dissatisfaction . . . a widespread, irretrievable breakdown in professional morale." But for this she often blamed *who* the women were in nursing as much as the system that oppressed them. She frequently equated intelligence with educational attainment and class, proclaiming:

The one essential in curing the ills of any profession is intelligence; and the worst thing which can happen to a profession is to have the intelligent mothers and fathers of the community decide that the profession is undesirable for their daughters.[51]

The working-class orgins of most nursing students, in Burgess's view, was a deterrent to professional achievement. These women, she noted in another speech, were not "high-grade material" but rather high school dropouts who "stayed out late at night and were slightly incorrigible." It was their concerned parents, urged on by high school principals, she contended, that suggested these women needed the "good stern discipline of the training school."[52]

Fearful that such women would find other solutions to the nursing situation, Burgess candidly declared:

These undereducated, unprepared women make trouble within the profession. Many of them are drawn from a social group which is not strictly professional in character. They are the ones who are talking trade unionism for nurses. It is natural that they should. Their fathers, brothers, and sweethearts are ardent members of trade unions. . . .

They are less and less inclined to accept leadership from other nurses whose academic and social backgrounds are better, and they are increasingly inclined to stand apart and work bitterly for what seems to them the only possible economic solutions for their difficulties.

Her conclusion bears emphasizing, for it baldly stated the reform effort's intentions to exclude:

Somehow these undereducated women, in inadequate social and academic background, must be kept out of the profession. Fortunately there is no longer any need for them. . . . Therefore, our first problem . . . How can women be kept out of nursing who manifestly have not the proper background to enter . . . ?[53]

The Grading Committee reports pointed toward the need for systematic change in nursing. In its aftermath, the nursing leadership faced two possible strategic choices that were not necessarily mutually exclusive. One was to continue to place the efforts at reform at the point of production of *nursing students* by pressuring hospitals to close down their schools and replace student labor with that of graduates. The other option was to reorganize at the point of production of *nursing care* by trying to reshape the distribution of nursing in the community and to assert control over all those who nursed for hire. In either case, the necessity to act swiftly and decisively was clear. Adelaide Nutting, tiring from so many years of endless discussion of the same problems, was gravely worried that the committee had spent so much money to come up with so little in terms of a powerful mechanism for change.[54] Similarly, in 1932 Janet Geister, the American Nurses' Association's executive director, forcefully stated:

It is my firm conviction that unless organized nursing takes hold of the treatment of its problems with the same interest and vigor it used in obtaining a diagnosis, much of the value of the diagnosis will be lost.[55]

Although failing to act decisively, the nursing leadership did act. They tried to keep the women Burgess had labeled of "inadequate social and academic background" out of the nursing schools. They refused to find solutions to the problems of the majority of the women already in the profession, other than to pressure them into becoming hospital staff nurses.

THE ABANDONMENT OF PRIVATE DUTY

In choosing to concentrate on encouraging collegiate nursing, voluntarily upgraded educational standards in hospital schools, and graduate service in hospitals, the nursing leadership consciously abandoned the nurses already working primarily in private duty. As the Goldmark and Grading Committee reports had documented, the crisis in nursing was one of both oversupply and underdemand. This was particularly true for the profession's majority still locked into private-duty work.[56] In the home market, private-duty nurses competed, increasingly unsuccessfully, with the cheaper services of the untrained nurse and the charitable services of the public-health nurse. And as more well-to-do patients began to use the hospitals, private-duty nurses began to find more of their employment, when they could, as "specials" for these patients in hospitals' private rooms and pavilions.[57]

Private duty, always an expensive service, was thus increasingly utilized by a smaller percentage of the population. By the late 1920s, nearly ten times as many families sought medical care as they did private-duty nursing care. Income, rather than medical or nursing needs, determined the demand: The 9 percent of the population with incomes over $5,000 a year received more than half the private-duty nursing services.[58] "The graduate nurse is in a continuous dilemma," medical economist C. Rufus Rorem told a nursing convention in 1933. "She cannot find employment as a private duty nurse in the home because more and more patients are going to hospitals. She cannot find employment as a staff nurse in the hospitals because the hospital patients are attended by undergraduate nurses."[59]

As the Depression deepened, the crisis of the early 1920s became a catastrophe. One reliable source reported that 60 percent of all nurses were unemployed by 1932–33. A New Jersey study found nurses working an average of fifty-seven days in 1932 and the market for private duty as "negligible." A nursing registry in Boston reported: "In 1931, members asked for work. By 1932 we received several requests for aid."[60] By the early 1930s, the ANA's own small relief fund was becoming overburdened by demand. Reports circulated of nurses applying for federal and state relief programs and having to be given shoes and clothes before they could begin work. At the ANA's biennial convention in 1932, executive director Janet Geister poignantly reminded delegates of the special problem of the "blight of unemployment" for nurses.

The outstanding evil is not the threat of loss of food and shelter but the destruction of morale that results from the slow, cumulative perception of not being needed. . . . In nursing its destructiveness is proportional to the intensity and universality of the original urge to be of use. But the many nurses who . . . "want work, not charity," are suffering quietly in a way perhaps we will never know.[61]

Various local "share-the-work" schemes were tried: lowered wage scales in the nursing registries to allow every nurse on the registry to make a minimal income; reduced hours for "specials" to provide extra shifts; charitable donations from work relief committees. Many nurses abandoned the field or found work in a variety of federal programs.[62]

Along with its economic emergency, nursing was facing a concomitant political and social crisis. The discontent and anger within nursing, as May Ayers Burgess feared, threatened to become more vocal. Private-duty nurses, left without jobs and belittled by those in leadership, grew increasingly bitter over their unemployment and more defensive about their lack of education and skills. Over half the private-duty nurses queried by the Grading Committee reported they would leave private duty if they could, except for older and less educated women for whom there was no place to go. "Have not been able to save enough money to do otherwise," another New York nurse wrote, "and am untrained for any other kind of work and now am too old to train."[63] As Burgess had so bluntly stated, the profession no longer needed such women. But at the same time, they were the majority in nursing and something had to be done to address their needs and quiet their discontent.

Janet Geister attempted to implement a series of plans that would have encouraged the reorganization of private duty from individual to group practice, both inside and outside the hospital.[64] Her vision entailed transforming the registry into something akin to a nursing group practice, and linking its work to that of a community's public-health nursing service. Aware of the need to introduce graduate nursing in the hospitals, she nevertheless felt something "drastic" had to be done for "those who are already in the field and will be there for years to come."[65]

But Geister's tactics and strategy brought her into conflict with the AMA's president and board, as well as with leading public-health nurses concerned with the encroachment of private duty into their arena. When Geister was forced by the board to resign in 1933, private-duty nurses lost their main leadership supporter. Curriculum planning, rather than reorganization of the registries, became the focus of the task forces and committees Geister left behind.[66] Apparently under Geister's urging, medical reformer Michael Davis wrote a politely worded, but stinging, criticism of the nursing leadership in 1939 for its failure to act on its awareness that nursing needs and services had to be matched.[67]

Geister's programmatic suggestions, even if they had been carried out, might not have helped private-duty nurses either find new modes of work in the community or stave off the forces that led to the growth of graduate staff nursing. Attempts by other groups of workers to form the kind of cooperatives she proposed did not often last in the face of the power of industrial capital. Similarly, the more powerful reformers with views compatible with hers on the Committee on the Costs of Medical Care lost out to the entrenched forces of the AMA when they advocated group practices and prepaid health plans.[68] Nor perhaps could the financing have been found at that time to pay for such ambulatory care, except in a few foundation-supported settings or small communities.[69] Nor, finally, is it certain that her strategy would have appealed to the majority of private-duty nurses who had become unwilling to provide home-based care. But in the absence of reorganization of the private-duty field, the vast unemployment of graduate nurses provided a pool of women increasingly and desperately in need of work.

As the Grading Committee's final report in 1934 succinctly saw the problem, there were still "too many yet too few trained nurses": too many who were "ill-prepared" and too few who were "broadly-experienced, professionally-minded."[70] The overproduction of nurses with very different skills had gone beyond the crisis stage.

The nursing leadership, with one eye focused on the physician's increasing power and professional autonomy, and the other on its own ill-trained and subordinate ranks, hoped that documentation of the issues and legitimation of its demands for educational improvements would become the basis for support of reform. The leaders continued to try to tighten the ring of protection around nursing and to plan, at best, for the needs of the very few. Unable, and often unwilling, to make bold moves, they made recommendations and waited as change swirled around them.[71] Caught between efforts to continue caring, and to create autonomy, nursing became stalled. Collaboration, as Nutting had so clearly noted, did not lead to real improvements.

The Depression did more than rob nurses of work, and often of hope. As Janet Geister had foreseen in 1926, the era of nursing equivalent to the solitary cobbler, at a bench, making a whole shoe or filling a contract for a customer, was coming to an end. Economic, social, scientific, and political forces were pressuring the hospitals and the nursing system. And without a viable alternative, by the mid-1930s, the old system of staffing hospitals primarily with nursing students began to crack.

10

Great transformation, small change

As the Depression deepened, the hospital seemingly beckoned both the patient and the nurse to step through its doors. Patients who could no longer afford the private care of physicians and nurses sought their charitable services in the hospitals.[1] The graduate nurse, desperate for work, reluctantly turned to the hospital for assistance and salvation. During the Depression years, nursing's "great transformation" from private duty to hospital staffing took place.

This change was neither inevitable nor easy. Often under protest, private-duty nurses gave up trying to work individually as patients' employees and began to staff hospitals' nursing services. Nurses were finally forced to accept the necessity for a greater division of labor in the hospital nursing work force. Hospitals, in turn, had to be convinced that graduate nurses, along with other subsidiary nursing workers, were a cheaper and more dependable, disciplined, and skilled work force than students.

The culmination of the nursing educational reform efforts, the technical changes in medical and nursing care, the economic pressures on the hospitals, and the severe financial straits of the nurses combined to make the change possible. This transformation in work site and role brought nurses new sources of authority and responsibility, but the old problem of how to obtain and keep the right to care remained unresolved.[2]

THE HOSPITAL IN TRANSITION

By the time of the stock market crash in 1929, hospitals had become big businesses in the American economy. By 1930, the building boom of the 1920s had left the nation with 6,719 hospitals with a capacity of 955,869 beds. This represented an increase in little over a decade of more than 25 percent in the number of institutions, and 56 percent in the number of beds. During the 1930s and 1940s, the number of patients every year in each hospital bed rose from sixteen to twenty-seven.[3] Hospitals were both more numerous and larger. In 1928 hospitals represented a $3 billion investment in plants and equipment, exceeded only by capital outlays in the iron and steel, textile, and food and kindred-products industries.[4]

By the 1920s and 1930s, changes in medical therapeutics and practice also were making hospital care more complex and specialized. Diabetic patients, for example, who traditionally had been treated by dietary changes alone, came to the hospital, by the end of the 1920s, to have their insulin intake standardized. The importance of blood typing for transfusions was known by 1910, but it was not until 1917 that a method for anticoagulation was developed to make transfusions possible and safe on a wide scale. Hospital clinical labs were established in three-quarters of all American hospitals by 1938. Thus, by the 1930s diagnostic techniques were becoming more complicated and required increasingly trained and educated personnel to use and interpret them.[5]

Specialization in medicine both caused these changes and grew because of them. Between 1917 and 1940, sixteen different approved medical specialty boards were incorporated, fourteen of them during the 1930s. Three-quarters of all American physicians in 1928 described themselves as being in general practice; by 1942 the percentage had dropped to just below half. Medical specialization brought about a demand for a similar division in hospital-based medical care as specialty clinics proliferated.[6] In his 1940 overview of changes in medicine, physician Iago Galdston observed that the patient with indigestion and pain might have in the past seen a doctor in the office for a few visits. "Today," he wrote,

such an individual may not have his condition diagnosed until he has had a gastro-intestinal x-ray series, a chemical analysis of his gastric secretions, and possibly one or more tests of his liver functions. . . . Should the diagnosis be, as it well might, duodenal ulcer, the treatment is likely to involve the hospitalization of the patient for a period ranging from one to three months. In addition, the patient may be subjected to numerous other tests to establish, among other things, his progress toward recovery.[7]

Such changes placed greater demands on the hospital's nursing service. The increased technical medical procedures physicians were "too busy" to perform were *added* to the nurse's other, more traditionally defined, tasks of bathing, monitoring, teaching, and comforting the patient.

The nursing care for a diabetic patient, for example, had become quite complicated by 1930. The nurse was expected to prepare the tray for a daily blood sample; not serve breakfast until the sample was taken; verify the amount of insulin given before each meal; coordinate with the diet kitchen to see that the food was served exactly ten to fifteen minutes after the insulin was injected; secure a twenty-four-hour specimen of all voided urine; and teach the patient how to give the insulin hypodermics and to estimate, weigh, and prepare his or her own diet. In the case of Galdston's hypothetical ulcer patient, a nursing text counseled that "a large part of the nurse's duties are combating depression and controlling diet."[8]

The increasing complexity of the care meant the added necessity for someone to coordinate the procedures. As a nursing educator pointed out:

> The intricate system of requisition and forms required by the modern hospital, the inventory of elaborate equipment, the responsibility for the upkeep and safekeeping of such equipment, the more exact and detailed keeping of clinical records and reports on patients, all have created many new duties for the nurse. These duties, too, have reduced the total number of hours per day the nurse may devote to the actual nursing care of the sick.[9]

The nurse by the 1930s was doing much more than monitoring fever or assisting at a delivery: She was becoming responsible for making sure that the complex system of hospital care actually was delivered. More and more, the nurse's job became that of a hospital supervisor. She had to guide and oversee patients and other hospital workers through the daily maze of activities, procedures, tests, and tasks. All of this became exceedingly difficult to accomplish with any degree of success. As students or graduate nurses rushed to complete these increasingly complex tasks, patients in search of individualized or consistent bedside care frequently had to hire their own "specials."

The increase and specialization of the hospital's medical and nursing services also caused an acute financial crisis. Hospital administrators and trustees, particularly in the voluntary institutions, worried as pay patients' occupancy rates fluctuated wildly. Hospital closings became common.[10] As in the earlier depressions, the question of costs, or more to the point, how to lower them and increase hospital income, was an overriding concern.

During the Depression, hospitals launched a two-pronged program of recovery by encouraging occupancy and regularizing their income source. Between 1932 and 1934, the American Hospital Association had a committee on public education that sought to "teach" the public the value of their hospitals. Hospitals were urged to hire public-relations consultants, to make speeches in their communities, to issue bulletins, give tours, etc. National Hospital Day, begun by the editor of *Hospital Management* in 1921, was touted as an excellent time to acquaint the community with the hospital through a well-managed public-relations campaign. Hospitals also sought to educate the public about regulations on admitting procedures, visiting hours, and bill paying to standardize the patient's relationship with the institution.[11]

A major effort was made to stabilize the hospital's source of income from patients. One administrator noted that cash in advance was a good principle on which to base administration but that it was difficult to achieve in practice. The public, he bemoaned, still perceived the hospital as a neighborhood "Ma and Pa" store where credit was available, rather than a cash-only supermarket. "A good Piggly Wiggly clinic or a great A&P hospital," he suggested, "are not quite possible at this time in the full sense of the idea."[12] Rather, third-party payments, in particular the Blue Cross plans, become the solution to the hospital's income dilemma. As one hospital official wrote later, "Blue Cross was sired by the depression and mothered by the hospitals out of desperate economic necessity." With amazing speed, Blue Cross was endorsed by the American Hospital Association and promoted throughout the country. By 1937 there were one million members and thirty-nine plans; by 1947 another twenty-six million people had joined.[13]

The problem of money, indeed the very survival of their institutions, made it possible and necessary for hospital administrators and trustees to discuss financial concerns and businesslike management much less apologetically than ever before. "Medical service is an expensive commodity," the *Modern Hospital* editorialized in 1931. "There is nothing unethical or inhumane in exercising business acumen and judgment in the administration of the hospital." It was argued, by denouncing the old evils of charity, that asking patients for payments kept them from "pauperizing themselves."[14] Costs had to be reconsidered as well. In 1938, a hospital administrator reflected that the "old days" of not worrying about costs because of the availability of charitable gifts had gone. "More recently, as the sources of such gifts have begun to disappear or dry up," he concluded, "hospitals have been compelled to turn their attention to internal problems of management."[15] As Frank Gilbreth had predicted in 1914, the hospital would attend to its management only when the fiscal "incentive" was present.[16]

TINKERING WITH CHANGE

The Depression and new technical needs inevitably forced hospitals to reexamine their nursing service. The pattern of having a student or attendant staff, a few graduate nurses as supervisors, and private-duty specials for those who could afford them came under increasing scrutiny. The old system was no longer working, but several different attempts were made at first to shore it up.

The private-duty special had always caused hospitals economic and disciplinary problems. A special worked *in* the hospital, but she was not *of* the hospital; she retained her position as an employee of the patient, not the hospital. She presented her bill for her services separately to the patient or had it itemized on the hospital charges. As medical economist C. Rufus Rorem pointed out, "The employment of a special nurse may often interfere with the payment of a hospital bill, and it is well known that "special nursing" fees often interfere with the payments of reasonable fees for the services of physicians." In an "average case," cited by Rorem, a family was billed sixty-seven dollars for hospital care and seventy-four dollars for the nursing. Private nursing, as well as private physicians, stood as "economically competing products," as Rorem labeled them, with hospital care.[17]

The special nurse was also a control problem since she was subject neither to the discipline of a wage worker nor to that of a student. Hospitals posted rules for special nurses and tried to keep the more "troublesome" ones off their registry lists, but the special was what the term implied – in a special position in the hospital hierarchy. Above all, she owed her loyalty to the patient, not the institution, and her nursing methods to her training school, not the hospital in which she worked.

Criticism of the special was common. A Florida nursing superintendent bemoaned the lack of loyalty and devotion on the part of specials and their unwillingness to work as hard as the students. The special nurse, she added, "is much given to telling the pupil nurses how things should be done. She indulges in much . . . criticism and shows lamentable lack of wisdom and dignity."[18] Boston City Hospital's nursing superintendent reported in 1928 that she had suspended two special nurses for listening to a radio in a doctor's room instead of caring for the patients and for being "insolent" when reprimanded. A year later, she eliminated screens around the private patients because special nurses used them, she charged, "to escape being detected sleeping."[19]

Nursing superintendents were particularly worried that specials would undermine their pupils' "ideals," teach them different methods, or disparage the hospitals. In one of the Grading Committee's surveys, a majority of the six hundred nursing superintendents queried had, or wanted, separate dining rooms for specials to keep them apart from the students during nonworking hours.[20] Other superintendents complained that specials brought in their own equipment or pilfered the hospital's, stored supplies in their patients' rooms, took linens home and returned them to the hospital's laundry when soiled, or raided the diet kitchens with impunity.[21]

To combat the problems, a number of hospitals began to experiment with a nursing system called "group nursing," halfway between special and graduate staff nursing. Hospital patients were "grouped" together in a special unit and cared for by a specific number of nurses. The system was not unlike what had been called "divisional specialing" during the nursing shortage of World War I where several patients shared a private nurse. In some ways it was a nursing subcontracting system under which the hospital paid the nurse's wages, but charged the patients directly for this service over and above their hospital bill. Group nursing differed from staff nursing in that the nurses could not be moved to other units, the hospital could charge extra for it, and the patients had to be grouped in specially designed rooms.[22]

Group nursing had several advantages for both the nurses and hospitals over the private-duty system. It made possible shorter hours because three nurses could do eight-hour shifts for two patients, instead of four nurses on twelve-hour shifts. The hospital could also make a surplus over expenses for housing and feeding the nurses by charging the patient. One group nursing advocate reported that after seven years the system "stabilized the nursing service and made for order and regularity in the hospital."[23] It was slightly cheaper for the patient than paying for a special, and it offered the private-duty nurse shorter hours, steady employment, and responsibility for the total care of several patients. Although the system made the nurse a member of the hospital's staff, her time was explicitly allocated only to a set number of patients, and her efforts were still paid for directly by the patient, not the hospital.[24]

In sum, it offered the nurse the autonomy and care giving of private duty, without its isolation and uncertainty. Commenting on a number of these plans in 1930, Janet Geister wrote with great hope: "Many nurses are prophesying that soon group nursing will be available at most hospitals of any size in the country. From all accounts it combines efficiency and service. What more can the twentieth century ask?"[25]

The answer to Geister's rhetorical query was *more* efficiency and service. Notable experiments in group nursing took place in several major hospitals. But it never became a widespread or viable system. By the early 1940s it was clear that nurses had offered this plan, but it had "not been accepted in the majority of hospitals."[26]

Several economic and political difficulties for patients, nurses, and hospitals cut short the use of group nursing. Although group nursing saved the patient money on specials, those who could afford a group nurse often had the means to pay for their own nurse. Those who needed the attention of a special nurse, but could not afford one, rarely could pay for a group nurse either.

Many in the nursing leadership saw group nursing as a stopgap measure that allowed hospitals to avoid their "responsibility" for the overproduction of nurses. Shirley Titus, the dean of Vanderbilt University's School of Nursing, was group nursing's most vocal critic. She reminded nurses that the system was invented in World War I at a time of nursing shortages and actually decreased, rather than increased, the number of graduate nurses employed by the hospitals.[27] By taking the pressure off the inadequate nursing care provided by students, group nursing allowed a hospital to continue its nursing school and to contribute to the surplus of nurses. Group nursing, she charged, "has delayed the complete breakdown in the old system of nursing the hospital sick with student nurses."[28]

Group nursing presented a number of disadvantages to the hospitals as well. It demanded an architectural arrangement most hospitals did not have since it required what now would be called semiprivate accommodations. Although this form of room usage became more prevalent during the Depression, most hospitals still had either private rooms or wards.[29] The group nursing scheme put pressure on the hospitals to keep such beds filled or to prolong patient stays. Hospitals could not shift nurses out of the unit to other locations to relieve student labor or fill in for missing graduates. The system solved none of the real staffing and control problems the institutions faced. As Titus had argued, group nursing did not improve general staff nursing in the hospital as a whole.

Whether as specials or as group nurses, graduates had increasing difficulty obtaining enough employment to survive. To relieve the suffering, a number of state nursing associations and alumnae groups began to organize to pressure hospitals to limit the hours of the shifts for graduate nurses as a way to share the work. The hope was that with eight-hour shifts, a patient needing twenty-four-hour care would hire three nurses instead of just one for the entire period, or only two on twelve-hour rotations.

This kind of change, however, was difficult to achieve. In 1932, two-thirds of all student nurses still worked more than an eight-hour day (or night), and private-duty nurses were excluded from even the minimal legislation that governed student labor. Less than twelve-hour duty was almost unheard of, and nearly 12 percent of the private-duty nurses surveyed by the Grading Committee in the late 1920s were working twenty-four-hour shifts.[30] Many nurses continued to believe that even a twelve-hour schedule was symptomatic of nursing's declining "service to the patient," or that limitations in hours would mean insufficient work.[31]

With the promulgation of the National Recovery Act (NRA) codes in 1933 covering employment conditions, the possibility that the eight-hour day might be imposed by outside forces arose. The American Hospital Association's executive secretary worked with what the association proudly called "record breaking speed" to exempt hospitals from the "blanket codes" covering hours and working conditions. His skills must have included more than just speed since the NRA office subsequently issued a statement of support to the association, declaring: "The banner of humanity flying over your hospital means more to our people than all of the blue eagles [signs of compliance with the NRA codes] you could hang in your windows."[32]

The question of the limitation of hours again placed the nursing leadership in a contradictory position. At the ANA it was feared that if an NRA code was applied to the hospitals, nurses might be exempted because they were "professional employees" and thus would be forced to do more of the work. At the same time, they did not want nurses to be classified as industrial workers subject to such codes. In a widely distributed leaflet, "The NRA and Nursing," the American Nurses' Association stated: "An attempt should be made to approach reasonable working conditions by encouraging, where possible in the interest of the patient as well as the nurse, an eight-hour day." But, they asserted, "an arbitrary limitation of hours controlled by law violates the whole spirit of nursing." Although the nursing organizations stood for "reasonable hours, adequate income and opportunity for growth," the *American Journal of Nursing* editorialized, "They do not stand for the application of trade union methods to professional service."[33]

On the state and local levels, nurses were much less willing to simply hope for better hours, and much less fearful of taking what appeared to be "trade unionist" actions. As early as 1929, District V of the California State Nurses' Association had begun organizing for an eight-hour day for both private-duty and general staff nurses. In Massachusetts, a group of Boston's Beth Israel Hospital graduate nurses, in conjunction with several nursing alumnae associations, began similar agitation in 1933. After long negotiations with the Boston Medical Superintendents' Club, the eight-hour plan was introduced in some of the major Boston hospitals in May 1934.[34]

Others in nursing had different hopes for hours limitations. At Massachusetts General Hospital in Boston, nursing superintendent Sally Johnson argued that the eight-hour day would "reduce parents' objections to nursing as a vocation for their daughters." With reasonable hours, she stated, repeating an old refrain, nursing schools would be able to attract "a larger number of young women who possess integrity of character, an acceptable social background, the attributes of a desirable personality, and a higher level of education."[35]

By the end of 1933, however, eight-hour days were in effect in only 2.3 percent of the nation's hospitals. Under the pressure of several state associations, in April 1934 the American Nurses' Association finally passed a resolution going on record "as approving an eight-hour day as the required working day of nurses."[36] The eight-hour day continued to make slow progress. By October 1937 it was mandatory or optional in less than a fifth of the country's hospitals. Fifty-hour weeks continued to be common until after World War II.[37]

Thus the movement to restrict nursing hours did very little to change the hospital nursing service system, or provide more work. The efforts to tinker with the nursing service through group nursing or hours restrictions, rather than to transform it, proved of little help to the hospitals, nurses, or patients. But the task of changing the service to one staffed by graduates and other subsidiary nursing workers was formidable.

THE RELUCTANT STAFF NURSE

The statistics suggest that the change to graduate staffing was a rapid fait accompli. Nearly 60 percent of all the hospital beds in the country in the late 1920s were in hospitals with nursing schools; of these, 73 percent had *no* graduate staff nurses and only 15 percent had four or more. "Attendants" predominated in the staff positions in the hospitals without schools. Between 1929 and 1940, however, the number of nursing schools dropped by 574. While the remaining schools often became larger, there was an explosive expansion in the number of graduates working in staff positions. The estimated figures suggest that the numbers rose from only 4,000 in 1929 to 28,000 in 1937 to over 100,000 by 1941. By 1941, there were more staff nurses than private-duty nurses and students combined.[38]

The statistics, however, do not reveal how difficult it was to make this transition. Many hospital officials regarded the idea that they pay for a nursing service as "unreasonable" and saw student service as an "inalienable right."[39] Similarly, many graduate nurses, though willing to serve as specials in the hospital, hated staff nursing. They associated hospital work with the discipline, regimentation, and exploitation of their student days. The kind of patient care that private duty and even group nursing allowed, with responsibility for the total care of individual patients, was often not possible to give in staff nursing. The organization of work and frequent understaffing required nurses to be task, rather than patient, oriented.[40]

With the dearth of employment in private duty, however, and the failure of such reforms as Geister's plans for a revival in home-based graduate nursing, group nursing, and hours restrictions, the graduate nurse had few choices if she wanted to stay in her field. Desperate for work, graduate nurses had to knock on the hospital's door and offer to accept very minimal wages or even just room and board. Many nurses thus found the relatively steady employment and their new skills and responsibilities a welcome change.[41]

Graduate staff nursing, or general floor duty as it was also labeled, still had to be "sold" to the hospitals. Blue Cross financing and reimbursements for what the hospitals labeled "reasonable costs" helped to solve some of the expense dilemmas. Hospitals could bury the cost of nursing in the hospital bill and pass it on to the insurer for reimbursement.[42] Furthermore, the ideological ground had already been prepared by the Goldmark and Grading Committee reports. A New York hospital superintendent admitted at a nursing gathering in 1934 that

a hospital superintendent is no longer considered a traitor to his brothers, when he admits that there is actually something to the long standing contention by your leaders that nursing merits a "New Deal" and that fundamental changes in the attitude of the hospital toward nursing and nursing education are necessary.[43]

Similarly, nursing leaders reminded hospitals of their "moral obligations" to their patients to provide both older nurses and more skilled nursing care.[44] Graduate nurses, they argued, did not have to leave patients to attend classes and could provide more continuous care, while freeing students to improve both their clinical and theoretical training. The Depression was clearly the crucial time to force the changes that had been advocated by nursing leaders for a generation. "This is the moment," the venerable seventy-four-year-old M. Adelaide Nutting urged in 1932, "– we shall never have a better."[45]

The nursing organizations still moved very slowly to take advantage of conditions. At Nutting's urging, the board of the National League of Nursing Education (NLNE) proposed that a letter be sent out from all three national nursing organizations to hospital officials, urging the employment of graduate nurses. Six months later, after many conferences to make the letter acceptable, it was finally mailed out, with accompanying suitable publicity, to over 6,000 hospital trustees and nursing and hospital superintendents.

An extremely cautious document after so many months of drafting, the letter offered assurances that both hospitals and nursing would benefit from better selection of students, introduction of tuition fees in the schools, and the employment of subsidiary workers and maids to do the routine work and graduate nurses to provide the skilled care. It even promised that graduate nurses were "available at relatively low salaries." The only hint of hostility in the letter was a concluding sentence that chided hospitals, reminding them that the nursing employment crisis was not simply due to the Depression but resulted from "the weakness of a system of accepting students primarily as workers in the hospital."[46] This rather polite request for aid in the face of an overwhelming crisis was reported on a back page of the *American Journal of Nursing* under the headline "Suggestions for Trustees," while *Modern Hospital* labeled it "an appeal."[47] This was hardly a bold move to confront a serious problem.

The stated purpose of the letter was to garner the hospitals' suggestions on how to improve nursing's condition. The *American Journal of Nursing*'s editors promised that replies would be divided by the ANA's staff into eight different categories.[48] Rather pathetically, the nursing organizations received only 115 answers to their written appeal for help. Ever hopeful, even the usually astute Janet Geister saw the meager replies as "favorable indications of interest and cooperation." But Adelaide Nutting, although she believed the letter was an "admirable . . . first step," angrily retorted:

Replies under 5% – number of replies the clearest possible evidence of the attitude toward nursing of these hospital officials – no attention need be paid to letter – why not the courtesy of a reply to so courteous an appeal – .[49]

The letter did suggest a major element of the graduate nurse's value to the hospital: She was supposedly no longer an expensive commodity. For nearly twenty years a number of comparative cost studies had been devised to try to prove to skeptical hospital officials that graduate nursing was cheaper than student labor, especially if the nursing school was brought up to decent standards. But the cost studies were very idiosyncratic and ideologically motivated. They proved only that the "cheapness" of the graduate service depended on how many students each graduate nurse replaced and how high the nursing care standards were in the hospital.[50]

Assessing the results of a small cost study it did in 1932, the Grading Committee found what the hospitals had been arguing all along: Of the hospitals in their survey, 82 percent concluded they could not afford to give up their nursing schools, even with the depression of graduate wages. It appeared that the use of graduates and maids might prove a saving primarily in small hospitals with fewer than fifty beds, or in hospitals that replaced 10 students with only 3.5 graduates.[51] More realistically, a study that defined a high level of nursing care concluded:

When student and general duty graduates are on duty in the same hospital there is little difference in the amount of work they do, the number of patients for which they care, or the amount of skill and responsibility involved. The student nurse works a slightly shorter week but does almost the same things. . . . Students get very little if any more supervision than the graduate floor duty nurses though they carry as heavy a nursing load.[52]

Hospitals that did not have such a high standard for nursing care found they could pressure the desperate graduate nurses to do more work than the students. There were still no recognized standards that determined a reasonable "nursing load."

Aware of this danger, in 1933 the NLNE issued "A Study on the Use of Graduate Nurses for Bedside Nursing in the Hospital" and then a joint study with the American Hospital Association in 1936 entitled "Manual of Essentials of a Good Hospital Service." In 1937, at the urging of the nursing associations, the American College of Surgeons agreed to begin to formulate plans for the first surveys of hospital nursing services under its hospital-standardization program. But such efforts could provide guidelines, not the ongoing pressure on individual institutions necessary to enforce improvements in actual nursing conditions.[53] As an NLNE study of the nursing service in fifty New York City hospitals concluded, "When the pressure of work becomes too great, quality of nursing is inevitably sacrificed."[54]

As graduate staff nursing became more common, nursing leaders continued to argue that the graduate nurse would bring greater skills to the hospital because she was older and more experienced, and greater loyalty because of her professionalism. However, this promise was exactly what the leaders themselves were bemoaning: Because of their training and education, graduate nurses had neither the skills nor the loyalty the hospitals demanded. More candidly, the editors of the *American Journal of Nursing* agreed that the difficulty with graduate service was what one superintendent called nurses' "almost worshipful" adherence to their own schools' methods and their failure to develop an "inclusive professional loyalty."[55] Citing this editorial, the Boston City Hospital Nursing School alumnae newsletter headlined an article on graduate service "Narrow Loyalties Threaten Success of Graduate Staff." Alumnae were warned: "If you get a job as a general staff nurse, remember to be loyal first to your profession. Graduate service is on trial in many hospitals."[56]

The trial ended in compromise: Many of the smaller hospitals did close their schools, but many others kept theirs open and instituted a mixture of graduates, subsidiary workers, and students in their nursing services. Boston's Long Island Hospital, for example, as a small chronic-care institution, had increasing difficulty attracting enough students who met the very minimal state-mandated educational requirements for entrance to training. In October 1936 their nursing school closed and their nursing service was staffed by graduates, attendants, and students brought over on affiliation from the training school at Boston City Hospital. The New England Hospital for Women and Children faced a similar crisis in the mid-1930s as it found it hard to staff its wards and fulfill curriculum requirements through affiliations. But the hospital continued its school while increasing the number of graduate nurses on its staff. Boston City, under attack by nursing educators for its low standards, tried both to upgrade its school and to increase its graduate service. Massachusetts General, after commissioning an accounting study that proved it could ill afford to lose its school, still cut the school's budget and increased its graduate service in the hospital.[57] Thus, although the system of student labor in the hospital did not die out, the graduate staff nurse by the end of the 1930s was becoming a familiar figure in the nation's hospitals.

EMPLOYMENT AND CONTROL AT A COST

The promise of cheapness, hard work, and loyalty had to be exacted from a work force at first thankful for work but quickly unwilling to be compliant, or to fulfill someone else's promises. More than shelter and overwork had to be exchanged if graduate nurses were to give hospitals the service and loyalty they demanded. Whenever the scarcity of jobs eased in particular communities, nursing registries reported increasing difficulty in getting nurses to take hospital staff positions. As a Detroit nurse reported in 1940, "There were unemployed private duty nurses and there were positions on staffs in hospitals that were going begging."[58]

Nurses, when they took staff positions, responded to the difficult conditions in the classic ways of all workers: Hospitals began to report increasing absenteeism and high turnover. At New England Hospital for Women and Children, for example, between 1938 and 1940, graduate nurses were slightly less likely to be ill than students, but twice as likely to be absent. They also quit to take positions in the larger hospitals where the pay was better. High turnover rates in staff positions were reported all across the country.[59]

Graduate nurses expected better working conditions and more control over patient care than did students. But this was precisely what the hospitals were unable, or unwilling, to give. Nursing leaders charged that area-wide wage agreements between hospitals, and hospital officials' pressure on community chests, kept nursing wages artificially low. Hospitals continued to expect their staff nurses to work split shifts and long hours, to move from ward to ward when needed, and to live and take their meals within hospital walls.[60] Nurses also reported dismissals, on short notice, when cheaper workers became available.[61]

The hospital nursing system that made it difficult for nurses to provide decent patient care and to be recognized for their efforts was continually attacked. Although economics underlay the problems, it was the social relations that most affected nurses. A 1936 survey of private-duty nurses concluded it was the "heavy patient load" that deterred them from taking staff positions. Forced to "neglect patients," nurses lamented their inability to give what they labeled "artistic nursing care" to their patients. Salary was of less importance to these nurses than their sense that hospitals neither recognized their service nor allowed them to care in appropriate ways.[62]

The status of many of the hospitals' nurses may have shifted from student to graduate, but hospitals' methods of control and their willingness to grant more autonomy did not change accordingly. More farsighted administrators warned that real labor trouble faced hospitals unless they instituted more cash salaries, adequate meals, pensions, job analysis, and promotion ladders to encourage greater loyalty. But very few hospitals made any real efforts to upgrade their personnel policies.[63]

Because hospitals held an oligopsonist position in the nursing labor market, they did not have to raise wages. Low pay, long hours, split shifts, authoritarian supervision, and rigid rules continued to plague hospital nursing. By 1946, for example, staff nurses were averaging 87 cents an hour and one in four received less than 75 cents. In contrast, a typist could earn 97 cents, or a bookkeeper $1.11, for much less arduous work.[64]

The major thrust of improvement efforts for nurses, as it had been for students, was in housing, but often as a way to keep absenteeism down. The New England Hospital nursing board, for example, noted that nurses living outside the hospital were absent more than eight times as many days as those who lived in the nurse's home. They perceived better housing as one of their most pressing needs. Massachusetts General Hospital in the late 1930s cut educational funds for its training school, while improving graduate and student housing.[65]

Aware of the very few attempts to change conditions, nursing organizations began to call for improvements in hours, shift schedules, staff education, and pensions.[66] But the nursing leadership appeared unable, or unwilling, to distinguish between staff nursing problems and educational reforms. In 1938, the ANA Board of Directors refused to create a separate section for graduate staff nurses apart from the section for graduate nurses involved in education. It was argued that they "should not be considered as separate groups, but should be regarded as being included with other nurses engaged in institutional work and concerned with education, as well as service programs, in such institutions."[67]

Two years later, under considerable pressure from local and state nursing groups, the ANA board finally agreed to give staff nurses their own section. As educators, the nursing leadership seemed to be thinking in terms of the need for continual character training, rather than organizing nurses to secure control over their work. Character and loyalty still defined the proper nurse.[68]

Hospitals continued to search for a cheaper way to staff their nursing services and still make sure all the technical and bureaucratic tasks were performed. In turn, the nursing leadership continued to argue that nursing students should not be forced to provide hospital nursing services, unless it was part of their supervised clinical training, and that graduates, as "professional" nurses, should not have to perform the hospital's dirtiest tasks.[69] The obvious solution, for both the hospital's management needs and nursing's professional quest, was to increase the number of lower-paid subsidiary nursing and housekeeping personnel. When several New Deal programs helped to make such workers available by providing some training, their presence in the hospitals seemed assured.[70]

Nursing was finally forced by circumstances to take a position on the critical question of how to control and use another level of nursing personnel: the issue it had struggled over since the 1890s. Many graduate nurses continued to protest against any acceptance of such workers, still fearful they would take away their jobs both inside and outside the hospitals. After much protest and debate, in 1936 the joint boards of the national nursing associations finally approved licensure for such workers a year after New York State passed the first mandatory licensure law for all nursing personnel.[71]

The acceptance by nurses of another kind of recognized and trained nursing worker was based on the demand that they be kept in lowly positions, while graduate nurses were guaranteed supervisory roles. Hospitals were reminded that such workers were to be seen as "employees, not students." Hospitals tacitly agreed in principle to pay such workers less than graduates and to assign them to nursing-generated lists of "non-nursing functions." An administrator promised that aides in a training program in a California hospital were told repeatedly "that they are not and will not be nurses."[72]

On a busy and chronically understaffed hospital floor, however, the bargains about roles were constantly being renegotiated among nurses, lower-level workers, and administrators. By 1939, the director of the American College of Surgeons' Hospital Standardization Program reported to the ANA that they "had been obliged" to lower the ratings of a number of hospitals because they were employing so many subsidiary workers who did much more than the housekeeping and bed-making functions.[73]

Nor were such workers content to carry bedpans. "They do much prefer to do nursing service rather than household duties," a California nurse complained.[74] One hospital administrator admitted behavioral training was becoming essential.

The fact that they are not and cannot become nurses is a handicap to their morale and enthusiasm. That must be overcome by teachers with sufficient vision and personality to inspire these students to make the most of their limited opportunities.[75]

Even more candidly, a report on an aide program in Cleveland noted disapprovingly that the workers, "eager, docile and pliable during training," soon began to resent their limited place and the "class distinctions in the hospital." Such a worker, the report concluded, had to be taught to limit her aspirations and to "be satisfied to continue to try to perfect herself in the skills her assignments permit, rather than to forge ahead to new accomplishments."[76] The old constraints in training were now being bequeathed to another kind of nurse.

The fiction of distinctions was maintained and became a weapon in the internecine hospital wars between nurses and aides. But the divisions were often crossed when there was understaffing, necessity, or a nurse willing to teach. Nurse's aide Lillian Roberts recalled the kindness of a nurse she worked under in the nursery at Chicago's Lying-In Hospital in the late 1940s.

So we got along very well. And I was able to relate to her asking her every day I wanted to learn something new. And so I would ask her about all kinds of deformities that we would see in the nursery: the color of a baby, and why this was happening and why the other thing was happening. And then I explored with her my own analysis of things. Sometimes I'd be right just in observing and putting some common sense into it. Before long, when the interns would come to examine the babies I could tell them what was wrong with every baby. I'd have them lined up for them. And they got so that they depended upon me, because I really got to know.

The administration recognized Roberts's skill and scheduled her in charge of the nursery whenever the nurse was off, but kept paying her an aide's salary. She always had to acknowledge the authority of both physicians and other nursing students who came into her terrain. Roberts reported:

I would very diplomatically have to direct them, although they resented the hell that I was both black and a nurse's aide. But I had to do it in such a way that they didn't feel that I was claiming to know more than they did. And I realized that.

Roberts and other aides were allowed to do the work but were constantly reminded that they were not nurses. Aides were almost never allowed to sit in on "shift reports," even though hearing about patient progress and planning would have helped them give better care. There was also no mechanism for them to upgrade their skills on the job or to become real nurses.[77] The ring of protection drawn around nursing, and the hospital's need for a divided and cheap work force, kept Roberts and other aides from such advancement. Nursing's "success" in its quest for greater control was built on the limiting and degrading of others.

BEDSIDE OR BARGAINING

By the late 1930s, and increasingly during the Second World War and immediate postwar years, nursing was moving farther away from the patient's bedside. Nurses had patient contact as they changed dressings, performed complex procedures, or prepared patients for the operating room. As care became more complicated, nurses did gain new technical skills and some bureaucratic authority.

Although many graduate nurses continued to make beds, feed patients, give backrubs, check supplies, and take vital signs, such tasks could be, and were, given over to others. As supervisor, the nurse spent more time coordinating patient activities, handing out medications, writing nursing notes, performing clerical duties, and organizing the work of an increasingly complex staff. The nurse became tied to the nurses' station, whereas patients became disembodied voices on an intercom system or a cup of pills on a medication chart.[78] When a patient buzzed for assistance, it was likely that an aide would appear at the door. The nurse may have gained more responsibility than she had in private duty, but in the hospital's structure and reward system, her authority was not commensurate with her responsibilities.[79]

Under these conditions, the nursing oversupply of the 1920s and 1930s became a widely heralded nursing shortage in the war and postwar years.[80] The war effort and better-paying war-industry jobs took thousands of nurses. Others married in the immediate postwar years and joined the forced exodus of white women to hearth and home. Declining enrollments in the training schools left hospitals bemoaning their short staffing. Even the formation of a Cadet Nurse Corps, in which the Public Health Service underwrote the education of nursing students in exchange for agreements to perform essential military or civilian nursing, did not meet the reported need.[81]

Hospitals increasingly turned to yet another new category of nursing worker, labeled the licensed practical or vocational nurse, as well as to nursing aides, both paid and volunteer. In 1942 the National Nursing Council for War Service, which coordinated nursing activities during the war, in conjunction with the Public Health Service and the American Red Cross, began to initiate more training programs for practical nurses and to approve the training of aides.[82] A *Hospital Management* poll in August 1945 reported that 85 percent of the administrators queried wanted practical nurses in their institutions, particularly when graduate nurses were not available. Although uncertain about the care they would provide, and the antipathy they would engender on the part of graduate nurses, administrators agreed that such a worker had a place if she were willing to take a "subservient position."[83]

As these changes swirled around them, private-duty nurses, as an embittered minority, felt themselves under constant attack for doing "luxury" or "nonprofessional" work and for not contributing enough to relieve war shortages.[84] Reports from the private-duty nursing section of the ANA emphasized nurses' increasing sense of their own marginality and estrangement from the nursing organizations. A 1943 summary of over one hundred letters to the ANA from private-duty nurses in thirty-one states underscored their distrust of the apparent power of the national organizations and the National Nursing Council: "In the opinion of these writers the ANA had done nothing to help them." By 1946, they requested that the ANA make a statement about the "essentiality" of their service, as they were reported to be "apprenhensive about the future" and particularly the role of "auxiliary" workers.[85] As Janet Geister had feared, private duty remained nursing's most chaotic, increasingly politically volatile, and conservative sector.

The disquiet in nursing went far beyond the private-duty ranks. The National Nursing Council was criticized by state nursing associations for its approval of practical nursing training.[86] Declining membership in the ANA reflected increasing estrangement of nurses from the professional associations. In the hospitals, the rapid turnover in staff nursing positions became endemic. When individual efforts to improve control over work on the hospital floor proved limited, inevitably, the solution May Ayers Burgess had feared – the need for unionization and collective bargaining among nurses – crept into the hospital.

There had been some unionization of nurses in hospitals since the early 1900s. But during the 1930s, such efforts spread while the open discussion of the possibility of unionization increased even more.[87] Unions like the American Federation of Government Employees, the Building Service Employees International Union, and the American Federation of State County and Municipal Employees, as well as more independent unions, gained contracts for nurses in selected hospitals. Although wages and hours often did improve under these contracts, the problems of governance and control over work continued.

Wary of these developments, the ANA's leadership created a committee on "Unions for Nurses" in January of 1937.[88] By June of that year, the ANA board voted against nurse membership in unions and urged nurses to use their professional associations "to improve every phase of their working and professional lives."[89] Clearly stating the ANA's position, its president declared: "We have spent many years in an effort to have our work designated a profession. Can it continue to be a profession if we join the labor unions?"[90]

Caught in the historical vise of pursuing professional goals without demanding real changes in social, economic, and gender relations, the ANA's leadership sought "collaboration." Gone by the end of the 1930s was the implicit, if not frequently explicit, antagonism to hospitals and doctors that characterized the political beliefs of nursing's first generation of leaders. A 1938 meeting of the ANA Advisory Council made clear this viewpoint. Reporting on her state association's struggles to counter the organizing efforts by unions in Seattle, the state representative from Washington explained:

We have felt our greatest strength was in our close working with the medical groups. . . . I think when we tie ourselves up definitely to these professional groups, that is the best defense we have against anything of that kind.[91]

At the same meeting Emma Nichols, the chair of the ANA's "union" committee, gave a rendition of labor history and contemporary labor struggles that emphasized the seemingly dangerous power thrust of modern unions. While expressing sympathy for the need of workers (and presumably nurses) to improve their conditions, Nichols condemned union tactics. Nichols's comments also revealed an incredible naïveté toward hospital–nursing relations. She criticized unions for their "back-door" approach to organizing. Instead, she declared:

How much better it would be if that organizer would go in the front door, approach the official who is in charge of the institution, and present the Union's plan for such an organization and let the man who is in charge of that institution present it to the members, if it is going to help in any way the professional and economic standing of that institution.[92]

With this kind of understanding and antagonism toward organizing, it is not surprising that the ANA did not consider that its members might serve as professional bargaining representatives, and it held off authorizing such a role for its state units. In 1938, although it expanded its earlier stand on the necessity for nurses to work for improvements through their associations, bargaining was not mentioned as one of the recommendations. Joint committees with the American Hospital and Catholic Hospital Associations were established instead.[93] A pamphlet entitled *The ANA and You*, first distributed in 1937 to explain the advantages of professional association membership, was reprinted. And in January 1940, the ANA Committee to Study the Question of Unions was rechristened the "Committee to Promote ANA Membership."[94]

While the ANA equivocated, graduate nurses began to join unions. The state associations could no longer wait for the national leaders to understand the situation. In California, under the leadership of Shirley Titus, the state nursing association agreed in 1943 to become a bargaining agent for nurses when more voluntary efforts to gain raises in salaries for staff nurses failed. By 1946, the ANA, while disassociating itself from "labor unionism," formally sanctioned the concept of collective bargaining by professional associations.

Slowly and reluctantly, the nurse as the hospital's employee, and the economic and social ramifications of that status, were being recognized.[95] Nearly a century of reform and institutional change led nurses – students, trained, partially trained, and untrained alike – into the hospitals. Continuing conflict between different nursing personnel was inevitable but the ideological and structural basis for unity was now possible.

Even when graduate nurses became increasingly ensconced within the hospitals' walls, and the real beginnings were made to separate nursing education from the nursing service, many of the profession's old dilemmas resurfaced in new forms. As nurses were forced further away from care giving, orders to provide "TLC" (tender, loving care) actually had to be *written* on patients' charts. Shortages and high turnover rates continued to plague hospitals. Division and resentment over aides and practical nurses persisted.[96] But new skills and the collective institutional strength of nurses augured change. The basis for demanding the right to care, rather than accepting it as a duty, was being created.[97]

Conclusion
Beyond the obligation to care

Nursing's long "apprenticeship to duty," to recall M. Adelaide Nutting's memorable phrase, continually thwarted the profession's advance, yet made transformation possible. Obligation to patients and work created a normative tradition that gave nursing a moral and practical basis for its authority.[1] Such a tradition provided individual nurses with the opportunity to express their desire to care and to empower others. But as long as the basis for caring remained a duty, it constrained nursing's efforts to control its own practice and occupational future.[2]

Nursing, as labor, began as women's work for families, friends, and community. As a form of caring, it was often taught by mother to daughter as part of female apprenticeship, or learned by a domestic servant as an additional task. Embedded in the seemingly natural or ordained character of women, it became an important manifestation of women's expression of love of others, and thus integral to the female sense of self.[3]

In the late eighteenth and early nineteenth centuries, the expanding economy of the Eastern coast cities made possible the conditions that allowed for the redefinition of bourgeois female virtue. Caring could be manifested by such women in ways other than nursing as mothering and other activities took on new emotional weight. Nursing as labor could thus be separated from nursing as the manifestation of familial love. With this kind of division, nursing could become a trade "professed" in the marketplace yet learned within the confines of the family. The permeable boundaries for women between unpaid and paid labor allowed nursing to pass back and forth when necessary. For many older middling- and working-class women, nursing beckoned as respectable community work.

Hospital nursing, however, had a very different cultural meaning. The assumed loathsomeness of the tasks, dissolution of the patients, and disorder of the institutions allegedly made caring impossible. The mainly working-class women who took up this labor continually tried to define their own sense of caring, even if it meant everything from sharing their liquor supply with male patients to managing a delivery on their own. In doing so, they confronted differing assumptions about the duties and obligations of those who offered care. Drawing on their own sense of the rights of working-class women, they pressed for a degree of control over their labor and seized a circumscribed form of power. But the nature of their onerous work, the paternalism of the institutions, and the lack of a defined ideology of caring undermined their efforts. Mere resistance to those above them, or contending assertions of rights, could not become the basis for nursing authority.

Beginning in the 1870s, the Nightingale-based reforms for nursing training were to have changed all that. Nursing was to have gained a theoretical justification from its duty to care and a political base from its female hierarchy. Modeled on the power women had developed through their antebellum reform activities, nursing relied on the language of duty to provide its basis for authority. Female character, built on the obligation to care, was to be exalted and honed in the creation of the new nurse. Autonomy became the required sacrifice on an altar of altruism in the hopes of greater reward.

The ethic of altruism, so rooted in the cultural soil of womanly duty, did not, in the case of nursing, create the rationale to give nursing rights over its own future. Paeans to altruism alone, whether based on spirituality, individual character, or educational preparation, could not become the basis for an ideological claim for control over the organization of nursing. As necessity and desire were pulling more young women into the labor force, and woman's-movement activists were placing women's rights at the center of cultural discussion, nursing's call to duty served as an attempt to use an increasingly antiquated language to shore up a changing economic and cultural landscape. Nursing became a type of collective female grasping for an older form of security and power in the face of rapid change.

The demands and ideology of duty continually constrained nursing reform and advancement. Duty at the bedside was translated by physicians and hospital authorities as duty in the broader political arena as well. Nursing was always struggling to gain the power to define itself or control entry into practice. Under these conditions, division became inevitable as nurses with conflicting class positions and sensibilities clashed over the appropriate definition of nursing, a coherent strategy for change, and the meaning of womanhood.

The particular female hierarchy within nursing further restricted the nurses' collective power. For many women, sisterhood and "homosocial networks" served to overcome the limits of the separate spheres of Victorian life. Sisterhood, at least in its fictive forms, underlay much of the female power that grew out of women's culture in the nineteenth century. But nursing, from its very beginnings, created a female hierarchy in which sisterhood was difficult to achieve when different class-based assumptions about behavior and work collided. Commonalities of the gendered experience could not become the basis for unity as long as hierarchical filial relations, not equal sisterhood, underlay nurses' lives.

Some nurses were able to create the very special safety and comfort of a women's culture. But nursing had neither the financial nor the cultural power to create the separate women's institutions that provided so much of the basis for women's reform and rights efforts.[4] Under these conditions, nurses found it very difficult to make the collective transition out of a woman's culture of obligation into an activist assault on the structure and beliefs that oppressed them. Nursing remained bounded by its ideology and its material conditions.

Nurses, as I have argued, were not merely silent in the face of these difficulties. Within the limits of their circumstances and understandings, many pressed in different ways for increasing autonomy and power. Ironically, the demand for autonomy based on the duty to care could not provide them with the ideological formulation needed. Such a demand appeared as an inherent contradiction and the essence of abandonment of obligation. Thus efforts by those in leadership to gain greater freedom and power for nursing through efficiency techniques, increased division of labor, and educational reform merely escalated conflict. Although such efforts brought about changes very slowly, and freed some nurses from hospital and physician paternalism, they also rebound much of the nursing work force in new strands of control. The language and strategies of change that had seemed to work so successfully for predominately male groups had differing consequences for this female work force. The social and ideological experience of gender and class continually thwarted nursing's efforts to lay claim to social power in this way.[5]

Some nurses did attempt to create a new vocabulary and tactics for change. Worker-nurses like "Candor" could sever caring from "self-immolation" because their class background and work experience gave them a differing basis for understanding the meaning and labor of nursing. Such women could create a viable nursing equivalent to the "shop floor" culture of other working-class groups that gave them some control over their daily work lives.[6] But the power of the ethic of duty, and the continual criticism by the nursing leadership, physicians, and much of the public, limited the overall effect of such workers' control. Isolated until the late 1930s in separate workplaces, organizing and the collective vocalization of an alternative understanding of nursing were difficult to achieve.

Nursing's history thus suggests a way to rethink the consequences and conditions of caring in women's lives. The effort to understand the meaning of caring runs deeply through Western philosophy, psychological and sociological theory, and women's studies scholarship. Philosophical debates have centered on the role of the emotions versus reason in moral judgment and the relative priority of altruism and autonomy. Psychologists and psychoanalysts have argued over the meaning of caring for the creation of gender identity. Sociologists have examined the effect of caring on patients and care givers. And women's studies scholars have explored caring as both the basis for women's strength and our oppression.[7]

Much of this literature runs the risk of universalizing caring as an element in female identity, or a human quality, separate from the cultural and structural circumstances that create it. But as policy analyst Hilary Graham argued, caring is not merely an identity, it is also work. Although Graham's analysis moved us beyond seeing caring as a psychological trait, her work focused primarily on women's unpaid labor in the home. She did not fully discuss how the forms of caring are shaped by the contexts in which they are practiced. Caring is not just a subjective and material experience, it is also a historically created one. Particular circumstances, ideologies, and power relations thus create the conditions under which caring can occur, the forms it will take, and the consequences it will have for those who do it.[8]

Nursing history demonstrates that the basis for caring also shapes its effects. As Carol Gilligan has attempted to argue in her study of moral reasoning, the "ethic of care" can grow out of very different and changing motivations. These differences have consequences for the actions people are willing to take and the meaning they give to these actions.[9] Whether one agrees that Gilligan has proved that gender affects one's moral "voice," her study underlines the importance of understanding the ethical frameworks that individuals, or by analogy, occupational groups, bring to the work of caring.[10]

Trained nursing began as an occupation based on the duty to care. Neither ethical dilemmas nor questions of role were anticipated because it was assumed that duty would make such conflicts impossible. The nurse as an individual, and nursing as an occupational group, were to conform to a given set of rules. Judgments as to the appropriate behavior and stance of nursing were to be based on the acceptance of orders. Thus nursing did not need a code of ethics, physician John Shaw Billings told nursing leaders at the turn of the century, because a good nurse should merely be told to be a good woman.[11]

The duty to care, however, was never that simple, even in the 1870s. Duties could not be made either "comprehensive or consistent."[12] There was continual conflict among physicians, nurses, and other providers over appropriate care, and thus the role of the nurse. Caring always requires individual flexibility and judgment. But their unbending adherence to rules earned nurses opprobrium.

Armed with this sense of their obligation to the work of caring, nurses did try to determine how they would satisfy this duty.[13] Whether at the bedside or at a legislative hearing on practice laws, however, the duty to care became translated into the demand that nurses merely follow doctors' orders. The acknowledgment of responsibilities so deeply ingrained in nursing and American womanhood, as nursing school dean Claire Fagin has noted, continually drowned out the nurse's assertion of the right to free herself from such constraints in order to fulfill her duties.[14] The tradition of obligation made it very difficult for nurses to speak about rights at all, or to articulate a vision of caring that acknowledged the need for the right to determine duty.

In order to obtain this right, nursing first had to assert its prior right to be "recognized as having a claim on rights."[15] Given the obligation to care and their position as a womanly occupation, nursing was kept from being given the moral standing with which to make this claim. Nursing's educational philosophy, ideological underpinnings, and structural position made it difficult to create the circumstances from which to gain such recognition. It was not so much a lack of vision that thwarted nursing as it was, and often continues to be, the power to give that vision substantive form.[16]

In the last forty years, the conditions necessary to achieve this power have begun to be created, although many of nursing's continual dilemmas have simply taken new forms. The separation of nursing education from the nursing service has slowly become a reality, fueled (until quite recently) as much by the federal largess that underlay the vast expansion of the health-care empires as the years of nursing's intensive struggle. Hospital-based diploma training is being rapidly replaced by nursing programs and schools in community colleges and universities.[17]

But as federal money for nursing education has become increasingly scarce, the less expensive community college programs are becoming the modern equivalents of diploma schools. As the nursing leadership attempts to legislate the baccalaureate degree as the entry-level credential for nursing practice, the question of what constitutes appropriate education continues to be one of nursing's most divisive political problems. At the core of this debate are still the issues of what counts as a nursing skill, how it is to be learned, and whether a nurse's character can be measured by educational criteria.[18]

Nor has the question of who should nurse been settled. The division of labor, established in the 1940s, among registered nurses, licensed practical nurses, and aides, has begun to crumble. In the immediate postwar years, many hospitals quickly substituted LPNs for RNs when they could. By the late 1960s the common wisdom was that the LPNs did at night what RNs were supposed to do during the day. Often only aides responded to the request for bedside care as nurses became increasingly tied to the "meds" cart, numerous monitors, and the nursing station.[19] With the decreasing pay differential between RNs and LPNs, the hospital's attempts to control spiraling labor costs, nursing discontent with being limited to the coordinating role, increasing conflict within "team nursing," and the growing technical nature of care giving, many hospitals are now returning to a form of "primary nursing" where individual nurses are given total responsibility for a set number of patients on any given shift. But other hospitals, in the name of cost savings, eliminate their most skilled nurses. A five-week strike in 1984 by 6,000 nurses against fifteen Minneapolis-St. Paul hospitals to protest the layoffs of more senior nurses suggests what may be in the future.[20] Or we may see the elimination of nursing workers below the RN level and a "speedup" and addition of what are now called "nonnursing functions" (e.g., carrying bedpans, moving furniture, cleaning up) to nurses' duties.

The increasingly technical and machine-aided nature of hospital-based health care has also affected nursing's situation. Nurses are now responsible for an array of new technologies and procedures from cardiac-monitoring devices to respiratory therapies. Even if the nurses do not actually run the new machinery, they must have "an ability to integrate and synthesize a volume of differentiated knowledge in order to translate that knowledge into coordinated, safe patient care."[21] Nursing, after all, is what is intensive about intensive-care units, as former nursing school dean Donna Diers has pointed out.[22] Many feel these technologies have given nurses a new sense of autonomy and skill.

Technical knowledge and skill do not directly translate into control over work, higher pay, or respect. Increasingly, the demands of the job have made many nurses feel as if they spend their time playing "beat the clock" as they run from task to task in an ever more complicated system, thereby losing their sense of caring.[23] As the predicted surplus of doctors of the 1990s puts nursing on a collision course with medicine over what counts as medical or nursing care, nurses may find it difficult to defend what they now do as nursing.

The abandonment of the hospital as the exclusive base of nursing education and the growing sophistication of nursing care have made certain changes possible. Whole generations of nursing students are becoming socialized into their professional identity on a theoretical level before they ever learn practical skills. New nursing leaders are attempting to instill in their students a renewed sense of pride in the caring skills of the nurse and their base in scientific and psychological theories. Nurses are being educated to believe in the autonomous arena of nursing care where rights are as important as responsibilities.[24] The fact that the very first legal case on comparable worth was brought by a group of Denver nurses suggests nursing's ongoing role in the political effort to have caring revalued.[25]

Contemporary feminism, as in the Denver case, has provided some

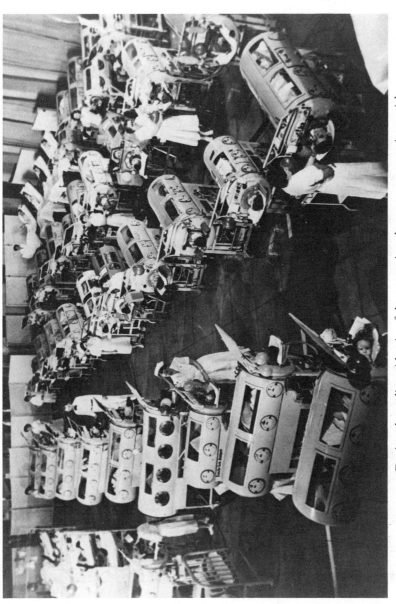

During the polio epidemic of the 1950s, iron lungs were set up in specialized units for respiratory care. Los Angeles County Hospital, Los Angeles, California, early 1950s. *Source:* Countway Library

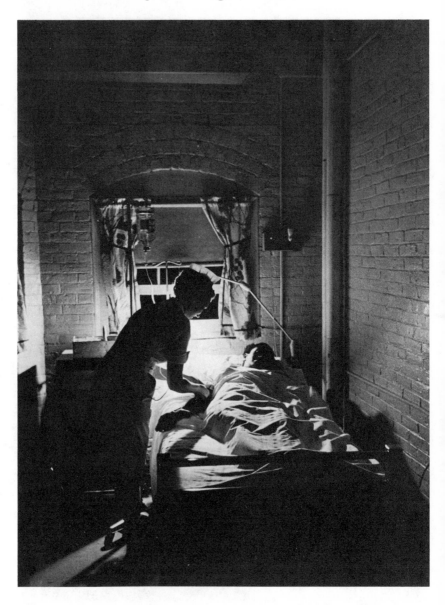

In a semi-lit basement room, a nurse inserts an IV and tries to comfort her patient. Boston Lying-in Hospital, Boston, Massachusetts, circa 1960. *Source:* Countway Library

nurses with the grounds on which to claim rights.[26] Feminism, in its liberal form, appears to give nursing a political language that stresses equality and rights within the given order of things. It suggests a basis for caring that stresses individual discretion, values, and equality. Just as liberal political theory undermined more paternalistic formulations of government, classical liberalism's tenets applied to women have much to offer nursing. The demand for the right to determine how to care challenges deeply held beliefs about gendered relations in the health-care hierarchy and the hierarchy itself.

The nature of the nursing experience, however, suggests the constraints on a liberal political effort to address the problems of caring. The individualism and autonomy of a liberal rights framework often fail to acknowledge collective social need, to provide a structure for discerning conflicts over rights, or to address the reasons for the devaluing of women's activities.[27] Thus nurses have often rejected liberal feminism, not just out of their oppression or some kind of "false consciousness," but because of some deep understandings of the limited promise of equality and autonomy in a health-care system they see as flawed and harmful. In an often inchoate way, such nurses recognize that those who claim the autonomy of rights often run the risk of rejecting altruism and caring itself.[28] Thus, a nursing school dean had to remind a graduating class, as I noted at the beginning of this book, that the value of caring need not be undervalued.

Several feminist psychologists have suggested that what women really want in their lives is "autonomy with connectedness."[29] In the case of nursing this will require the creation of the conditions under which it is possible to value caring and to understand that the empowerment of others does not have to involve self-immolation.[30] To achieve this, nurses will have to create a new political understanding for the basis of caring and find ways to gain the power to implement it. Nursing can do much within itself to bring this about, as the examples I give in this book demonstrate, but nurses cannot do it alone. The dilemma of nursing is too tied into the broader problems of gender and class in our society to be solved solely by the political efforts of one occupational group.

Nor are nurses alone in benefiting from such an effort. If nursing can create the vision of autonomy and altruism as linked qualities, and achieve the power to forge this unity, all of us have much to gain. Nursing has always been a much conflicted metaphor in our culture, reflecting all the ambivalences we give to the meaning of womanhood.[31] Perhaps in the future it can give this metaphor, and ultimately caring, new value in all our lives.

Appendix

Quantitative analysis of student records can help the historian create a composite portrait of the women who entered nursing through training. To do this, a sample was taken from the student records for the three Massachusetts nursing schools at Boston City Hospital (BCH), Somerville Hospital, and Long Island Hospital for students entering between 1878 and 1939. For a discussion of these data see Chapter 5.

The BCH student records are in the BCH School of Nursing Papers at the Nursing Archives, Mugar Library, Boston University. The Somerville and Long Island records are respectively in the basement record room of the Somerville Hospital School of Nursing in Somerville, Massachusetts, and the Office of the Director of Nursing, Long Island Hospital, Squantum, Massachusetts. All the records were kept alphabetically regardless of the student's entry date. The sample for Long Island and BCH was selected by taking every fifth case. If the fifth case was outside the sample years, the next case was selected and the fifth after that, etc. Because the record group was smaller at Somerville (the records of students entering between 1893 and 1903 were kept incompletely in one notebook), every available case was taken. There were 231 cases in the BCH sample, 175 in the Somerville, and 103 in the Long Island.

The BCH records span the years 1878–1939, but at the time of the coding, the records for the earlier years were much more complete and therefore comprise most of the data for the nineteenth-century years. The Somerville and Long Island records ran from 1903 to 1939 and 1899 to 1939, respectively. In the case of the Somerville and BCH records, only women who completed training were used; the Long Island records included women who dropped out. There was, however, no statistically significant difference between the groups in either the Long Island sample or in an additional test run on extra records taken from the files of dropouts at Somerville.

In cross-tabulations run on the data, a significance level of .05 or better was taken to accept statistical significance. Data were recoded into twenty- and thirty-year intervals so that the number of cells in the chi-square would not affect statistical outcome significantly. The data were, however, also run in decade and school subsamples so that trends could be established more finely.

The application forms provided the following information for students from all three schools: age, birthplace, marital status, parity, family responsibilities, education, occupation, previous hospital experience, entry and graduation years, current addresses, parents living or dead. Unfortunately, only the Somerville application asked for the student's religion. For the 152 women for whom religious affiliations was given, a third were Catholic, 3 percent were Jewish, and nearly two-thirds were from various Protestant denominations. Because of the existence of Catholic hospital training schools, however, the Somerville data are not enough to provide a reliable sample of the religious backgrounds of the students. Catholic students would more likely be trained in Catholic hospitals (see Nursing Student Records, Office of the Nursing Director, St. Margaret's Hospital, Dorchester, Massachusetts).

The major unfortunate loss during the process of collecting the data was the student records for the Waltham Training School for Nurses in Waltham, Massachusetts. Although I had made contact with the Waltham Graduate Nurses' Association and had begun a very preliminary survey of their records in 1977, in 1978 when I returned to Waltham to begin the coding, the records had been thrown out because they were deemed no longer "important." Because of the non–hospital-based nature of the school, and its explicit effort to reach women working in the Waltham Watch factory, these records would have made an excellent contrast to those of the other schools. The historian in search of quantitative records outside the census and city directory is often one step ahead of, or in this case, one step behind, the garbage collector. One last box of a few applications, and applications to the nurses' aide program at Waltham, was saved, and I have placed these records in the Waltham collection at Mugar Library. The numbers were too small, however, to be of use in this sample.

Table A.1. *Address upon application to training of nursing students in the Boston training schools sample, by size of community (in %)*

Address	Period entering training			
	1878–99	1900–19	1920–39	All
Rural/small town	26.5	29.2	33.5	30.0
Medium towns	32.4	35.6	31.0	33.3
Urban	41.2	35.2	35.5	36.5
(N = 507)				

Source: Nursing student records from Boston City, Somerville, and Long Island hospitals, 1878–1939.

Table A.2. *Comparison of birthplace and address of nursing students in the Boston training schools sample, by size of community (in %)*

Size of community	Birthplace	Address
Rural/small town	50.1	30.0
Medium towns	23.3	33.3
Urban	26.6	36.5
(N = 507)		

Source: See Table A.1.

Table A.3. *Comparison of birthplace and address of nursing students in the Boston training schools sample, by location of community (in %)*

Location of community	Birthplace	Address
Boston	6.7	8.1
Boston suburbs	20.3	45.6
New England	19.5	17.3
Rest of the U.S.	8.9	4.9
Maritimes	29.6	17.7
Rest of Canada	5.1	6.3
Rest of the world	9.9	0.2
	(N = 507)	(N = 509)

Source: See Table A.1.

Table A.4. Cross-tabulation of birthplace by address of nursing students in the Boston training schools sample (in %)

Birthplace/ location of community	Address/location of community						
	Boston	Boston suburbs	New England	Rest of the U.S.	Maritimes	Rest of Canada	Rest of the world
Boston	44.1	52.9	2.9	0.0	0.0	0.0	0.0
Boston suburbs	2.9	87.4	6.8	1.0	1.0	1.0	0.0
New England	5.1	28.3	62.6	0.0	1.0	3.0	0.0
Rest of the U.S.	4.4	33.3	11.1	42.2	2.2	4.4	2.2
Maritimes	6.7	29.3	5.3	0.0	56.7	2.0	0.0
Rest of Canada	3.8	15.4	0.0	3.8	3.8	73.1	0.0
Rest of the world	10.0	62.0	10.0	6.0	2.0	8.0	2.0
(N = 507)							

Source: See Table A.1.

Table A.5. *Comparison of addresses of nursing students in the Boston training schools sample to population of Massachusetts and northeastern states (in %)*

Population	Rural	Urban[a]
1878–99		
Sample	26.5	73.5
Massachusetts	21.7	78.3
Northeast	45.1	54.9
1900–19		
Sample	29.2	70.8
Massachusetts	12.5	87.5
Northeast	31.1	68.9
1920–39		
Sample	33.5	66.5
Massachusetts	9.9	90.1
Northeast	23.5	76.5

[a]Urban in the census definition is a population of 2,500 or more.

Source: Percentages calculated from Boston training schools sample; U.S. Department of Commerce, Bureau of the Census, *Historical Statistics of the United States,* Part I, Series A (Washington, D.C.: Government Printing Office, 1976), pp. 172–94, 195–209.

Table A.6. *Highest education level obtained by nursing students in the Boston training schools sample (in %)*

Education level	Period entering training			
	1878–99	1900–19	1920–39	Totals
Common school	51.0	43.0	16.0	36.3
Some high school	40.2	53.0	80.8	58.9
Special training or college	4.9	3.2	3.2	3.5
Normal school	3.9	0.8	0.0	1.2
	(N = 102)	(N = 251)	(N = 156)	(N = 509)

Source: See Table A.1.

Table A.7. *Previous occupations for nursing students in the Boston training schools sample, by school (in %)*

| Occupational category | Nursing school | | | |
	Boston	Somerville	Long Island	Total
At home	28.6	41.1	36.3	34.4
Professionals	16.0	5.7	4.9	10.2
White collar	14.3	25.1	13.7	17.9
Proprietors	0.4	0.0	0.0	0.4
Skilled workers	7.8	0.6	5.9	4.9
Service workers	14.3	14.3	16.7	14.8
Semiskilled	8.7	1.7	8.8	6.3
Domestics	10.0	11.4	13.7	11.2
	(N = 231)	(N = 175)	(N = 102)	(N = 508)

Source: See Table A.1.

Table A.8. *Previous occupations for nursing students in the Boston training schools sample, by entry year (in %)*

| Occupational category | Period entering training | | | |
	1878–99	1900–19	1920–39	Totals
At home	26.5	33.1	41.9	34.4
Professionals	18.6	11.2	3.2	10.2
White collar	5.9	17.5	26.5	17.9
Proprietors	0.4	0.0	0.0	0.4
Skilled workers	9.8	6.0	0.0	4.9
Service workers	17.6	12.4	16.8	14.8
Semiskilled	4.9	10.0	1.3	6.3
Domestics	16.7	10.0	9.7	11.2
	(N = 102)	(N = 251)	(N = 155)	(N = 508)

Source: See Table A.1.

Notes

LIST OF ABBREVIATIONS IN NOTES

Institutions and Organizations Cited

AHA   American Hospital Association
AMA   American Medical Association
ANA   American Nurses' Association
BCH   Boston City Hospital
BML   Boston Medical Library
HAW   Home for Aged Women
MGH   Massachusetts General Hospital
MNA   Massachusetts Nurses' Association
NLNE   National League for Nursing Education
NOPHN   National Organization for Public Health Nursing

Journals, Proceedings, and Transactions Cited

AJN   *American Journal of Nursing*
BHM   *Bulletin of the History of Medicine*
HM   *Hospital Management*
JAMA   *Journal of the American Medical Association*
MH   *The Modern Hospital*
NHR   *National Hospital Record*
PCNJ   *Nurses Journal of the Pacific Coast*, 1905–1907; thereafter *Pacific Coast Nursing Journal*
SS   *Reports and Proceedings of the American Society of Superintendents of Training Schools in the United States*
TAHA   *Transactions of the American Hospital Association*
TNHR   *The Trained Nurse*, 1888–93; thereafter *The Trained Nurse and Hospital Review*

INTRODUCTION The dilemma of caring

1 Gregory Witcher, "Last Class of Nurses Told: Don't Stop Caring," *Boston Globe*, May 13, 1985, pp. 17–18.
2 For a further discussion of the division between autonomy and altruism see *Toward a New Psychology of Women* (Boston: Beacon Press, 1976), p. 71. See also Larry Blum et al., "Altruism and Women's Oppression," in *Women and Philosophy: Towards a Theory of Liberation*, ed. Carol C. Gould and Marx W. Wartofsky (New York: Putnam, 1976), pp. 222–47; Linda J. Nicholson, "Feminist Theory: The Private and the Public," in *Beyond Domination: New Perspectives on Women and Philosophy*, ed. Carol Gould (Totowa, N.J.: Rowman and Allanheld, 1984), pp. 221–30; and Carroll Smith-Rosenberg, *Disorderly Conduct* (New York: Knopf, 1985).

3 Hilary Graham, "Caring: A Labour of Love," in *A Labour of Love: Women, Work and Caring,* ed. Janet Finch and Dulcie Groves (Boston/London: Routledge and Kegan Paul, 1983), p. 13.

4 The clearest direct commandments on caring can, of course, be found in the many writings of Florence Nightingale, in particular her *Notes on Nursing* (New York: Appleton, 1860). The contemporary relationship of nurse to patient is covered in various ethics texts; see, for example, James L. Muyskens, *Moral Problems in Nursing* (Totowa, N.J.: Rowman and Littlefield, 1982). For a discussion of the problem in terms of actual nursing practice, see Patricia Benner, *From Novice to Expert* (Reading, Mass.: Addison-Wesley, 1984).

5 Nancy Tomes, "Little World of Our Own: The Pennsylvania Hospital Training School for Nurses, 1895–1907," in *Women and Health in America,* ed. Judith Walzer Leavitt (Madison: University of Wisconsin Press, 1984), pp. 467–81.

6 See Smith-Rosenberg, *Disorderly Conduct,* and Susan Levine, "Labors in the Field: Reviewing Women's Cultural History," *Radical History Review* 35 (1986): 25–48.

7 For overview discussions and bibliographies on this growing area of historical scholarship see Joan Jacobs Brumberg and Nancy Tomes, "Women in the Professions: A Research Agenda for American Historians," *Reviews in American History* 10 (June 1982): 275–96. For a critique of the reigning paradigm on women's culture, see Nancy Hewitt, "American Women's History in the 1980s," *Social History* 10 (October 1985): 299–322.

8 I have used the term "middling classes" rather more often than "middle class" since it is the label used in the nineteenth century and more clearly reflects what historian Barbara Epstein called a "disparate grouping rather than a homogeneous whole. This grouping included professionals, shopkeepers and other tradespeople, independent artisans, possibly skilled workers, . . . people who were neither wealthy nor desperately poor" (*The Politics of Domesticity: Women, Evangelism and Temperance in Nineteenth-Century America* [Middletown, Conn.: Wesleyan University Press, 1981], p. 3).

9 See M. Adelaide Nutting, "Apprenticeship to Duty," a speech to the students of the Vassar Training Camp, September 9, 1918, and printed in *A Sound Economic Basis for Schools of Nursing* (1926; reprint, New York: Garland, 1984), pp. 350–64. See Carroll Smith-Rosenberg, *Religion and the Rise of the American City* (Ithaca, N.Y.: Cornell University Press, 1971); Joan Jacobs Brumberg, *Mission for Life: The Story of the Family of Adoniram Judson* (New York: Free Press, 1980); and Anne Firor Scott, "On Seeing and Not Seeing: A Case of Historical Invisibility," *Journal of American History* 71 (June 1984): 7–21.

10 For a discussion of the differences between rationality and capitalist rationality see Herbert Marcuse, "Industrialization and Capitalism in the Work of Max Weber," in *Negations: Essays in Critical Theory* (Boston: Beacon, 1968), pp. 201–26.

    By rationalization, I mean the process of using a variety of methods to formalize, standardize, and routinize work that was previously governed by custom, and to create a more specialized division of labor. I share the perspective of a number of recent scholars that rationalization was a broad process encompassing a variety of techniques that were often very industry- and time-specific. My thinking on rationalization was primarily influenced by the work of Susan Porter Benson. See her " 'The Clerking Sisterhood': Rationalization and the Work Culture of Saleswomen in American Department Stores, 1890–1960," *Radical America* 12 (March-April 1978): 41–55, and *Counter Cultures: Saleswomen, Managers, and Customers in American Department Stores* (Urbana: University of Illinois Press, 1986).

11 On male nurses, see brief discussion in Jane Mottus, *New York Nightingales* (Ann Arbor, Mich.: University Microfilms Books, 1981). See Darlene Clark Hine, ed., *Black Women in the Nursing Profession: A Documentary History* (New York: Garland, 1985); Darlene Clark Hine, "From Hospital to College: Black Nurse Leaders and the Rise of Collegiate Nursing Schools," *Journal of Negro Education* 51 (Summer 1982): 222–37, and "Mabel K. Staupers and the Integration of Black Nurses into the Armed Forces," in *Black Leaders of the 20th Century,* ed. John Hope Franklin

and August Meier (Urbana: University of Illinois Press, 1982), pp. 241–57; and Patricia Sloan, "Black Hospitals and Nurse Training Schools: The Formative Years" (Paper presented at the Fifth Berkshire Conference on the History of Women, Vassar College, Poughkeepsie, N.Y., June 1981). Both Sloan and Clark Hine are working on book-length studies. For the major older studies, see Adah B. Thoms, ed., *Pathfinders: A History of the Progress of Colored Graduate Nurses with Biographies of Many Prominent Nurses* (1929; reprint, New York: Garland, 1985), and Mabel Keaton Staupers, *No Time for Prejudice: A Story of the Integration of Negroes in Nursing in the United States* (New York: Macmillan, 1961).

The major survey of the religious sisterhoods remains Ann Doyle, "Nursing in Religious Orders in the United States," *American Journal of Nursing* 29 (July 1929): 775–86; (August 1929): 959–69; (September 1929): 1085–95; (October 1929): 1197–1207; (November 1929): 1331–43; (December 1929): 1446–84. See discussion in Joan Lynaugh, *The Community Hospitals of Kansas City, Missouri, 1875–1915* (New York: Garland, 1987).

12 JoAnn Ashley, *Hospitals, Paternalism and the Role of the Nurse* (New York: Teachers College Press, 1976). See also Susan Reverby, "Review of Ashley," *Social Science and Medicine* 11 (April 1977): 443.

13 See Susan Armeny, "Nurses, Women Philanthropists, and the Intellectual Bases for Cooperation Among Women," in *Nursing History: New Perspectives, New Possibilities*, ed. Ellen Condliffe Lagemann (New York: Teachers College Press, 1983), pp. 13–46. A history of the relationship of nursing to feminism still has to be written.

14 Barbara Melosh, *"The Physician's Hand"* (Philadelphia: Temple University Press, 1982).

15 For a debate on the relationship between women's culture and feminist politics, see Ellen DuBois, Mari Jo Buhle, Temma Kaplan, Gerda Lerner, and Carroll Smith-Rosenberg, "Politics and Culture in Women's History: A Symposium," *Feminist Studies* 6 (Spring 1980): 26–64. See also Smith-Rosenberg, *Disorderly Conduct;* and Nancy Cott, "Feminism in the 1920's" (Paper presented at the Feminist Theory Colloquium Series, Northeastern University, Boston, Mass., November 9, 1986).

16 See, for examples, Susan Reverby and David Rosner, eds., *Health Care in America: Essays in Social History* (Philadelphia: Temple University Press, 1979); Celia Davies, ed., *Rewriting Nursing History* (Totowa, N.J.: Barnes and Noble, 1980); Melosh, *"The Physician's Hand"*; Lagemann, ed., *Nursing History: New Perspectives, New Possibilities;* Judith Leavitt and Ronald Numbers, eds., *Sickness and Health in America*, 2d ed. (Madison: University of Wisconsin Press, 1985), and Janet Wilson James, "Writing and Rewriting Nursing History: A Review Essay," *Bulletin of the History of Medicine* 58 (Winter 1984): 568–84.

CHAPTER 1 *"Professed" nursing: from duty to trade*

1 On women's work see Mary P. Ryan, *Womanhood in America,* 3d ed. (New York: Franklin Watt, 1983), pp. 2–74; Nancy F. Cott, *The Bonds of Womanhood* (New Haven, Conn.: Yale University Press, 1977); Laurel Thatcher Ulrich, *Good Wives: Image and Reality in the Lives of Women in Northern New England, 1650–1750* (New York: Oxford University Press, 1983); Mary Beth Norton, *Liberty's Daughters* (Boston: Little, Brown, 1980), and "The Evolution of White Women's Experience in Early America," *American Historical Review* 89 (June 1984): 593–619; Linda Kerber, *Women of the Republic* (Chapel Hill: University of North Carolina Press, 1980).

2 Catherine Beecher, *Domestic Receipt-Book* (New York: Harper, 1846), p. 214; see also Cott, *Bonds of Womanhood,* pp. 63–100. For a discussion of the importance of this work in women's lives, see Gerda Lerner, ed., *The Female Experience* (Indianapolis: Bobbs-Merrill, 1977), pp. 151–201.

3 Ibid.; see also Eliza W. Farrar, *The Young Lady's Friend – by a Lady* (Boston: American Stationer's, 1837); William Alcott, *The Young Woman's Guide to Excellence* (Bos-

ton: George Wright, 1841 ed.), pp. 301–2; Martha Verbrugge, "The Social Meaning of Personal Health: The Ladies' Physiological Institute of Boston and Vicinity in the 1850s," in *Health Care in America: Essays in Social History,* ed. Susan Reverby and David Rosner (Philadelphia: Temple University Press, 1979), pp. 45–66.

4 Farrar, *The Young Lady's Friend,* p. 57. For an example of a physician who was advised to leave her practice to care for her mother, see Lerner, *The Female Experience,* p. 179.

5 Kathryn Kish Sklar, *Catharine Beecher: A Study in American Domesticity* (New Haven, Conn.: Yale University Press, 1973), p. 214; Faye Dudden, *Serving Women: Household Service in Nineteenth-Century America* (Middletown, Conn.: Wesleyan University Press, 1983), pp. 30, 130–31.

6 Stowe quoted by Cott, *Bonds of Womanhood,* p. 57; Huntington quoted by Barbara Berg, *The Remembered Gate: Origins of American Feminism* (New York: Oxford University Press, 1978), p. 121; Ednah Cheney, ed., *Louisa May Alcott: Her Life, Letters and Journals* (Boston: Robert Bros., 1889), p. 224.

7 S. Weir Mitchell, *Doctor and Patient,* 3d ed. (Philadelphia: Lippincott, 1888), pp. 122–27.

8 William Alcott, *Young Woman's Guide,* p. 305.

9 *Godey's Lady's Book,* February 1840, p. 95. I am grateful to Carol Lasser for this reference. The historiography on changes in the antebellum women's sphere is rapidly growing. See, for example, Norton, "The Evolution of the White Women's Experience in Early America"; Ruth H. Bloch, "American Feminine Ideals in Transition: The Rise of the Moral Mother," *Feminist Studies* 4 (Summer 1978): 102–8; Berg, *The Remembered Gate;* Mary P. Ryan, *The Empire of the Mother* (New York: Haworth, 1982).

10 For the contemporary views, see Catharine E. Beecher, *Miss Beecher's Housekeeper and Healthkeeper* (New York: Harper and Brothers, 1876), and Sarah Josepha Hale, *The Good Housekeeper,* 7th ed. (Boston: Otis Bros., 1844). See also Susan Strasser, *Never Done: A History of Housework* (New York: Pantheon, 1982).

11 For a discussion of the expansion of urban domestic service see Dudden, *Serving Women;* Julia Cherry Spruill, *Women's Life and Work in the Southern Colonies* (Chapel Hill: University of North Carolina Press, 1938); and David M. Katzman, *Seven Days a Week: Women and Domestic Service in Industrializing America* (New York: Oxford University Press, 1978), especially p. 59.

12 Janet Lynn Golden, "From Breast to Bottle: The Decline of Wet Nursing in Boston, 1869–1927" (Ph.D. diss., Boston University, 1984).

13 The best easily available primary source on colonial midwifery is the "Diary of Martha Moore Ballard, 1785–1912," *The History of Augusta* [*Maine*], ed. Charles Elventon Nash (Augusta, Me.: Charles Nash and Sons, 1904). For secondary sources on midwives see Ulrich, *Good Wives,* pp. 126–38; Catherine M. Scholten, "On the Importance of the Obstetrick Art: Changing Customs of Childbirth in America, 1760–1825," *William and Mary Quarterly* 3d ser., 34 (1977): 426–45; Charlotte Borst, "Midwives in Early New England 1620–1820: From Healers and Community Authority to Quack and Outsider" (M.A. thesis, Department of History, Tufts University, 1977); Judy Barrett Litoff, *American Midwives 1860 to the Present* (Westport, Conn.: Greenwood, 1978); Jane B. Donegan, *Women and Men Midwives* (Westport, Conn.: Greenwood, 1978). On Southern midwives see Marie Campbell, *Folks Do Get Born* (1946; reprint, New York: Garland, 1984); and Spruill, *Women's Life and Work in the Southern Colonies.*

14 Litoff, *American Midwives,* p. 17. See also Alfred Worcester, *Monthly Nursing* (Boston: Mason, 1886). "Monthly" became the generic term for obstetrical and neonatal nursing care.

15 See Dudden, *Serving Women.*

16 "Mrs. B.," a monthly nurse, told Virginia Penny: "When food is to be prepared, the child's clothes washed, or anything of that kind done, she rings a bell and gives orders to a servant." Virginia Penny, *The Employments of Women: A Cyclopedia of Women's Work* (Boston: Walker, Wise, 1863), p. 420.

17 See Alex Berman, "The Heroic Approach in Nineteenth-Century Therapeutics," in *Sickness and Health in America,* ed. Judith Walzer Leavitt and Ronald L. Numbers (Madison: University of Wisconsin Press, 1978), pp. 77–86; Ronald L. Numbers, "Do-It-Yourself the Sectarian Way," in ibid., pp. 87–96; and Charles E. Rosenberg, "The Practice of Medicine in New York a Century Ago," in ibid., pp. 55–74.

18 For examples of both viewpoints see Ednah Dow Cheney, "Woman in Philanthropy – Care of the Sick," in *Woman's Work in America,* ed. Annie Nathan Meyer (1891; reprint, New York: Arno, 1972), pp. 346–58; Alfred Worcester, *Nurses and Nursing* (Cambridge, Mass.: Harvard University Press, 1927), pp. 4–5; Elizabeth Cady Stanton, *Eighty Years and More* (1898; reprint, New York: Shocken, 1971); Victor Robinson, *White Caps: The Story of Nursing* (Philadelphia: Lippincott, 1946); John Duffy, *The Healers: A History of American Medicine* (Urbana: University of Illinois Press, 1979).

19 "The Shortage of Nurses: Reminiscences of Alfred Worcester '83," reprint from the *Harvard Medical School Alumni Bulletin* (April and June 1949), n.p., Alfred Worcester Papers, Countway Library, Harvard Medical School, Boston, Mass.

20 Louisa May Alcott, *Life, Letters and Journals,* p. 352.

21 The terms "permanent" and "transient" have to be used gingerly. Turnover was quite rapid in household servants. See Dudden, *Serving Women,* pp. 193–235.

22 In 1825, nurses in Massachusetts reportedly were paid $2.00 a week, whereas maids averaged $1 to $1.50. In 1868, a New York nurse received from $1 to $2 a day; women in the sewing trades were averaging $8 a week and young servant women only $2.22. Wages in Massachusetts were similar. See Stanley Lebergott, *Manpower in Economic Growth: The American Record since 1800* (New York: McGraw-Hill, 1964), pp. 281, 284, and 542, and Helen L. Sumner, *History of Women in Industry in the United States* (reprint, New York: Arno, 1974; originally vol. 10, *Report on Condition of Women and Child Wage Earners in the U.S.* [Washington, D.C.: Government Printing Office, 1910]), pp. 185 and 262; "Introduction and Statistical," *3rd Annual Report of the Bureau of the Statistics of Labor, Massachusetts 1872* (Boston: Wright and Potter, 1872), p. 68, and *16th Annual Report of the Bureau of the Statistics of Labor, Massachusetts 1885* (Boston: Wright and Potter, 1885), p. 253.

23 Penny, *Employments of Women,* p. 421.

24 Cheney, ed., *Alcott, Life, Letters and Journals,* p. 173. For an example of the attempt to allude to the nobility of nursing for the middle-class woman, see the *New York Daily Tribune,* September 30, 1845, p. 1, quoted in Alice Kessler-Harris, *Out to Work* (New York: Oxford University Press, 1982), p. 57. There are difficulties in gaining accurate data for the nineteenth-century nurse. The printed census data on the employment of women are very uneven. The nursing category, in addition, is very inexact. Some years it includes trained nurses, untrained nurses, and midwives under the title "nurse." In other years, nurses were counted with domestic servants. Only in twentieth-century censuses are the trained and untrained separated. For examples of the statistics in Boston and Massachusetts see Lemuel Shattuck, *Report to the Committee of the City Council . . . Census of Boston for . . . 1845 . . .* (Boston: John Eastburn, 1846), p. 41; Secretary of the Commonwealth of Massachusetts, *Census of the Commonwealth of Massachusetts, 1885 . . . by Carroll D. Wright,* vol. I, *Population and Social Statistics, Part 2* (Boston: Wright and Potter, 1888), pp. 342–43; Secretary of the Commonwealth of Massachusetts, *Census . . . 1905,* vol. II, *Occupations and Defective and Social and Physical Conditions* (Boston: Wright and Potter, 1909), pp. 9, 30, 114, 495.

It is also difficult to be certain of nativity of nurses because of the ways they were enumerated in the census. In Boston in 1880, for example, Irish women filled the ranks of domestic service while native-born women held on to nursing; see Carroll D. Wright, *The Working Girls of Boston* (Boston: Wright and Potter, 1889), pp. 6–7. The national nativity figures for 1880 suggest, however, that Boston's nursing market may have been unusual for excluding Irish women. In the U.S. figures, 71.2 percent of the nurses were native-born, and 11.6 percent were Irish.

The figures for domestics were 76.4 and 12.4 percent, respectively. U.S. Census Office, *Statistics of Population of the U.S., 10th Census 1880,* vol. I, *Population* (Washington, D.C.: Government Printing Office, 1883), p. 756.

25 See Georgia L. Sturtevant, "Personal Recollections of Hospital Life before the Days of Training Schools," *Trained Nurse and Hospital Review* 57 (November 1916): 260; Rosenberg, "The Practice of Medicine in New York," p. 56; Worcester, "The Shortage of Nurses"; Cheney, "Woman in Philanthropy."

26 U.S. Census, *12th Census of the United States, 1900, Special Report on Occupations,* ccxxii, reprinted in Sumner, *History of Women in Industry in the United States,* p. 248.

27 The label "state of affliction" was awarded to widows by Cotton Mather; see *The Widow of Nain* (Boston: 1728), pp. 10–11, cited by Alexander Keyssar, "Widowhood in 18th Century Massachusetts: A Problem in the History of the Family," *Perspectives in American History* 8 (1974): 83–122; see also Carole Haber, *Beyond Sixty-Five: The Dilemma of Old Age in America's Past* (Cambridge: Cambridge University Press, 1983).

28 Case no. 18, "Admissions Committee Records," vol. I, Box 11, Home for Aged Women (HAW) Collection, Schlesinger Library, Cambridge, Mass. Data on nurses admitted to the home were also found in "Records of Inmates, 1858–1901," "Records of Admission, 1873–1924," and "Records of Inmates, 1901–1916," all in Box 11. I am grateful to Carol Lasser and Brian Gratton for guiding me through these records.

29 *First Annual Report of the Association for Relief of Aged Indigent Females, 1851,* HAW Collection, Box 10, p. 10. For the historical relationship between the old and the poorhouse, see Michael Katz, "Poorhouses and the Origins of the Public Old Age Home," *Health and Society/Milbank Memorial Fund Quarterly* 62 (Winter 1984): 110–40.

30 *Board of Managers Minutes and Annual Meetings,* May 5, 1859, HAW Collection, Box 10.

31 Ibid., July 21, 1859.

32 "Admissions Committee Records," HAW Collection, Box 11, vol. I, cases 2 and 135. I analyzed the demographic and work histories in the admissions records of all nurses ($N = 132$) applying to the home between 1850 and 1912. On most variables, there was no statistically significant shift over time (significance level .05 or better). I have particularly focused on the years between 1850 and 1886 because of the availability of a comparative study by Carol Lasser on all the women in the home, primarily domestics; see " 'The World's Dread Laugh': Singlehood and Service in Nineteenth-Century Boston," in *The New Labor History and the New England Working Class,* ed. Donald Bell and Herbert Gutman (Urbana: University of Illinois Press, 1984).

The occupational categories are those found in Stephan Thernstrom, *The Other Bostonians* (Cambridge, Mass.: Harvard University Press, 1973), appendix B. My recoded categories followed the job titles in the Thernstrom appendix. In addition, I have added the separate category of farmer because of the rural origins of many of these women.

33 Lasser, " 'The World's Dread Laugh.' " For general discussion on marriage patterns, see Peter R. Uhlenberg, "A Study of Cohort Life Cycles: Cohorts of Native-Born Massachusetts Women, 1830–1920," *Population Studies* 23 (November 1969): 411.

34 Lasser calculates migration age by subtracting the number of years a woman claimed to have been in Boston from her age upon application to the home. The figures obtained are, of course, only approximations since they do not consider if the women might have stretched the truth to make their applications more acceptable to the home trustees. Similarly, given the enormous rate of in- and out-migration to Boston in the nineteenth century, it is probable that the women (as many of them noted in their applications) moved in and out of the city.

35 See, for example, Carol Groneman, " 'She Earns as a Child: She Pays as a Man': Women Workers in a Mid-Nineteenth-Century New York City Community," in

Class, Sex and the Woman Worker, ed. Milton Cantor and Bruce Laurie (Westport, Conn.: Greenwood, 1977), pp. 83–100. Groneman's study of Irish and German women's work in New York's Sixth Ward in 1855 gives a slightly different picture. She found "the younger widows worked as seamstresses, milliners, and cap makers, while those over forty years of age turned to laundering and housekeeping" (p. 96). She found no nurses in her sample, although it is possible some of those listed as housekeepers were also doing some nursing.

36 "Admission Committee Records," HAW Collection, vol. I, cases 186, 121, and 207.

37 Ibid., cases 37, 135, and 205.

38 Penny, *Employments of Women,* p. 420.

39 Sturtevant, "Personal Recollections," p. 260; see also Alfred Worcester, *Training Schools for Nurses in Small Cities* (Boston: George Ellis, 1893), p. 1.

40 William Alcott, *Young Woman's Guide,* p. 305.

41 See, for example, James Jackson, MD, *Another Letter to a Young Physician* (Boston: Ticknor and Fields, 1861), p. 121.

42 Dorothy Deming, *The Practical Nurse* (New York: Commonwealth Fund, 1947), p. 28.

CHAPTER 2 *Order and chaos in hospital nursing*

1 The social history of the American hospital has gained the interest of a number of historians in recent years. See Leonard Eaton, *New England Hospitals 1790–1833* (Ann Arbor: University of Michigan Press, 1957); Charles E. Rosenberg, "And Heal the Sick: The Hospital and the Patient in Nineteenth-Century America," *Journal of Social History* 10 (June 1977): 428–47, "From Almhouse to Hospital: The Shaping of the Philadelphia General Hospital,," *Milbank Memorial Fund Quarterly/ Health and Society* 60 (Winter 1982): 108–54, and *The American Hospital: The Formative Years* (in press); Morris J. Vogel, *The Invention of the Modern Hospital* (Chicago: University of Chicago Press, 1979); David Karl Rosner, *A Once Charitable Enterprise: Health Care in New York and Brooklyn, 1890–1915* (Cambridge: Cambridge University Press, 1982); Rosemary Stevens, "Sweet Charity: Pennsylvania and the Voluntary Hospitals, 1870–1910," *Bulletin of the History of Medicine (BHM)* 58 (Winter 1984): 474–95.

2 J. M. Toner, "Statistics of Regular Medical Associations and Hospitals of the United States," *Transactions of the American Medical Association* 24 (1873): 288–333. As Vogel (*Modern Hospital,* p. 137) points out, Toner listed 178 hospitals, but 58 were identified as insane asylums.

3 "Suggestions on the subject of providing, training and organizing nurses for the sick poor in workhouse infirmaries" (letter to Sir Thomas Watson Bart, member of the committee appointed by the President of the Poor Law Board, London, January 19, 1867, p. 1), quoted in Brian Abel-Smith, *A History of the Nursing Profession in Great Britain* (New York: Springer, 1960), p. 5. Catholic nuns or members of Protestant nursing orders also became nurses in some hospitals, but this is another history beyond the scope of the present work.

4 Vogel, *Modern Hospital,* p. 1.

5 Copy of January 22, 1875, entry in Massachusetts General Hospital Trustees, *Annual Report for 1875,* Massachusetts General Hospital (MGH) Nursing Records, Box 13, Folder 2B, Countway Medical Library, Rare Books Room, Harvard Medical School, Boston, Mass.; see also, Vogel, *Modern Hospital,* pp. 5–28.

6 There appears to have been some difference in the patient class mix between hospitals in the East and those in the West and Northwest as the latter tended to be less ubiquitously lower working class (personal communication from Charles Rosenberg based on his forthcoming book on the history of the hospital). For a history of Southern community hospitals see Peter Buck and Barbara Rosenkrantz, *Healthy, Wealthy and Wise* (in press). For an older overview on this topic see George Rosen, "The Hospital: Historical Sociology of a Community Institution,"

in Rosen, ed. *From Medical Police to Social Medicine* (New York: Science History Publications, 1974), pp. 274–303. Not all public institutions were outgrowths of almshouses or intended to serve only the lumpen proletariat; see Vogel, *Modern Hospital,* pp. 29–58, on the founding of Boston City Hospital.

Proprietary hospitals, that is, institutions owned by individuals, groups, or a company intended to make a profit, began to appear in the nineteenth century. There were only thirty-nine such hospitals in 1873 when Toner made his survey. There is no history of proprietary hospitals, although some discussion of their developments can be found in Bruce Steinwald and Duncan Neuhauser, "The Role of the Proprietary Hospital," *Law and Contemporary Problems, Health Care* 35 (Autumn 1970): 811–38, and David A. Steward, "The History and Status of Proprietary Hospitals," *Blue Cross Reports Research Series* 9 (March 1973): 2–9.

7 A historian of the Boston Lying-In Hospital made a clear distinction as to whom the hospital served: "In Boston, poor women who were respectable were accepted at the Lying-In Hospital; those who were poor but not respectable were sent to the House of Industry"; Frederick C. Irving, *Safe Deliverance* (Boston: Houghton Mifflin, 1942), p. 70. See also David Rosner, "Health Care for the 'Truly Needy,' 19th Century Origins of the Concept," *Milbank Memorial Fund Quarterly/Health and Society* 60 (Summer 1982): 355–85.

8 On moral stewardship see Clifford S. Griffin, *Their Brothers' Keepers: Moral Stewardship in the United States 1800–1865* (New Brunswick, N.J.: Rutgers University Press, 1960), and Nathan I. Huggins, *Protestants against Poverty: Boston's Charities 1870–1900* (Westport, Conn.: Greenwood, 1971); On class relations see "Fireside," *Boston Evening Transcript,* January 22, 1879, cited by Morris J. Vogel, "Patrons, Practitioners and Patients: The Voluntary Hospital in Mid-Victorian Boston," in *Victorian America,* ed. Daniel Walker Howe (Philadelphia: University of Pennsylvania Press, 1976), p. 130. For a discussion of the overlay of deference and class language, see Asa Briggs, "The Language of 'Class' in Early Nineteenth-Century England," in *Essays in Labour History in Memory of G. D. H. Cole,* ed. Asa Briggs and John Saville (London: Macmillan, 1960), pp. 43–73.

9 On the home model, see Susan Lynne Porter, "The Benevolent Asylum – Image and Reality: The Care and Training of Female Orphans in Boston, 1800–1840" (Ph.D. diss., Boston University, 1984).

10 Boston City Hospital, *25th Annual Report, 1888,* p. 33; Rosenberg, "And Heal the Sick," p. 433. For a theoretical discussion of the nature of authority under paternalism, see Richard Sennett, *Authority* (New York: Knopf, 1980), pp. 50–83.

11 Nathan Bowditch, *A History of the Massachusetts General Hospital, to August 5, 1851,* 2d ed. with a continuation to 1872 (Boston: Trustees from the Bowditch Fund, 1872), pp. 398–99; Eliza Higgins, "Matron's Journals," 4 vols., 1873–89, Rare Books Room, Countway Medical Library, Harvard Medical School, Boston, Mass. These journals provide insight into the daily life of a late nineteenth-century small hospital. I am indebted to Laurie Crumpacker for this source and to the staff of the Public Relations Office of the Brigham and Women's Hospital for allowing me to use the journals when they were not yet in the library.

12 Figures calculated from Bowditch, *History of the Massachusetts General,* p. 703; Boston Lying-In Hospital, *Annual Reports 1873–1889;* and Toner, "Statistics of Hospitals."

13 See discussion in Eaton, *New England Hospitals,* p. 112, and Charles E. Rosenberg, "Inward Vision and Outward Glance," *Bulletin of the History of Medicine* 53 (Fall 1979): 346–91. For discussion on women trustees, see "The Boston Lying-In Hospital: Why Women Are Not on Its Board of Trustees or Employed as Physicians," *Boston Evening Transcript,* February 6, 1888, clipping laid in Higgins, "Matron's Journals," vol. IV; Marion Hunt, "Women and Childsaving: St. Louis Children's Hospital, 1879–1979," *Missouri Historical Society Bulletin* 36 (January 1980): 65–79; and Virginia G. Drachman, *"Hospital with a Heart": Women Doctors and a Century of Separatism at the New England Hospital for Women and Children, 1862–1968* (Ithaca, N.Y.: Cornell University Press, 1984).

14 Higgins, "Matron's Journals," vol. IV, May 26, 1885.
15 Ibid., vol. IV, July 9, 1889. Both Rosenberg ("And Heal the Sick" and "Inward Vision") and Rosner (*A Once Charitable Enterprise*) discuss the tensions between trustees, stewards, superintendents or matrons, and physicians.
16 Higgins, "Matron's Journals," vol. III, August 20, 1880.
17 See Rosenberg, "And Heal the Sick" and "Inward Vision." For a discussion of the ambiguities of authority in nineteenth-century medicine see Barbara Rosenkrantz, "The Search for Professional Order in 19th Century American Medicine," in *Sickness and Health in America*, 2d ed., ed. Judith Walzer Leavitt and Ronald Numbers (Madison: University of Wisconsin Press, 1986).
18 Henry C. Wright, *Report of the Committee of Inquiry into the Departments of Health, Charities and Bellevue and Allied Hospitals in the City of New York* (New York: City of New York Board of Estimate, 1913), p. 78.
19 Higgins, "Matron's Journals," vol. I, January 9, 1875, February 22, 1875; vol. II, March 29, 1878. See also vol. I, June 16, 1875; vol. III, September 10, 1882.
20 On the difficulties for poor women, see Christine Stansell, "Women, Children, and the Use of the Streets: Class and Gender Conflict in New York City, 1850–1860," *Feminist Studies* 8 (Summer 1982): 309–35, and "The Origins of the Sweatshop: Women and Early Industrialization in New York City," in *Working Class America*, ed. Michael H. Frisch and Daniel J. Walkowitz (Urbana: University of Illinois Press, 1983), pp. 78–103.
21 Higgins, "Matron's Journals," vol. II, July 1, 1880.
22 See discussion in Georgia Sturtevant, "Personal Recollections of Hospital Life before the Days of Training Schools," *TNHR* 52 (November 1916): 255–60; (December 1916): 321–27; 53 (February 1917): 67–71, (March 1917): 127–31; and Emily Elizabeth Parsons, *Memoir of Emily Elizabeth Parsons* (1880; reprint, New York: Garland, 1984).
23 Higgins, "Matron's Journals," vol. I, June 1, 1874; vol. II, November 11, 1878.
24 Ibid., vol. II, December 3, 1878. On the hiring of relatives, see vols. I, March 6, 1873; II, April 30, 1878, and December 22, 1879; III, April 30, 1882. Rosenberg ("And Heal the Sick") also discusses the hiring of relatives in the hospital.
25 Higgins mentions at least four different nurses who were called away when their children became ill; see vols. I, January 19, 1874; II, March 15, 1878; III, September 16, 1882; and IV, April 10, 1888.
26 Ibid., vols. I, June 16, 1875, and II, September 10, 1882.
27 Ibid., vol. II, June 3–July 19, 1879.
28 Georgia L. Sturtevant came to the Massachusetts General in 1862 as an assistant nurse and stayed for thirty-three years; she finally retired in 1895, having become the hospital's matron. Her four-part memoirs were published in *Trained Nurse and Hospital Review*, twice, once right after her retirement in 1895 and again in 1916. "Personal Recollections," November 1916, pp. 259–60.
29 The turnover figures were calculated from Higgins's recording of the entry and departing dates of her nursing staff.
30 Sturtevant, "Personal Recollections," December 1916, p. 321; Linda Richards, *Reminiscences of Linda Richards* (Boston: Thomas Todd, 1911), p. 7.
31 See, for example, Sturtevant, "Personal Recollections," November 1916, p. 257, and Higgins, "Matron's Journals," vol. IV, January 1 and February 26, 1889.
32 Many hospital annual reports listed patient occupations. For an all-too-brief discussion of the number of domestic servants among the female patients at the Massachusetts General and Boston City Hospitals, see Vogel, *Modern Hospital*, pp. 11–12. For discussions of the work see Richards, *Reminiscences*, p. 6; Higgins, "Matron's Journals," vol. III, April 29, 1883; and typescript of interview with Mary Elizabeth Norris by Ruth Sleeper, August 11, 1936, Massachusetts General Hospital Nursing Records, Box 13, Folder 2B, Countway Medical Library, Harvard Medical School.
33 Sturtevant, "Personal Recollections," December 1916, p. 332; Higgins, "Matron's Journals," vols. I, March 12, 1875, and III, June 4, 1883.

34 Higgins, "Matron's Journals," vol. IV, July 28, 1888. For further discussion of medical authority see Rosenkrantz, "The Search for Professional Order."
35 Higgins, "Matron's Journals," vol. IV, July 28, 1888.
36 Ibid., May 21, 1884, March 24, 1885, and July 28, 1885; vol. III, April 12, 1884.
37 For examples, see ibid., March 7, 1880, October 7, 1883; vol. IV, July 28, 1885, July 25, 1888. For further discussion of behavioral expectations based on gender see the next chapter.
38 Typescript copy of excerpt from Oliver Wendell Holmes, "An Introductory Lecture Delivered before the Medical Class of Harvard University," November 6, 1867, p. 39, in Massachusetts General Hospital Nursing Records, Box 13, Folder 2B, Countway Medical Library.
39 Sturtevant, "Personal Recollections," November 1916, p. 258.
40 Ibid., December 1916, p. 323.
41 On the nature of rituals, see Victor Turner, *The Ritual Process: Structure and Anti-Structure* (Ithaca, N.Y.: Cornell University Press, 1969), and Clifford Geertz, "Ritual and Social Change: A Javanese Example," *The Interpretation of Cultures* (New York: Basic, 1973), pp. 142–69. For a discussion of the importance of female-deference rituals in societies where women play an important economic role see Betty S. Denich, "Sex and Power in the Balkans," in *Women, Culture and Society,* ed. Michelle Z. Rosaldo and Louise Lamphere (Palo Alto, Calif.: Stanford University Press, 1974), pp. 243–62. For more contemporary analysis of rituals of deference between physicians and patients, see Charles L. Bosk, *Forgive and Remember: Managing Medical Failure* (Chicago: University of Chicago Press, 1979), and P. M. Strong, *The Ceremonial Order of the Clinic* (Boston and London: Routledge and Kegan Paul, 1979).
42 See Norris interview and Higgins, "Matron's Journals," vol. I, October 2, 1873, October 13, 1873, April 11, 1873, December 13, 1874. The issue of whether employees or employers could set the pace for the working day was continually fought over in numerous different industries during the nineteenth century. The exertion of employer power over this aspect of work was one of the great transformations of these years; see David Montgomery, "Workers' Control of Machine Production in the Nineteenth Century," *Labor History* 17 (Winter 1976): 485–509.
43 Higgins, "Matron's Journals," vol. II, January 11, 1876, and July 1, 1876.
44 Ibid., June 3, 1875, and IV, May 7, 1887.
45 Ibid., vol. II, May 22, 1879. Five days later when Higgins placed an ad for a nurse, again in the Boston papers, she asked for "a respectable, intelligent woman . . . Protestant." What kind of role religious and ethnic tensions played at the hospital is difficult to assess from Higgins's memoirs. She herself was an English Protestant. From the Irish last names of many of the nurses, I suspect they were probably Catholics. Higgins does not mention this as an issue, but the ad for a Protestant nurse does seem to hint at this kind of underlying tension. This was certainly true in other Boston hospitals, especially between Irish Catholic patients and Boston elite Protestant doctors.
46 Ibid., vols. II, December 22, 1879, and IV, October 2, 1884: Lucy Hubbard Kendall was registered with the Boston Medical Library Directory for Nurses, a registry that sent out private nurses in the New England area; see Susan Reverby, " 'Neither for the Drawing Room nor for the Kitchen': Private Duty Nursing in Boston 1880–1914," in *Women and Health in America,* ed. Judith Walzer Leavitt (Madison: University of Wisconsin Press, 1984), pp. 454–66. Kendall was also traced in the *Boston City Directory,* 1881–87.
47 "Matron's Journals," vol. IV, May 7, 1887. For more on the sexual norms and behavior of working-class women, see Christine Stansell, *City of Women, 1789–1860* (New York: Knopf, 1986).
48 Sturtevant, "Personal Recollections," December 1916, p. 323. Rosenberg ("And Heal the Sick") comes to a similar conclusion.
49 Montgomery, "Workers' Control." I have discussed the manifestation of this behavior in other women workers; see "Commentary on Women's Strikes" (Paper

given at the Third Berkshire Conference on Women's History, Bryn Mawr, Pa., June 1976); see also Susan Porter Benson, *Counter Cultures.*

CHAPTER 3 *Character as skill: the ideology of discipline*

1 Elizabeth Christophers Hobson, *Recollections of a Happy Life* (New York: Putnam, 1916), p. 140. Hobson's chapter on Bellevue was reprinted in *A Century of Nursing* (New York: Putnam, 1950). For a more recent history of Bellevue's training school see Jane Mottus, *New York Nightingales: The Emergence of the Nursing Profession at Bellevue and New York Hospitals, 1850–1920* (Ann Arbor, Mich.: University Microfilms Books, 1981).

2 Morris Vogel, *The Invention of the Modern Hospital* (Chicago: University of Chicago Press, 1979).

3 Ibid; see also David Rosner, *A Once Charitable Enterprise* (Cambridge: Cambridge University Press, 1982); Frederick D. Keppel, "The Modern Hospital as a Health Factory," *Modern Hospital* (*MH*) 3 (October 1916): 304; "The Hospital as a Factor in Modern Society," *MH* 1 (September 1913): 33; and Del T. Sutton, "Three Years of Growth in the Hospital Field," *National Hospital Review* (*NHR*) 4 (October 1901): 30–33.

4 See Lynn Weiner, *From the Working Girl to the Working Mother* (Durham: University of North Carolina Press, 1984), and Mari Jo Buhle, "The Nineteenth-Century Women's Movement: Perspectives on Women's Labor in Industrializing America" (Cambridge, Mass.: Bunting Institute, 1979).

5 Barbara Ehrenreich and Deirdre English, *Witches, Midwives and Nurses: A History of Women Healers* (Oyster Bay: Glass Mountain Pamphlets, 1972), p. 34. This pamphlet, which describes nurses as the occupational end result of an attempt to take power away from women healers, became an underground minor classic, selling over 75,000 copies. Their view of nursing history has shaped an entire generation of women's understanding of the field, and it is therefore imperative that its limitations be examined and understood. For another view, see Margaret Connor Versluysen, "Old Wives Tales? Women Healers in English History," in *Rewriting Nursing History*, ed. Celia Davies (Totowa, N.J.: Barnes and Noble, 1980), pp. 175–99.

6 The Nursing Archives at Boston University has the largest collection in the United States of Nightingale letters. The extant Nightingalia is enormous. For a beginning see the two major, but older, biographies, Edward Cook, *The Life of Florence Nightingale*, 2 vols. (London: Macmillan, 1913), and Cecil Woodham-Smith, *Florence Nightingale* (London: Constable, 1950). See also W. J. Bishop and Sue Goldie, *A Bio-Bibliography of Florence Nightingale* (London: Dawsons, 1962). For more recent interpretations see Charles E. Rosenberg, "Florence Nightingale on Contagion: The Hospital as Moral Universe," in *Healing and History*, ed. Charles Rosenberg (New York: Science History Publications, 1979), pp. 116–35, and Donald R. Allen, "Florence Nightingale: Toward a More Psychohistorical Interpretation," *Journal of Interdisciplinary History* 6 (Summer 1975): 23–45.

7 For a negative and controversial recent biography see F. B. Smith, *Florence Nightingale: Reputation and Power* (New York: St. Martin's, 1982). For more feminist interpretations see Elaine Showalter, "Florence Nightingale's Feminist Complaint: Women, Religion and *Suggestions for Thought*," *Signs* 6 (Spring 1981): 395–412; Eva Gamarnikow, "Sexual Division of Labour: The Case of Nursing," in *Feminism and Materialism: Women and Modes of Production*, ed. Annette Kuhn and AnnMarie Wolpe (London and Boston: Routledge and Kegan Paul, 1978), pp. 96–123; Sandra Holten, "Feminine Authority and Social Order: Florence Nightingale's Conception of Nursing and Health Care," *Social Analysis* (August 1984): 59–72; Lois A. Monteiro, " 'On Separate Roads': Florence Nightingale and Elizabeth Blackwell," *Signs* 9 (Spring 1984): 520–33; and Anne Summers, "Ladies and Nurses in the Crimean War," *History Workshop Journal* 16 (Autumn 1983): 33–56. As a complex and powerful historical figure, Nightingale can be read and taught many different

ways; see Elvi Whittaker and Virginia Olesen, "The Faces of Florence Nightingale: Functions of the Heroine Legend in an Occupational Sub-Culture," in *Anthropology and the American Life,* ed. Joseph G. Jorgensen and Marcello Truzzi (Englewood Cliffs, N.J.: Prentice-Hall, 1974), pp. 307–22.

8 See Rosenberg, "Florence Nightingale"; Gamarnikow, "Sexual Division of Labour"; and Holton, "Feminine Authority."

9 Anna Jameson, *Sisters of Charity Abroad and at Home and The Communion of Labour; Two Lectures on the Social Employment of Women* (London: Longman, Brown, Green, Longman and Roberts, 1859); Caroline H. Dall, *Women's Right to Labour; or, Low Wages and Hard Work* (Boston: Walker, Wise, 1860); Virginia Penny, *The Employments of Women* (Boston: Walker, Wise, 1863); see discussion in Gamarnikow, "Sexual Division of Labour"; Mari Jo Buhle, "The Nineteenth-Century Women's Movement"; and Martha Vicinus, *Independent Women; Work and Community for Single Women, 1850–1920* (Chicago: University of Chicago Press, 1985), pp. 85–120.

10 Kathryn Kish Sklar, *Catharine Beecher: A Study in American Domesticity* (New Haven, Conn.: Yale University Press, 1973).

11 *Notes on Nursing: What It Is, and What It Is Not* (1860; reprint, Philadelphia: J.P. Lippincott, 1946), p. 134.

12 Nightingale, "Sick Nursing and Health Nursing," *Nursing of the Sick 1893,* ed. Isabel Hampton et al. (New York: McGraw-Hill, 1949), p. 24.

13 For an exposition of her medical ideas, see Rosenberg, "Florence Nightingale"; Holton, "Feminine Authority"; and Florence Nightingale, *Notes on Hospitals,* 3d ed. (London: Longmans, Green, 1863).

14 See Monteiro, " 'On Separate Roads.' "

15 John D. Thompson and Grace Goldin, *The Hospital: A Social and Architectural History* (New Haven, Conn.: Yale University Press, 1975), pp. 155–69, 231.

16 Woodham-Smith, *Florence Nightingale,* p. 348. Kathryn Sklar's summation of Beecher's mission could equally apply to Nightingale if, in the following quote, "hospital" were substituted for "society." Sklar concluded that Beecher intended that "women would first themselves be made over and then they would reshape the society" (*Catharine Beecher,* p. 101).

17 Charles J. Stille, *History of the U.S. Sanitary Commission* (Philadelphia: Lippincott, 1866), pp. 17–37. The impact of the Nightingale reforms was initially felt by Northern charity reformers. Although there are memoirs of Southern Civil War nurses, there is not yet a modern history of the effect of the Civil War and the Nightingale reforms on nursing in the South.

18 See Agatha Young, *The Women and the Crisis* (New York: McDowell, Obolensky, 1959), p. 9. There is a vast literature of memoirs and secondary books on women during the Civil War. For a good, if slightly controversial, view with useful bibliographic footnotes, see Ann Douglas Wood, "The War within a War: Women Nurses in the Union Army," *Civil War History* 18 (September 1972): 197–212; see also Anne L. Austin, *The Woolsey Sisters of New York* (Philadelphia: American Philosophical Society, 1971).

19 Victor Robinson, *White Caps: The Story of Nursing* (Philadelphia: Lippincott, 1946), pp. 130–47.

20 Louisa May Alcott, *Hospital Sketches* (1863; reprint, New York: Garland, 1984), p. 3; Katharine Prescott Wormeley, *The Other Side of the War with the Army of the Potomac* (Boston: Ticknor, 1888–89), p. 43; "All Our Women Are Florence Nightingales," *New York Herald,* April 15, 1864, quoted by Mary Elizabeth Massey, *Bonnet Brigades* (New York: Knopf, 1966), p. 350.

21 Walt Whitman, *Specimen Days* (1882; reprint, Boston: Godine, 1971).

22 Wormeley, *Other Side of the War,* p. 102.

23 Georgeanna Woolsey, *Three Weeks at Gettysburg* (New York: Randolph, 1863), p. 208.

24 See Alcott, *Hospital Sketches,* p. 94.

25 Wood, "The War within a War," and Jane Swisshelm, *Half a Century* (Chicago: Jansen, McClurg, 1880), p. 359.
26 Dorothea Dix's difficulties with male authorities make this abundantly clear; see Francis Tiffany, *Life of Dorothea Lynde Dix* (New York: Houghton Mifflin, 1891), and Helen E. Marshall, *Dorothea Dix* (Chapel Hill: University of North Carolina Press, 1937).
27 Jane Stuart Woolsey, *Hospital Days* (New York: Van Nostrand, 1868), p. 41; Katharine Wormeley, *The United States Sanitary Commission: A Sketch of Its Purposes and Its Work* (Boston: Little, Brown, 1863), p. 24. For more on the Sanitary Commission see George M. Fredrickson, *The Inner Civil War: Northern Intellectuals and the Crisis of the Union* (New York: Harper and Row, 1965), pp. 99–112; William Quentin Maxwell, *Lincoln's Fifth Wheel: The Political History of the United States Sanitary Commission* (New York: Longmans, Green, 1956); and Stille, *History of the U.S. Sanitary Commission*. For the Sanitary Commission's ideals and its impact on nursing, see also Susan Armeny, "Organized Nursing, Women Philanthropists, and the Intellectual Basis for Cooperation Among Women," in *Nursing History: New Perspectives, New Possibilities,* ed. Ellen Condliffe Lagemann (New York: Teachers College Press, 1983), pp. 13–46.
28 For a general discussion of the impact of the war experience on such women see Sheila Rothman, *Woman's Proper Place* (New York: Basic Books, 1978), pp. 63–77; see also Buhle, "The Nineteenth-Century Women's Movement," and Janet Wilson James, "Women and the Development of Health and Welfare Services in Industrial America, 1870–90" (paper presented at the Third Berkshire Conference on the History of Women, Bryn Mawr College, Bryn Mawr, Pa., June 1976).
   For a good introduction to the thinking of women reformers see Abby Howland Woolsey, "Hospitals and Training Schools," report to the Sanitary Commission on Hospitals, State Charities Aid Association, New York, May 24, 1876, in *A Century of Nursing* (New York: Putnam, 1950), pp. 3–133.
29 Rothman, *Woman's Proper Place,* p. 72, and Sara E. Parsons, *History of the Massachusetts General Hospital Trained School for Nurses* (Boston: Whitcomb and Barrows, 1922), pp. 25–27; Hobson, *Happy Life;* Austin, *Woolsey Sisters.*
30 The history of these early schools has been retold many times in the standard nursing histories. For more recent views, see James, "Women and the Development of Health and Welfare Services"; Mottus, *New York Nightingales;* and Dorothy Sheahan, "The Social Origins of American Nursing and Its Movement into the University: A Microscopic Approach" (Ph.D. diss., New York University, 1980).
   "Training" women for nursing had been suggested before 1873. In 1798, Dr. Valentine Seaman had given a series of lectures to nurses at New York Hospital, traditionally considered the first example of such kind of "training." There were other sporadic attempts at training in the pre–Civil War years, but nothing was sustained. In 1868 the eminent Pennsylvania physician Samuel Gross became the chairman of a "committee of one" in the American Medical Association to study the necessity for systematic nursing education. He urged local medical societies to become involved in the organization of nurse's training, but his fellow physicians did not immediately heed his advice. In 1872, Dr. Susan Dimock at the New England Hospital for Women and Children began a training program for nurses consisting of twelve lectures by the hospital's visiting medical staff and some minimal bedside instruction.
   It is therefore somewhat ironic that Linda Richards is given the title of "America's first trained nurse," although she graduated from the program at the New England Hospital for Women and Children. The major nursing histories, however, written by nurses, give the title of first training *schools* to those programs that followed the Nightingale model. Only Victor Robinson, a physician and medical historian (*White Caps,* pp. 238–40), emphasizes the importance of the New England Hospital training school. See also Linda Richards, *Reminiscences of Linda Richards* (Boston: Thomas Todd, 1911), and Richards Papers, Nursing Archives, Boston University; and Virginia Drachman, *"Hospital with a Heart"* (Ithaca, N.Y.: Cornell University Press, 1984).

31 For an excellent discussion of physician authority in the nineteenth century, see Barbara Gutmann Rosenkrantz, "The Search for Professional Order in Nineteenth Century American Medicine," in *Sickness and Health in America*, 2d ed., ed. Judith Walzer Leavitt and Ronald L. Numbers (Madison: University of Wisconsin Press, 1986).

32 See Regina Markell Morantz, Cynthia Stodola Pomerleau, and Carol Hansen Fenichel, *In Her Own Words* (Westport, Conn.: Greenwood, 1982), and Drachman, *"Hospital with a Heart."*

33 See Mary A. Clymer, "Diary 1887–1889," Hospital of the University of Pennsylvania School of Nursing, Alumnae Association Office. I am grateful to Diana Long for sharing this source with me. See also E. B. Lowry, *The Home Nurse* (Chicago: Forber, 1914), and Minnie Goodnow, *The Technic of Nursing* (Philadelphia: Saunders, 1926).

34 Dr. Cook, comments on paper by Dr. G. S. C. Badger, "The Ideal Curriculum for a Training School," read at the Third Semi-Annual Meeting of the New England Association for the Education of Nurses, Boston, 1906, and printed in *Trained Nurse and Hospital Review (TNHR)* 36 (May 1906): 272, and "The Nurse's Limitations," *NHR* 9 (March 1906): 8.

35 Alfred Worcester, *Training Schools for Nurses in Small Cities* (Boston: Ellis, 1893), p. 838. On the similar promise for domestic service and the Lowell mill work, see Faye E. Dudden, *Serving Women* (Middletown, Conn.: Wesleyan University Press, 1983); Thomas Dublin, *Women at Work: The Transformation of Work and Community in Lowell, Massachusetts* (New York: Columbia University Press, 1979); Margaret Gibbons Wilson, *The American Woman in Transition: The Urban Influence 1870–1920* (Westport, Conn.: Greenwood, 1979); Susan L. Porter, "Mother/Mistress, Servant/Child: The Orphan as Indentured Servant in the Early Victorian Family" (Paper presented at the Fourth Berkshire Conference on the History of Women, Mt. Holyoke College, South Hadley, Mass., August 1978); Louise A. Tilly and Joan W. Scott, *Women, Work and Family* (New York: Holt, Rinehart and Winston, 1978).

36 Stanley Schultz, *The Culture Factory* (New York: Oxford University Press, 1973), p. 66. See also discussion in Rothman, *Woman's Proper Place*, and Lynn W. Weiner, *From Working Girl to Working Mother*. For further discussion on the social origins of nursing students, see Chapter 5.

37 M. Adelaide Nutting, "Apprenticeship to Duty," in *A Sound Economic Basis for Schools of Nursing* (1926; reprint, New York: Garland, 1984).

38 "Probationers Rules, Massachusetts General Hospital School of Nursing," n.d., probably 1919–20, Massachusetts General Hospital School of Nursing Papers, Box 13, Folder 2 AC, Countway Medical Library, Rare Books Room, Harvard Medical School, Boston, Mass.

39 Louise Darche, "Trained Nursing – Employments for Women – No. 2," *The Delineator* 43 (June 1894): 667–78.

40 Alma Revelle O'Keefe, president of the Kansas State Nurses' Association, quoted in Mary E. Marksman, *Triennial Report, Alumnae Association, St. Joseph's Hospital Training School for Nurses* (Kansas City, Mo.: n.p., 1913), quoted in Joan Lynaugh, "Nurses and Hospitals in Transition, 1875–1915" (Unpublished paper, 1984). I am grateful to Professor Lynaugh for making her work available. For examples of the necessary virtues, see *Student Record Book, Somerville Hospital School of Nursing, 1898–1929*, Somerville Hospital, Nursing School Director's Office Files, Somerville, Mass. Whether because of lack of imagination, or emphasis, in addition to "womanly" the most commonly listed virtues were "kind, gentle, quiet, conscientious, tactful, and dignified." For discussion of the use of the term "manly," see Burton J. Bledstein, *The Culture of Professionalism: The Middle Class and the Development of Higher Education in America* (Cambridge: Cambridge University Press, 1979), pp. 9–18. For a contemporary discussion of the link between nursing and womanliness, see Claire Fagin and Donna Diers, "Nursing as Metaphor," *New England Journal of Medicine*, July 14, 1983, 116–17.

41 Quoted in Isabel Stewart, *The Education of Nurses* (New York: Macmillan, 1943), p. 169.

42 Quoted in U.S. Bureau of Education, *Training Schools for Nurses,* Circulars of Information, no. 1 (Washington, D.C.: Government Printing Office, 1879), p. 14.

43 Thomas Le Duc, *Piety and Intellect at Amherst College* (New York: Columbia University Press, 1946), p. 99; Stanley Schultz, *The Culture Factory* (New York: Oxford University Press, 1973); George F. Peterson, *The New England College in the Age of the University* (Amherst, Mass.: Amherst College Press, 1964); James McLachlan, *American Boarding Schools* (New York: Scribner, 1970); Daniel Howe, "American Victorianism as a Culture," *American Quarterly* 27 (December 1975): 527–29, and "The Social Science of Horace Bushnell," *Journal of American History* 70 (September 1983): 305–22. See also Mary Kelley, *Private Woman, Public Stage: Literary Domesticity in 19th Century America* (New York: Oxford University Press, 1984), esp. pp. 67 and 103. I am grateful to Barbara Solomon for helping me think through this section. See her book, *In the Company of Educated Women* (New Haven, Conn.: Yale University Press, 1985).

44 M. Adelaide Nutting, *Proceedings of the Fifth Annual Meeting of the American Society of Superintendents of Training Schools for Nurses* (1898; reprint, New York: Garland, 1984), p. 49.

45 See Bledstein, *Culture of Professionalism,* and Daniel Rodgers, *The Work Ethic in Industrial America* (Chicago: University of Chicago Press, 1978).

46 Rosenkrantz, "The Search for Professional Order."

47 Isabel Hampton Robb, *Nursing Ethics: For Hospital and Private Use* (Cleveland: Savage, 1901), p. 66.

48 Julia Wells, "Do Hospitals Fit Nurses for Private Nursing?" *TNHR* 10 (March 1890): 97.

49 Lavinia Dock, "The Relation of Training Schools to Hospitals," in *Nursing of the Sick 1893,* Isabel Hampton et al., p. 17.

50 Dr. William Richardson, *Address on the Duties and Conduct of Nurses in Private Nursing,* delivered at the Boston Training School for Nurses, June 18, 1886 (Boston: Ellis, 1886). The speech was printed as a pamphlet and reprinted in both the *TNHR* and *NHR.*

51 Lavinia L. Dock and Isabel M. Stewart, *A Short History of Nursing,* 2d ed. (New York: Putnam, 1925), p. 41.

52 John Allen Hornsby and Richard E. Schmidt, *The Modern Hospital* (Philadelphia: Saunders, 1913), p. 330.

53 "The Relation of Training Schools to Hospitals," p. 16.

54 Anna M. Fullerton, "The Science of Nursing – A Plea," *17th Annual Report of the Conference on Charities and Corrections, 1890* (Boston: Ellis, 1890), pp. 135.

55 Ibid., p. 136.

56 Georgiana Sanders, "Report of the Massachusetts General Hospital Training School Committee, November 23, 1909," Massachusetts General Hospital Invoices Book, 1909–10, Massachusetts General Hospital Papers, Countway Medical Library, Rare Books Room, Harvard Medical School, Boston, Mass. See also, "Rules for Nurses," *New York Herald,* September 12, 1904, reprinted in *TNHR* 34 (October 1904): 251–52.

57 "The Nurse – Laborer or Professional?" *MH* 8 (April 1917): 269; Amy Beers, "How Nurses May Contribute Towards a Hospital's Success," *MH* 3 (November 1914): 302–3; *Constitution and By-Laws and Regulations of the Brooklyn Homeopathic Hospital* (Boston: Eagle Book and Job Printing, 1890), p. 1; Nina Dale, "The Hospital Family – Cooperation in Domestic Management," *MH* 3 (September 1914): 187–89.

58 Somerville Hospital School of Nursing Student Records, Somerville Hospital, Somerville, Mass.

59 Anna Maxwell and Amy Pope, *Practical Nursing: A Textbook for Nurses and a Hand-Book for All Who Care for the Sick* (New York: Putnam, 1908), p. 74. Vicinus (*Independent Women,* p. 91) suggests that in British schools the family metaphor

came later in the nineteenth century, after the military one. In the United States they were united.

60 Lucy Drown to David Baldwin, July 16, 1908, Boston City Hospital Correspondence Book, Marion Parsons Papers, Nursing Archives, Boston University, Boston, Mass. See also "A Symposium on Hospital Discipline," *NHR* 8 (June 1905): 30.

61 Nightingale, "Sick Nursing and Health Nursing," p. 27; Robb, *Nursing Ethics,* p. 61; Dock, "The Relation of Training Schools to Hospitals," p. 16.

62 Woodham-Smith, *Florence Nightingale,* p. 348. See also Christopher Maggs, *The Origins of General Nursing* (London: Croom Helm, 1983).

63 For a discussion of the work of the nursing student, see Chapter 4.

64 Robb, *Nursing Ethics,* pp. 61 and 68; Lucy Catlin, "The Training School Problem," *NHR* 11 (December 1907): 42.

65 Helene K. Stewart, Boston City Hospital Student Records, Box 5, Folder 1, Student 2, Marion Parsons Papers, Nursing Archives.

66 Parsons, *Massachusetts General Hospital Training School,* p. 26. See also Janet Wilson James, "Isabel Hampton and the Professionalization of Nursing in the 1890s," in *The Therapeutic Revolution,* ed. Morris J. Vogel and Charles E. Rosenberg (Philadelphia: University of Pennsylvania Press, 1979), pp. 201–44, and Nancy Tomes, " 'Little World of Our Own': The Pennsylvania Hospital Training School for Nurses, 1895–1907," *Journal of the History of Medical and Allied Sciences* 33 (October 1978): 507–30.

67 Nursing Committee to Dr. Emily Pope, December 7, 1888, New England Hospital for Women and Children Papers, Box 6, Folder 1863, Sophia Smith Archives, Smith College, Northampton, Mass.

68 Augusta Elizabeth Jones, Boston City Hospital Student Records, Box 22, Folder 1, Student 3; Lucy Drown to John McCollum, December 1, 1908, Boston City Correspondence Book, Nursing Archives, Mugar Library, Boston University; Mary Morris testimony, *Majority and Minority Reports on Investigations of Boston Almshouse and Hospital at Long Island* (Boston: Ellis, 1890), p. 842.

69 Edith P. Michaels, Boston City Student Records, Box 5, Folder 8, Student 1; Madeline R. Carnes, Long Island Hospital Student Records, Nursing Director's Office, Long Island Hospital, Boston, Mass.; Emma Nichols to Mr. R. I. McLaren, May 12, 1911, Boston City Correspondence Book; Claudia Frances Kern, Boston City Student Records, Box 23, Folder 6, Student 4.

70 Women's Education Association Industrial Committee, Board of Directors of the Boston Training School for Nurses, *Minutes,* vol. 1, October 29, 1873, Massachusetts General Hospital, Records, Box 15, Folder 3c–10, Countway Medical Library, Rare Books Room, Harvard Medical School, Boston, Mass.

71 See Celia Genoud's testimony at the Long Island hearings, *Majority and Minority Reports . . . Long Island,* p. 780.

72 Lucy Jefferson, Boston City Student Records, Box 1, Folder 3, Student 3.

73 Agnes Bell, ibid., Box 15, Folder 3, Student 2.

74 Somerville Hospital Student Record Book and Student Records, and Lucy Drown to John McCollum, June 25, 1908, Boston City Hospital Correspondence Book.

75 Josephine W. Moore, Boston City Student Records, Box 26, Folder 6, Student 3.

76 Emma Nichols to Mrs. Harriet Know, August 10, 1911, Boston City Correspondence Book.

77 Nora Anna McDonough, Boston City Student Records, Box 5, Folder 1, Student 3, and Grace Francis Barnes, Box 2, Folder 8, Student 5.

78 See discussion of the nurses' reaction to Isabel Hampton Robb in James, "Isabel Hampton." For a playful rhyme on this issue, see S. Virginia Lewis, "Limericks for Nurses," *TNHR* 39 (September 1907): 151.

79 Records of dismissed students, Boston City Correspondence Books and Records; Long Island Hospital Student Records; *Conference Committee Minute Book, 1876–86,* New York Hospital Archives, New York Hospital, New York.

80 Emma Nichols to P. L. Dolliver, October 6, 1910, Boston City Correspondence

Book; Boston City Student Records, Box 21, Folder 8, Student 3, and Box 22, Folder 7, Student 3.
81 Nichols to Know, Lucy Drown to Emily L. Brennan, October 21, 1908, Boston City Correspondence Book.
82 Mary E. Caldwell and Celia Genoud testimony, *Majority and Minority Reports . . . Long Island*, pp. 768–82.
83 Mary Agnes Snively, "What Manner of Women Ought Nurses to Be?" *American Journal of Nursing* 4 (August 1904): 838. See also Nancy Tomes, " 'Little World of Our Own' "; Barbara Melosh, "*The Physician's Hand*" (Philadelphia: Temple University Press, 1982); and Susan Armeny, " 'We Were the New Women' ": A Comparison of Nurses and Women Physicians, 1890–1915" (Paper presented at the American Association for the History of Nursing Conference, University of Virginia, Charlottesville, Va., October 1, 1984).
84 Dorothy Sheahan, "The Influence of Occupational Sponsorship on the Professional Development of Nursing" (Paper given at the Rockefeller Archives Conference on the History of Nursing, May 1981, Tarrytown, N.Y.), p. 12.
85 I. Menzies, "A Case Study in the Functioning of Social Systems as a Defense against Anxiety," *Human Relations* 13 (May 1960): 95–121, is the classic psychoanalytic explanation for this problem; see also Virginia Walker, *Nursing and Ritualistic Practice* (New York: Macmillan, 1967). For further discussion on this question, see Chapter 4. Martha Vicinus (*Independent Women*) comes to a similar conclusion about the British schools.
86 Nancy Cott, *The Bonds of Womanhood* (New Haven, Conn.: Yale University Press, 1977), p. 204.

CHAPTER 4 *Training as work: the pupil nurse as hospital machine*

1 See Barbara Solomon, *In the Company of Educated Women* (New Haven, Conn.: Yale University Press, 1985).
2 U.S. Bureau of the Census, *Historical Statistics of the U.S. from Colonial Times to 1957* (Washington, D.C.: Government Printing Office, 1959), ser. B, pp. 192–94, 235–36.
3 "Nursing in the Small Hospitals," in *Educational Standards for Nurses*, ed. Isabel Hampton Robb (Cleveland: Koeckert, 1907), pp. 78–79.
4 L. R., letter to the editor, *Trained Nurse and Hospital Review* (*TNHR*) 14 (March 1895): 158.
5 Bureau of the Census, *Benevolent Institutions 1910* (Washington, D.C.: Government Printing Office, 1913), pp. 42, 75. Calculations of the number of hospitals with training schools are based on Massachusetts figures in this census report.
6 Mary Riddle, "How to Obtain Greater Uniformity in Ward Work," *SS 1898*, 60.
7 *Report of the Somerville Hospital, Period Ending April 30, 1897*, p. 4.
8 *Boston City Hospital Annual Report, 1879*, p. 19.
9 "Report of the Meeting of the New England Association for the Education of Nurses, December 10, 1909," *TNHR* 47 (March 1910): 185.
10 Averages from Jane Hodson, ed., *How to Become a Trained Nurse*, 3d ed. (New York: Abbatt, 1911), and M. Adelaide Nutting, *Educational Status of Nursing*, Bureau of Education Bulletin no. 7, 1912, whole no. 475 (Washington, D.C.: Government Printing Office, 1912).
11 *Majority and Minority Reports on Investigation of Boston Almshouse and Hospital at Long Island* (Boston: Municipal Printing Office, 1904), p. 1187.
12 Alpha, letter to the editor, *TNHR* 14 (April 1895): 228.
13 "2nd Annual Report of Long Island Hospital," in *Annual Report of the Pauper Institutions*, Trustees of the City of Boston (Boston: Municipal Printing Office, 1899), p. 47; see also Dr. Cox's testimony, *Majority and Minority Reports . . . Long Island*, p. 1601.
14 Dr. Alfred Worcester, *Small Hospitals: Establishment and Maintenance* (New York: Wiley, 1900), p. 42. Even the Catholic hospitals discovered that a professional

nurse would cost them a minimum of ten dollars a week but that a training school "would avert lavish expenditure" and alleviate the problem of chronic understaffing. Douglass Shand Tucci, *The Second Settlement, 1875–1925* (Boston: Trustees of St. Margaret's Hospital, 1974), p. 20, and Nursing Student Records, Office of the Nursing Director, St. Margaret's Hospital, Boston, Mass. See also Dr. W. E. Taylor's testimony, *Majority and Minority Reports . . . Long Island*, p. 1131.

15 See *10th Annual Report of Somerville Hospital, 1903*, p. 43. This was a common practice.

16 Boston City Hospital Student Records, Nursing Archives, Mugar Library, Special Collections, Boston University; *Somerville Hospital Annual Report for 1897*, n.p.; Mary Morris's testimony, *Majority and Minority Reports . . . Long Island*, p. 818.

17 Calculated from raw figures in Hodson, *How to Become a Trained Nurse*, pp. 133–49.

18 "The Obligations of Opportunity," originally given as a speech in 1916 and reprinted in Nutting's collection of essays, *Sound Economic Basis for Schools of Nursing* (1926; reprint, New York: Garland, 1984), p. 224. In the Somerville Hospital records, for example, a payroll for the mid-1890s lists the nursing students as "nurses." Somerville Hospital Records, Office of the President, Somerville Hospital.

19 Christine R. Kefauver, "What Is the Matter with the Training School?" *TNHR* 65 (August 1920): 119.

20 Adelaide Nutting, *Educational Status of Nursing*, p. 30, and "Statistical Report," p. 231.

21 Stella Goostray, *Memoirs: Half a Century in Nursing* (Boston: Boston Nursing Archive, Boston University Mugar Library, 1969), pp. 2–3; Medical Board Minutes, December 1, 1893, vol. IV, New England Hospital Papers, Box 4, Smith College.

22 A. T. Bristow, "The Training School Problem," *THNR* 38 (October 1907): 214; *A Study of the Incidence and Costs of Illness among Nurses* (New York: ANA, NLNE, and AHA, 1938); Kefauver, "What Is the Matter with the Training School?" p. 119; calculation of reasons for dropouts, Boston City Hospital Student Records, Nursing Archives, Mugar Library, Boston University, and Somerville Hospital Records, Somerville Hospital.

23 "Extracts from the Journal of a Pupil Nurse," *TNHR* 39 (February 1908): 99. The problem of poor living conditions was discussed frequently by nursing educators, and the plans for new homes, when they began to be built in the 1920s, fill the pages of the nursing journals.

24 See "The Ideal Curriculum of the Theoretical Part of a Nurse's Training"; see also the routines noted in the *Annual Report of the New England Hospital for the Year Ending September 30, 1891*, p. 11.

25 Letter to the editor, *TNHR* 10 (July 1890): 41. For a discussion of ritual behavior as protection see Everett Hughes, "Mistakes at Work," *Canadian Journal of Economics and Political Science* 17 (August 1951): 320–27.

26 See Bristow, "The Training School Problem," p. 151; discussion of Alice Twitchell's "The Discipline of the Nurse," *SS 1902*, p. 59; letter to the editor, *TNHR* 56 (November 1919): 423; and discussion at the New England Association for the Education of Nurses' Semi-Annual Meeting on "The Present Curriculum from the Point of View of the Nurse," *TNHR* 37 (April 1907): 226.

27 Eleanor H. Abbott, *The White Linen Nurse* (New York: Century, 1913), pp. 58–59, 69. For a general discussion of the nurse in fiction see Barbara Melosh, ed., *Nurses in Fiction* (New York: Garland, 1984).

28 Lucy Drown to Jessie Davies, June 4, 1908, Boston City Hospital Correspondence Book, Parsons Papers, Nursing Archives, Mugar Library, Boston University. See also Evelyn Wood, "The Head Nurse," *Pacific Coast Journal of Nursing* 10 (March 1914): 109.

29 Clara Weeks, *A Text-Book of Nursing* (1889; reprint, New York: Garland, 1984), p. 33.

30 For similar complaints see letters to the editor, *TNHR* 10 (July 1890): 44; 10 (November 1890): 236; and *TNHR* 46 (January 1911): 40.

31 Anna Mitchell, June 2, 1918, Boston City Hospital Student Records, Box 8, Folder 4, Student 4.
32 Minnie Callahan, September 11, 1908, ibid., Box 23, Folder 6, Student 1.
33 See Carroll Smith-Rosenberg, "The Female World of Love and Ritual," *Signs* 1 (Autumn 1975): 1–30.
34 Isabel Hampton Robb, *Nursing Ethics* (Cleveland: Savage, 1901), p. 138.
35 Ibid; see also Martin Duberman, " 'I Am Not Contented': Female Masochism and Lesbianism in Early Twentieth-Century New England," *Signs* 5 (Summer 1980): 825–41; Nancy Sahli, "Smashing: Women's Relationships before the Fall," *Chrysalis* 8 (1979): 17–22; and Leila Rupp, " 'Imagine My Surprise': Women's Relationships in Historical Perspective," *Frontiers* 5 (1981): 61–70. For an overview on the transition, see Carroll Smith-Rosenberg, "The New Woman as Androgyne," in *Disorderly Conduct* (New York: Knopf, 1985), pp. 245–96.
36 Mabel Jacques, "The Right of Vindication," *TNHR* 46 (January 1911): 9–11.
37 See Barbara Melosh, "*The Physician's Hand*" (Philadelphia: Temple University Press, 1982), and Martha Vicinus, *Independent Women* (Chicago: University of Chicago Press, 1985), pp. 85–120.
38 Letter to the editor, *TNHR* 5 (November 1890): 236.
39 "Extracts from the Journal of a Pupil Nurse," p. 99.
40 David Montgomery, "The 'New Unionism' and the Transformation of Workers' Consciousness in America, 1909–22," in *Workers' Control in America* (Cambridge: Cambridge University Press, 1979), p. 93.
41 "Nurses' Strikes," *TNHR* 24 (September 1902): 236; "The Striking Nurse," *TNHR* 52 (February 1915): 98.
42 For a slightly different discussion of the control in British schools, see Vicinus, *Independent Women*, pp. 85–120.
43 See Charles Rosenberg, "Inward Vision and Outward Glance: The Shaping of the American Hospital, 1880–1914," *BHM* 53 (Fall 1979): 356–91. The dates for these changes varied widely among different hospitals.
44 George H. M. Rowe, "Observations on Hospital Organization," *Transactions of the Association of Hospital Superintendents, 1902*, p. 65, and reprinted in *National Hospital Review (NHR)* 6 (December 1902): 3–10. For examples see Stephen Smith, "Report on the Committee on Hospitals, Dispensaries, and Nursing," *2nd New York State Conference of Charities and Corrections, 1902;* George P. Ludlam, "The Organization and Control of Nursing Schools," *New York Medical Journal* 83 (April 1906): 851.
45 L. L. Dock, "Hospital Organization," *American Journal of Nursing (AJN)* 3 (March 1903): 413–21.
46 "The Relationship of Training Schools to Hospitals," in Isabel Hampton et al., *Nursing the Sick, 1893* (New York: McGraw-Hill, 1959), p. 83. See also Estelle Freedman, "Separatism as Strategy: Female Institution Building and American Feminism, 1870–1930," *Feminist Studies* 5 (Fall 1979): 512–29.
47 Quoted in Dock, "Hospital Organization," p. 414. I have gone into detail on this debate because it reveals much about the two sides on the question of "hospital organization" and because JoAnn Ashley in *Hospitals, Paternalism and the Role of the Nurse* (New York: Teachers College Press, 1976), pp. 19–20, describes Rowe's position but not the nursing response to it. Dock's paper was also printed in the *NHR* 6 (February 1903): 10–13.
48 Dock, "Hospital Organization," *AJN* version, pp. 413–21. All quotes in text are from this article. For more on Lavinia Dock, see Janet Wilson James, ed., *A Lavinia Dock Reader* (New York: Garland, 1985).
49 See Thorstein Veblen, *The Engineers and the Price System* (New York: Heubsch, 1921).
50 Francina Freese–Adelaide Nutting Correspondence, June 1905, M. Adelaide Nutting Papers, File II, Drawer 2, Teachers College, Columbia University, New York.
51 "Can Insert Male Catheter," was considered, for example, an *extra* skill of gradu-

ate nurses who registered for private-duty work with the Boston Medical Library Directory for Nurses; see Chapter 6.
52 Freese to Nutting, June 1905; Eva G. Beecroft, "Seeking Institutional Positions – Traps for the Unwary," *TNHR* 55 (September 1918): 151.
53 Lucy Drown to Superintendent of Nurses, Victoria General Hospital, Halifax, April 22, 1908, Boston City Hospital, Correspondence Book, Nursing Archives, Mugar Library, Boston University.
54 Medical Board Minutes, April 2, 1886, and May 7, 1886, New England Hospital Papers, vol. II, Box 4, Smith College. See also Virginia Drachman, *"Hospital with a Heart"* (Ithaca, N.Y.: Cornell University Press, 1984).
55 Medical Board Minutes, May 7, 1886; vol. IV, April 2, 1897, September 3, 1897.
56 Eva Beecroft, "Seeking Institutional Positions," p. 153.
57 See, for example, James, "Isabel Hampton and the Professionalization of Nursing in the 1890s," and Nancy Tomes, " 'Little World of Our Own': The Pennsylvania Hospital Training School For Nurses, 1895–1907," *Journal of the History of Medicine* 33 (October 1978): 507–30. For further discussion of differences among schools, see Chapter 5.
58 Nutting, *Educational Status of Nursing*, p. 49.

CHAPTER 5 *"Strangers to Boston": who becomes a nurse*

1 There is a growing literature on changes in working women's options at the turn of the twentieth century. For overviews see Alice Kessler-Harris, *Out to Work* (New York: Oxford University Press, 1982), and Sarah Eisenstein, *Give Us Bread But Give Us Roses* (Boston: Routledge and Kegan Paul, 1983); and Lynn W. Weiner, *From the Working Girl to the Working Mother* (Durham: University of North Carolina Press, 1985).
2 Boston City Hospital Training School Records (hereafter cited as BCH Student Records), Boston City Hospital Training School Papers, Nursing Archives, Mugar Library, Boston University. These records come from a sample of the graduates of Boston City Hospital's training school (see discussion of this sample in the Appendix). The names have been changed, but the record numbers are retained. See Box 4, Folder 4, Student 4, February 14, 1880; Box 14, Folder 7, Student 3, January 17, 1899; Box 24, Folder 4, Student 1.
3 See Cindy S. Aron, " 'To Barter Their Souls for Gold': Female Clerks in Federal Government Offices, 1862–1890," *Journal of American History* 67 (March 1981): 835–53.
4 Julia Wells, "Do Hospitals Fit Nurses for Private Nursing?" *TNHR* 3 (March 1890): 98. The reasons why women entered nursing are obviously complex and different. For an examination of students entering the training schools at Johns Hopkins and Pennsylvania hospitals, respectively, see Janet Wilson James, "Isabel Hampton and the Professionalization of Nursing in the 1890s," in *The Therapeutic Revolution*, ed. Morris Vogel and Charles E. Rosenberg (Philadelphia: University of Pennsylvania Press, 1979), pp. 201–44, and Nancy Tomes, " 'Little World of Our Own': The Pennsylvania Hospital Training School for Nurses, 1895–1907," *Journal of the History of Medicine* 33 (October 1978): 507–30. For a comparison of a group of nursing *leaders* and women physicians, see Susan Armeny, " 'We Were the New Women': A Comparison of Nurses and Women Physicians, 1890–1915" (Paper presented at the American Association for the History of Nursing Conference, University of Virginia, Charlottesville, October 1984).
5 See Jane Hodson, ed., *How to Become a Trained Nurse* (New York: Abbatt, 1898), p. 145. This volume is a valuable source of both qualitative and quantitative information on training schools in the United States at the end of the nineteenth century.
6 Florence Nightingale to Dr. Farr, September 13, 1866, quoted in Cecil Woodham-Smith, *Florence Nightingale* (London: Constable, 1950), p. 483; Virginia M. Dunbar, "The Origin and Development of Two English Training Schools for Nurses"

(Master's thesis, University of London, 1936), p. 22. See also Christopher Maggs, *The Origins of General Nursing* (London: Croom Helm, 1983), for an excellent discussion on the class background of British nurses.

There was also a two-class system in the Nightingale system in England, based on class and ability to pay for training. There were separate categories of "probationers" and "lady-pupils." Lady-pupils from the upper and upper-middle classes were given special treatment and training and were expected to take the more superior hospital positions. The "daughters of small farmers and domestic servants" became the nursing rank and file in both hospital and private-duty work. In January 1875, for example, Alice Fisher, the daughter of a noted astronomer and educator, entered the Nightingale School at St. Thomas's Hospital in London as a lady-probationer, while her maid Emma entered as a nurse-probationer. Fisher went on to be enshrined in nursing history as the first nursing superintendent at the Pennsylvania Hospital in Philadelphia; the nursing histories do not yet record Emma's last name or her fate. See Victor Robinson, *White Caps: The Story of Nursing* (Philadelphia: Lippincott, 1946), p. 258.

7 Lucy Catlin, "The Training School Problem," *NHR* 11 (December 1907): 42.

8 For a methodological discussion, see the Appendix.

9 For information on students at Massachusetts General, albeit only for 125 women entering between 1888 and 1891, see Janet James, "Isabel Hampton and the Professionalization of Nursing in the 1890s." For similar data on nursing students at the Pennsylvania Hospital, see Tomes, " 'Little World of Our Own.' " Jane Mottus devotes a sixty-page chapter of her book to the students who entered the program at Bellevue and New York Hospitals; see *New York Nightingales: The Emergence of the Nursing Profession at Bellevue and New York Hospitals, 1850–1920* (Ann Arbor, Mich.: University Microfilms Books, 1981). All of these schools were more elite, however, than the hospital training programs under consideration in this sample. Thus these schools had stricter entrance requirements, more educational components to their training, and attracted a higher number of educated women.

10 Under pressure from nursing leaders, trained nursing was finally separated from untrained nursing and midwifery in the national census by 1900. However, it makes comparisons of nativity *before* the twentieth century difficult. See John D. Durand, *The Labor Force in the United States, 1890–1960* (New York: Social Science Research Council, 1948), pp. 209–16; Abba M. Edwards, *16th Census of the U.S.: 1940 Population, Comparative Occupation Statistics for the U.S., 1870–1940* (Washington, D.C.: Government Printing Office, 1943), p. 166.

11 John Murray Gibbon and Mary S. Mathewson, *Three Centuries of Canadian Nursing* (Toronto: Macmillan of Canada, 1947). In a mail survey of nursing students in ten states (including Massachusetts) done for nursing's Grading Committee survey in 1927, nurses were asked about their father's birthplace. The responses were then compared to census figures for white males of voting age in the United States in 1900. Twelve percent of the sample had Canadian-born fathers, as compared to 3 percent in the male 1900 population; 17 percent had fathers born in the British Isles, as compared to 7 percent in the general population. The figures did not differentiate between Irish and British births, nor did it take into account whether the British and Irish daughters had been raised in the United States or Canada; see Grading Committee, *Nurses, Patients and Pocketbooks* (1928; reprint, New York: Garland, 1984), p. 240. There is no study of this migration pattern, although its existence has been noted by nursing historians.

For more on this Maritime migration to Boston, see D. J. McDonald, *Population Migration and Economic Development in the Atlantic Provinces* (Fredericton, New Brunswick: Atlantic Provinces Economic Council, 1968), p. 34; S. A. Saunders, *The Economic History of the Maritime Provinces* (Ottawa, 1937); Gregory Kealey et al., "Canada's 'Eastern Question': A Reader's Guide to Regional Underdevelopment," *Canadian Dimension* 13 (1978): 37–40; David Frank, "The Nine Myths of Regional Disparity," ibid.: 18–19; Alan Brookes, "Out-Migration from the Maritime Provinces, 1860–1900," *Acadiensis* 5, 2 (1976): 42.

12 This information on McLaughlin (a pseudonym) is taken from her student records at Waltham (which I was able to examine preliminarily before they were destroyed; see the Appendix) and my interview with her in Somerville, Massachusetts, January 27, 1980. Student records often included recommendation letters that stated the woman was from "a very respectable country family" or "good country stock." For a very similar work history, see records of Margaret Corey (pseud.), Somerville Hospital, 1918–21, Somerville Hospital School of Nursing Records.

13 BCH Student Records, Box 10, Folder 7, Student 1; Box 5, Folder 8, Student 4; and Box 21, Folder 1, Student 1. In the latter case, the student was from Ontario, and the assistant superintendent who made the comments, Mary Riddle, had grown up on an Iowa farm.

    For a discussion of the male side of the country myth see E. Richard Wohl, "The 'Country Boy' Myth and Its Place in American Urban Culture: The Nineteenth-Century Contribution," ed. Moses Rischin, *Perspectives in American History* 3 (1969): 86.

14 The census at the time used populations of 2,500 or over to designate an urban area. However, such a population figure obscures the question of whether nursing students came from small towns and cities. I have therefore used the population-density characteristics as has Tomes in " 'Little World of Our Own.' " In Tables 5.2 and 5.4, "urban" should be read as referring to areas with populations over 10,000.

15 Yet a small comparison to the nursing sample to a group of women clerical workers in Boston suggests that the nurses were more rural in origin. In a sample drawn from the 1880 and 1900 census for Boston, historian Carol Srole found that slightly over 50 percent of the clerical workers in both censuses had been born in Boston. This is clearly much higher than for all the nurses in the Boston training schools sample. Of the 143 nursing students in the Boston schools sample who had previously worked in some kind of clerical occupation, less than 10 percent were born in Boston and only 30 percent had been born in other urban areas. There was no statistically significant shift over time. As with the rest of the nursing school sample, nearly a third of these former clerical workers were born in the Maritimes.

    The data on clerical workers were provided by Srole (Carol Srole to Susan Reverby, March 12, 1980) from her dissertation, " 'A Position That God Has Not Particularly Assigned to Men': The Feminization of Clerical Work, Boston, 1869–1915" (Ph.D. diss., Department of History, University of California at Los Angeles, 1984). The number of former clerical workers in the nursing sample was too small to usefully draw only those from 1880 and 1890, and I have therefore used all 143 in the entire sample.

    For further demographic and class information on clerical workers see Roslyn L. Feldberg and Evelyn Nakano Glenn, "Who Sits behind the Desk: An Exploration of Class Origins of Women Clerical Workers" (Unpublished paper, February 1978, Department of Sociology, Boston University). An earlier version of the paper was given at the American Studies Association Annual Meeting, October 1977.

16 See Bengt Ankerloo, "Agriculture and Women's Work: Directions of Change in the West, 1700–1900," *Journal of Family History* 4 (Summer 1979): 111–20; Roberta Balstad Miller, *City and Hinterland: A Case Study of Urban Growth and Regional Development* (Westport, Conn.: Greenwood, 1979), pp. 110–29; and Stephen Thernstrom, *The Other Bostonians* (Cambridge, Mass.: Harvard University Press, 1973), p. 17. The nursing student records can tell us if a student moved from her birthplace to somewhere else before she applied for training, but not much more about her migration. Such information would entail very precise record linkages beyond the scope of this current work. For an example of such a study, see Thomas Dublin, "The Social Origins and Consequences of Urban Migration: Migrants and Nonmigrants from Three New Hampshire Towns" (Paper presented at the annual meeting of the Social Science History Association, Cambridge, Mass., November 1979). I am grateful to Tom Dublin and Johnny Faragher for help in this section.

17 Richard Hofstadter, *The Age of Reform* (New York: Knopf, 1955), p. 23. Ruralness may have had more meaning in other parts of the country. A 1927 survey of rural women working in Richmond, Virginia, and Durham, North Carolina, suggests this pattern in the twentieth century. Directors of the training schools in the two cities were asked about their students. In Durham, the superintendents reported that three-quarters of their students came from areas of "open country and from very small villages and towns." Only one out of ten hospital schools in Richmond reported that an appreciable proportion of its students were from the city. O. Latham Hatcher, *Rural Girls in the City for Work* (Richmond, Va.: Garrett and Massie, 1930), p. 59.

18 Adelaide Nulting, *Educational Status of Nursing*, U.S. Bureau of Education Bulletin no. 7, 1912, whole no. 475 (Washington, D.C.: Government Printing Office, 1912), pp. 70–73.

19 Ibid.

20 Grading Committee, *Nurses, Patients and Pocketbooks*, pp. 251–53.

21 Mary Cawalader Jones, "The Training of a Nurse," *TNHR* 6 (January 1891): 16.

22 Anon., "The Present Curriculum from the Point of View of the Nurse," from the Semiannual Meeting of the New England Association for the Education of Nurses, *TNHR* 22 (April 1907): 221. Hatcher's interviews in 1930 with rural-born working women in Richmond and Durham revealed that nearly all of those who had wanted to do something else had wanted to be nurses (*Rural Girls in the City for Work*, p. 38). The necessity of giving up income to train or fear of the training blocked these women from reaching this goal.

23 See, for example, Lucy Drown to Margaret Hopkins, September 22, 1909, BCH Correspondence Book, Parsons Papers, Nursing Archives.

24 BCH Student Records, Mugar Library, Boston University, Box 5, Folder 8, Student 4; Box 2, Folder 4, Student 2.

25 Ibid., Box 2, Folder 8, Student 3.

26 Similarly, Cindy Aron's sample of 354 women in federal clerical positions as listed in the 1880 census similarly found that 44.9 percent had fathers who were deceased (Aron to Susan Reverby, February 25, 1980).

27 W. Gill Wylie, *Hospitals: Their History, Organization and Construction* (New York: Appleton, 1877), p. 79; Lavinia L. Dock and M. Adelaide Nutting, *A History of Nursing*, vol. 2 (New York: Putnam, 1912), p. 398; Sara E. Parsons, *History of the Massachusetts General Hospital Training School for Nurses* (Boston: Whitcomb and Barrows, 1922), pp. 19–20. For a more modern history of Bellevue, see Jane Mottus, *New York Nightingales*, and on the Massachusetts General school, see Sylvia Perkins, *A Centennial Review* (Boston: School of Nursing, Nurses' Alumnae Association, 1975).

28 James, "Isabel Hampton and the Professionalization of Nursing in the 1890s," p. 214; Mottus, *New York Nightingales*, p. 216.

29 Roslyn Feldberg and Evelyn Nakano Glenn conclude an examination of the class origins of clerical workers between 1900 and 1920 with the comment that "overall, what is striking about clerical workers is not the level of their class origins (they are somewhat less middle class than the descriptive literature suggests), but that their origins span so wide a range of the class structure" (p. 18). These findings are consonant with mine on nurses and raises again the difficulty of using occupation as an index of class, particularly in women's occupations because of "crowding" due to sex segregation. Thus, generalizations about the class background of nursing students will have to consider the *range* and the differences among schools. To try to portray a "typical" student, therefore, often conceals as much as it might reveal.

30 Mottus, *New York Nightingales*, p. 209. These differences between the Boston sample and New York Hospital also hold in the comparison to other elite schools, although such samples were done for much shorter time spans. James's analysis of students between 1889 and 1893 at Johns Hopkins revealed that "most were simply restless, tired of domestic responsibilities . . . or hard work . . . in such genteel

occupations as teaching and giving lessons in music and language, or serving as companions and housekeepers to the aged" ("Isabel Hampton and the Professionalization of Nursing," pp. 214–15). At the training school at Pennsylvania Hospital in the decade 1898–1909, Tomes found that only half the students had worked. Of the remaining women (N = 102), 45 percent had been teachers, 21 percent clerical workers, and 5 percent had worked in the sewing trades (" 'Little World of Our Own,' " p. 519). In contrast, for the comparable decade at BCH (1900–9, N = 87), less than a third of the students came to training directly from home. Although the number of clerical workers was comparable to Pennsylvania, only 22 percent of the BCH women had been teachers, and a much larger number had worked in the sewing trades.

31 Mottus, *New York Nightingales,* p. 211. In the Boston sample, there were only two domestic servants and eighteen housekeepers.

32 Mary Riddle, *Boston City Hospital Training School for Nurses* (Boston: City Hospital Alumnae Association, 1928), pp. 17–21. See also, "Memorial to Rosa McCormick," *TNHR* 20 (April 1898): 217.

33 BCH Student Records, Box 12, Folder 4, Student 2; Annette Fiske, *The First Fifty Years of the Waltham Training School for Nurses,* Waltham Papers, Nursing Archives, Mugar Library, Boston University (New York: Garland, 1985).

34 Domestic service did not become as much a black woman's occupation in Boston because there were relatively fewer blacks, and more Irish, than in other urban areas; see David Katzman, *Seven Days a Week: Women and Domestic Service in Industrializing America* (New York: Oxford University Press, 1978).

35 Somerville Hospital School of Nursing Student Records, Somerville, Mass.

36 John Mack Faragher, "Sister Carrie's Sisters: White Country Girls in the City of Chicago, 1880–1930" (Unpublished paper, Mt. Holyoke College, 1984). I am grateful to this author for sending me his paper.

37 Conference Committee Minute Book, December 30, 1882, New York Hospital Archives.

38 Christine R. Kefauver, "What Is the Matter with the Training Schools?" *TNHR* 64 (August 1920): 114.

39 Mary Riddle, "How to Obtain, Keep and Properly Instruct the Nurse," *AJN* 12 (December 1911): 180.

40 Christine Russell, letter to the editor, *AJN* 7 (June 1907): 716; "Romance Is Gone in Nursing the Sick," *Boston Herald,* June 9, 1907, clipping in MGH Scrapbook, Massachusetts General Hospital papers, Countway Library, Harvard Medical School, Boston, Mass.

41 Albert Wolfe, *The Lodging House Problem in Boston* (Cambridge: Harvard University Press, 1913), p. 82; Anna S. Richardson, *The Girl Who Earns Her Own Living* (New York: Dodge, 1909), p. 282, quoted in Sheila Rothman, *Woman's Proper Place* (New York: Basic, 1978), p. 43. On the general question of the cultural concern with the young working woman in the city see Weiner, *From the Working Girl to the Working Mother;* Faragher, "Sister Carrie's Sisters"; and Joanne J. Meyerowitz, "Holding Their Own: Working Women Apart from Family in Chicago, 1880–1930" (Ph.D. diss., Stanford University, 1983).

42 A Superintendent, "A Few Joys in Store for the Pupil Nurse," *NHR* 12 (January 15, 1908): 25–26.

43 Charlotte Aikens, "Some Opportunities for Young Women Outside the Nursing Field," *NHR* 13 (April 1, 1908): 3–4, and (April 15, 1908): 3–4. On the advantages of the nurses' homes, see Hampton, *Educational Standards for Nurses,* p. 25.

44 *End of the Road,* by Katherine Bemont Davis, Washington, D.C., National Archives; for a discussion of the film see Allan M. Brandt, *No Magic Bullets: A Social History of Venereal Disease* (New York: Oxford University Press, 1985).

45 On the issue of sexuality and nursing, particularly as viewed in the wider culture, see Barbara Melosh, *"The Physician's Hand"* (Philadelphia: Temple University Press, 1982).

46 See M. Adelaide Nutting, "How Can We Attract Suitable Applicants to Our

Training Schools for Nurses," in her *A Sound Economic Basis for Schools of Nursing* (New York: Putnam, 1926), pp. 154–85; Kefauver, "What Is the Matter with the Training Schools," discussion, *SS 1912*, p. 136; Mary L. Keith, "Report of the Sub-Committee on Training of Nurses," *NHR* 11 (February 1908): 6–11.

47 Christine Russell, letter to the editor, *AJN* (June 1907): 716. Twenty years later, nursing's Grading Committee concluded: "It is unfortunate that the public sometimes regards the nursing school as a sort of respectable reform school, where its mental or disciplinary cases can be sent. When a girl won't mind her mother, is beginning to stay-out late at night, refuses to go on with her high school work, and in general becomes a family problem, not infrequently the school authorities say to the mother: 'Why don't you put your daughter into a hospital training school? The girls are kept under very careful supervision there, and the discipline is just the thing she needs' " (*Nurses, Patients and Pocketbooks*, p. 441). The schools had now become the female equivalent of being sent into the army.

48 Kefauver, "What Is the Matter with the Training Schools?" p. 16. For a general discussion of the problem reformers had in getting young working women to accept their protection, see Weiner, *From Working Girl to Working Mother;* Margaret Gibbons Wilson, *The American Woman in Transition* (Westport, Conn.: Greenwood, 1979); Faragher, "Sister Carrie's Sisters"; and Sarah Eisenstein, *Give Us Bread But Give Us Roses* (Boston: Routledge and Kegan Paul, 1983).

49 "Romance Is Gone in Nursing the Sick," clipping. For a discussion of this change for college-educated women, see Carroll Smith-Rosenberg, "The New Woman as Androgyne," in *Disorderly Conduct* (New York: Knopf, 1985), pp. 245–96.

50 On the *Ladies' Home Journal* article, see "Are Hospital Nurses Underfed?" *NHR* 10 (October 1906): 48–49, and letters to the editor, November 1906, pp. 49–50 and December 1906, p. 15; "Romance Is Gone in Nursing the Sick," clipping.

51 Dorothy Dunbar Bromley, "The Crisis in Nursing," *Harper's Magazine,* July 1930, reprinted in *AJN* 30 (July 1930): 913–14.

52 Nutting, *Educational Status of Nursing,* p. 26. See also "Floating Nurses" (editorial) *NHR* 8 (September 1904): 6–7.

53 "Publicity for the Training Schools," *TNHR* 63 (November 1918): 298.

54 Nutting, "Some Problems of the Training Schools," *NHR* 12 (November 1908): 6. See also James, "Isabel Hampton and the Professionalization of Nursing," p. 234.

55 See Isabel Hampton Robb's discussion of the paper by Mary A. Samuel, "Economy in Hospital Work," *AJN* 5 (June 1905): 577; Evelina MacRae, letter to the editor, *TNHR* 66 (March 1921): 247; "The Character Requirement of the Nurse," *TNHR* 66 (April 1921): 433; St. Thomas, letter to the editor, *TNHR* 67 (January 1924): 72.

CHAPTER 6 *Nursing as work: divisions in the occupation*

1 Gertrude Harding, *The Higher Aspects of Nursing* (Philadelphia: Saunders, 1919), p. 109; Sara E. Parsons, *Nursing Problems and Obligations* (Boston: Barrows, 1916), p. 115. Much of this section draws on my article, " 'Neither for the Drawing Room nor for the Kitchen': Private Duty Nursing in Boston, 1873–1914," in *Women and Health in America,* ed. Judith Walzer Leavitt (Madison: University of Wisconsin Press, 1984), pp. 454–66. See also Barbara Melosh, *"The Physician's Hand"* (Philadelphia: Temple University Press, 1982), pp. 77–111.

2 Charlotte Aikens, *Studies in Ethics for Nurses* (Philadelphia: Saunders, 1916), p. 291; Isabel Hampton Robb, *Nursing Ethics: For Hospital and Private Use* (Cleveland: Savage, 1901); Anne Hintz, "On Business Principles," *TNHR* 15 (July 1895): 1–3.

3 See E. B. M., letter to the editor of the *Transcript,* October 24, 1881, clipping in vol. B, *Boston Medical Library (BML) Directory for Nurses' Records,* Rare Books Room, Countway Library, Harvard Medical School, Boston.
  Information on the work histories of private-duty nurses was drawn from a sys-

tematic sample of 539 nurses, 313 trained nurses and 226 untrained nurses, who registered at the BML Directory between 1880 and 1914. This directory, except in its closing years, represented anywhere from one-third to three-quarters of the nurses in Boston as accounted for by the census. The directory registered 4,550 nurses during its thirty-four years of existence. For further discussion of this sample, see " 'Neither for the Drawing Room nor for the Kitchen.' "

4 *Nursing Ethics*, p. 32. I am particularly grateful to Joan Brumberg for her thoughtful comments on this section.

5 These statements are based on a random sample of 100 patients who hired nurses through the *BML Directory* between 1880 and 1914. The occupations of the male patients, or males in the family of the patient, were obtained from the *Boston City Directory* for the appropriate years. The class base of those who used the services of private-duty nurses continued to be an issue in nursing and health care. For further discussion of the problem, see Chapter 9.

6 *BML Directory for Nurses Records;* Jane Mottus, *New York Nightingales: The Emergence of the Nursing Profession at Bellevue and New York Hospitals, 1850–1920* (Ann Arbor, Mich.: University Microfilms Books, 1981), pp. 289–90. It is difficult to calculate how much private-duty nurses actually made a year because they were notoriously bad at keeping such records. How much they made, of course, was directly related to how many cases they could get and how long the cases lasted.

7 Brennan Gill, *The Trouble of One House* (Garden City, N.Y.: Doubleday, 1950), p. 142. This quotation was given to me by Barbara Melosh.

8 Dr. J. Madison Taylor, letter to the editor, *AJN* 4 (May 1904): 659; Emily Stoney, *Practical Points in Nursing for Nurses in Private Practice,* 2d ed. (Philadelphia: Saunders, 1897), p. 24. For a parallel discussion of domestic service, see Faye Dudden, *Serving Women* (Middletown, Conn.: Wesleyan University Press, 1983).

9 Philadelphia, letter to the editor, *TNHR* 8 (September 1892): 278.

10 William L. Richardson, *Address on the Duties and Conduct of Nurses in Private Nursing* (Boston: Ellis, 1886), p. 10. Richardson's address must have been very popular because it was printed and widely circulated.

11 Annie E. Hutchison, "Practical Nursing in Private Practice," *TNHR* 37 (August 1906): 83. "Don't imagine that you can discipline a patient in his own home as you would in a hospital ward. It can't be done," the *Trained Nurse* cautioned. "Don'ts for the Private Duty Nurse," *TNHR* 47 (October 1911): 202.

12 Katherine Dewitt, *Private Duty Nursing* (Philadelphia: Lippincott, 1917), p. 70.

13 Hutchinson, "Practical Nursing," p. 84.

14 This is discussed more fully later in this chapter. The lack of wage differentiation between graduates was probably a function of both the difficulty of finding an equitable basis for evaluating skill and the efforts to differentiate between trained and untrained nurses. Where a registry was not a factor, doctors' choices often determined the nurse who received the most work.

15 Janet M. Geister, "Hearsay and Fact in Private Duty," *AJN* 26 (July 1926): 520. For further discussion of Geister, see my " 'Something Besides Waiting': The Politics of Private Duty Nursing Reform in the Depression," in *Nursing History: New Perspectives, New Possibilities,* ed. Ellen Condliffe Lagemann (New York: Teachers College Press, 1983).

16 See letter and newspaper clippings in the volumes of the BML Directory of Nurses Records.

17 This is not to suggest that the untrained nurses willingly did whatever the family wanted. One such nurse, for example, complained that families expected her to do the "spring housecleaning" along with the nursing. A Graduate of the Training School of Life, letter to the editor, *TNHR* 51 (March 1916): 369.

18 "The Path of Duty," *AJN* 4 (October 1904): 2.

19 Mottus (*New York Nightingales:* p. 262) contends that her data do not support the assertion by other historians that by the 1890s nursing was overcrowded and nurses were looking for other work. Less than 2 percent of her graduates left nursing for other work. Although these graduates may still have defined them-

selves as nurses, this does not obviate the issue of overcrowding as perceived by the women at the time, as a cursory reading of *Trained Nurse* in these years attests. Mottus has let the quantitative evidence blind her to the qualitative sources on this question. There was, for example, a precipitous drop in the demand for nurses during the initial years of the 1890s depression in the BML Directory (figures calculated from the raw data on the number of nurses requested each month, 1891–1914, in the *BML Directory Letterbook* BML Directory for Nurses Papers).

20 Data on the number of nurses available to work, by type of training, were compared to the number, by type of training, who actually did the work, for the years 1889–93. The raw data for this calculation can be found in the *BML Directory Letterbook*. Using the entire sample, there was also a statistically significant difference between training and the total number of cases received throughout the directory at the 0.01 level.

21 B. H. Giles to the directory, March 10, 1895, vol. F, *BML Directory of Nurses Records*, p. 176. For examples of letters that also reflect the nurses' bitterness at the lack of work, see Emilie Neale to Dr. Brigham, January 8, 1894; Dr. Putnam to Miss MacBrien, February 24, 1900, *BML Directory Letterbook*.

E. M. Walsh, for example, wrote Miss MacBrien at the directory in 1896: "I am discouraged staying in waiting for something to do. I have had only a few weeks on a cheap case since before Thanksgiving so you can see how much employment I have in a year" (Walsh to MacBrien, March 6, 1891, *BML Directory Letterbook*).

22 Letter to the editor, *PCNJ* 10 (March 1914): 130. In contrast, however, Waltham Graduate Nora Connolly spent nineteen years with one Boston family; see Annette Fiske, compiler, *A History of the Graduates of the Waltham Training School for Nurses* (Waltham: Waltham Graduate Nurses' Association, 1937), p. 130. I am grateful to Mrs. Virginia Bird of the Waltham Graduate Nurses' Association for lending me her copy of this history, an invaluable source of the short biographies of nearly all of the school's 776 graduates. It is now in the Waltham Training School Papers in the Nursing Archives, Mugar Library, Boston University, Boston, Mass.

23 These case rates were calculated from averages in the *BML Directory* sample. On the Cleveland nurse's experience, see James H. Rodabaugh and Mary Jane Rodabaugh, *Nursing in Ohio* (Columbus: Ohio State Nurses' Association, 1951), pp. 199–200.

24 Monthly deployments were calculated from figures in the *BML Directory Letterbook*. Massachusetts data for 1890 were compiled from the 1890 census and given to me by Alex Keyssar from his study of unemployment in Massachusetts; see Alexander Keyssar, *Out to Work: The First Century of Unemployment in Massachusetts* (Cambridge: Cambridge University Press, 1986). Unemployment frequency was calculated by dividing the total unemployed by the total number in the occupation. Unfortunately, these numbers include both untrained and trained nurses, as well as midwives.

25 Louise Marion Bosworth, *The Living Wage of Women Workers* (New York: Longmans, Green, 1911), pp. 33–39.

26 Letter to the editor, *PCNJ* (March 1914): 130; see also Fiske, *Waltham Training School for Nurses*, and letters in the *BML Directory for Nurses Records and Letterbook*.

27 Nursing educator Lavinia Dock, for example, lectured nurses: "We must not undersell; that is treachery to fellow workers." Quoted in A. S. Kavanaugh, "The Indispensable Combination in Hospital Work," *TNHR* 37 (January 1914): 75.

A private-duty nurse who secured her own cases did not, of course, have to adhere to an agreed wage rate. But it was considered a "breach of faith" with the directory for a nurse to overcharge the patients when she had agreed on one price (see Morton Prince to Miss C. C. MacBrien, February 12, 1901, *BML Directory Letterbook*). However, such overcharging was not uncommon. (See also ibid.; An Independent Nurse, letter to the editor, *TNHR* 43 [January 1908]: 58; Florence LaFleur in vol. R, p. 66, and L. M. B. Russell in vol. I, p. 58, *BML Directory for Nurses Records*.)

28 A Graduate, letter to the editor, *TNHR* 15 (January 1895): 43.
29 On blacklists, see memo from Dr. George H. M. Rowe, superintendent of Boston City Hospital to the directory, no date; numerous other letters in 1892, *BML Directory Letterbook.*
30 Letter to the editor, *TNHR* 23 (February 1904): 103.
31 "Private Duty Problems," *TNHR* 73 (July 1924): 57–58.
32 For further discussion of the registry problem and possible solutions, see Reverby, " 'Something Besides Waiting.' "
33 Committee on the Grading of Nursing Schools, *Nurses, Patients and Pocketbooks* (1928; reprint, New York: Garland, 1984), p. 361.
34 Lavinia Dock, "Overcrowding in the Nursing Profession," *TNHR* 21 (July 1898): 8–13.
35 Lucy Drown to Dr. Brigham, October 18, 1899, *BML Directory Letterbook.*
36 William Abbott, "Where the Superintendents Come From," *NHR* 1 (May 1898): 4. Abbott based his figures on data in Jane Hodson, ed., *How to Become a Trained Nurse* (New York: Abbatt, 1898). See further discussion later in this chapter on the effect of different schools on career options.
37 The biographies of such nursing leaders as Isabel Hampton, Adelaide Nutting, Irene Sutcliffe, S. Lillian Clayton, and Laura Logan confirm these patterns; see Meta Pennock, ed., *Makers of Nursing History* (New York: Lakeside, 1940).
38 "Vocational Opportunities for Nurses," *TNHR* 56 (February 1916): 107.
39 *Nurses, Patients and Pocketbooks*, pp. 364–72.
40 Ibid., p. 374; "Vocational Opportunities for Nurses"; Mottus, *New York Nightingales*, pp. 289–90.
41 Pennock, *Makers of Nursing History*, pp. 100–1. Goodnow is best remembered for her nursing history text, which went through numerous editions; see *Outlines of Nursing History* (Philadelphia: Saunders, 1916). Her last superintendency was at the Somerville Hospital School of Nursing.
42 Margaret West and Christy Hawkins, *Nursing Schools at the Mid-Century* (New York: National League for Nursing, 1950).
43 Adelaide Nutting, "American Hospital Association," *TNHR* 28 (October 1909): 242; "Conference on the Training of Hospital Administrators," called by the Officers of the Rockefeller Foundation, Hotel Commodore, New York, February 27, 1920, M. Adelaide Nutting Papers, Teachers College Archives, Columbia University, Cabinet X, Drawer 4.
44 C. J. Parnell, "The Selection and Organization of Hospital Personnel," *TAHA, 1920*, p. 101.
45 W. L. Babcock et al., "Proposed Method for Training Hospital Administrators: A Report to the American Hospital Association," *MH* 1 (March 1913): 176–78.
46 Michael Davis, *Hospital Administration: A Career* (New York: n.p., 1929), p. 35.
47 Michael Davis, "The Nurse in Hospital Administration," *AJN* 36 (June 1936): 561–63.
48 "Charlotte Aikens – One of *Trained Nurse*'s Own Editors," *TNHR* 123 (December 1949): 279. Unfortunately, there is no history of the replacement of women and nurses by male administrators. The occasional photographs of the delegates to the American Hospital Association meetings give some sense of the shifting percentage of women and men in the field over the years. For a more recent examination of women administrators, see Jerry L. Weaver and Sharon D. Garrett, "Sexism and Racism in the American Health Care Industry: A Comparative Analysis," *International Journal of Health Services* 8 (1978): 691–92.
49 Aikens, "Institutional Nursing," *TNHR* 45 (August 1910): 105–6; (September 1910): 181–82; (October 1910): 36–39; "Vocational Opportunities for Nurses."
50 Charles Emerson, "The American Hospital Field," in *Hospital Management*, ed. Charlotte Aikens (1911; reprint, New York: Garland, 1985), p. 63.
51 Dr. Brigham to Dr. Putnam, November 3, 1899, *BML Directory Letterbook*. For the nurses' complaints about this, see Alice Lincoln to Dr. E. W. Taylor, October 23, 1899, and Frances Norse to E. W. Taylor, January 1, 1899, *Long Island Hospital*

Letterbook, volume I, Long Island Hospital Collection, Rare Books Room, Countway Library, Harvard Medical School, Boston, Mass.

52 Minutes of the Medical Staff, New England Hospital Papers, Box 6, Folder 18, Sophia Smith Archives, Smith College, Northampton, Mass.

53 Emma Nichols to Dr. Francis Kenny, September 11, 1911, and Ellen C. Daly to Dr. John J. Dowling, January 1, 1920, *Boston City Hospital School of Nursing Correspondence Book,* Marion Parsons Papers, Nursing Archives, Mugar Library, Boston University.

54 Grading Committee, *Nurses, Patients and Pocketbooks,* p. 281. See also similar comments on p. 278.

55 Ibid., pp. 270–75. However, because the survey did not differentiate between levels of nurses in institutional work, it is impossible to discern if these opinions are those of staff nurses or women in positions of more authority.

56 Report of the Training School Committee, July 25, 1906, Secretary-Treasurer's Papers, New York Hospital Archives, New York. For other complaints, see Theodore MacClure, "Problems in the Management of Small Hospitals," *TAHA, 1908,* p. 206; Grading Committee, *Nurses, Patients and Pocketbooks,* p. 410.

57 Grading Committee, *Nurses, Patients and Pocketbooks,* p. 412.

58 Ellen C. Daly to Dr. John J. Dowling, November 9, 1928, *Boston City Hospital School of Nursing Correspondence Book.*

59 Daly (ibid.), for example, suggested such nurses' wages should be raised to $90 a month for the first year, $95 for the second, and $110 for those with five years of continuous service. See also, "Vocational Opportunities for Nurses."

60 Miss C. E. S. Somerville, "District Nursing," in Isabel Hampton et al., *Nursing the Sick 1893* (New York: McGraw-Hill, 1949), p. 120. Two contemporary histories of public-health nursing are Ysabella Waters, *Visiting Nursing in the United States* (Philadelphia: Fell, 1909), and Mary Gardner, *Public Health Nursing* (New York: Macmillan, 1915). The latter book underwent two revisions, reflecting changes in the issues within public-health nursing.

   More recent histories of this practice field include M. Louise Fitzpatrick, *The National Organization of Public Health Nursing* (New York: National League for Nursing, 1975); Karen Buhler-Wilkerson, "False Dawn: The Rise and Decline of Public Health Nursing" (Ph.D. diss., University of Pennsylvania, 1984); Barbara Melosh, "*The Physician's Hand,*" pp. 113–58.

61 Gardner, *Public Health Nursing,* p. 20.

62 Harriet Fulmer, "History of Visiting Nurse Work in America," *AJN* 2 (March 1902): 412. This is the best survey of visiting nurse work in the country at the time. See also Buhler-Wilkerson, "False Dawn."

63 Mabel Reid, "1938 Census of Public Health Nurses," *Public Health Nursing* 30 (November 1938): 632–35; Karen Buhler-Wilkerson, "False Dawn: The Rise and Decline of Public Health Nursing in America," in Lagemann, *Nursing History,* pp. 89–106.

64 For a brief discussion of the problem of practice models, see Karen Buhler-Wilkerson and Susan Reverby, "Can a Time-Honored Model Solve the Dilemma of Public Health Nursing?" guest editorial, *American Journal of Public Health* 74 (October 1984): 1081–82.

65 Grading Committee, *Nurses, Patients and Pocketbooks,* p. 264.

66 Ibid., p. 305; "Vocational Opportunities for Nurses," *TNHR* 56 (March 1916): 163.

67 Fulmer, "History of Visiting Nurse Work in America," p. 415.

68 Grading Committee, *Nurses, Patients and Pocketbooks,* p. 210.

69 For a discussion of why public-health nursing did not grow, see Buhler-Wilkerson, "False Dawn."

70 The Grading Committee's figures in 1928 are the first nationally available data on where the nurses were working. The figures here are thus estimates of the various nursing schools. See also Mottus, *New York Nightingales,* Chapter 6, and Susan

Armeny, "Resistance to Professionalization by American Trained Nurses, 1890–1905" (Paper presented at the Fourth Berkshire Conference on the History of Women, Mt. Holyoke College, South Hadley, Mass., August 25, 1978), p. 5. Armeny suggests in the 1890s that between 75 and 80 percent of all nurses were working in private duty. See also "Vocational Opportunities for Nurses," *TNHR* 56 (February 1916): 107–8, and (March 1916): 163–64.

71 Grading Committee, *Nurses, Patients and Pocketbooks*, p. 250.
72 Fiske, *Waltham Training School for Nurses*, pp. 7, 58–59, 64.
73 Quoted in "Who Started It?" *TNHR* 49 (November 1912): 298–99.
74 Philip A. Kalisch and Beatrice J. Kalisch, *The Advance of American Nursing* (Boston: Little, Brown, 1978), p. 191.
75 Until 1900, trained and untrained nurses were enumerated together. However, the 1900 figures did not give trained nurses' age or marital status separately. See Janet Hooks, "Women's Occupations through Seven Decades," *Women's Bureau Bulletin,* no. 218 (Washington, D.C.: Government Printing Office, 1947), pp. 149 and 163. BML data are from the sample.
76 See discussion in Barbara Harris, *Beyond Her Sphere: Women and the Professions in American History* (Westport, Conn.: Greenwood, 1978), pp. 101–2; Sheila M. Rothman, *Woman's Proper Place* (New York: Basic Books, 1978), pp. 44–47, 85–90, 221–24.

    In its survey in the late 1920s, the Grading Committee compared nurses' marriage rates to those of college graduates. Overall, 41 percent of nurses married compared to 45 percent of the college graduates. Nurses were more likely to marry during the first four years after graduation, but from the fifth year on the percentage married was higher in the college group; see Grading Committee, *Nurses, Patients and Pocketbooks*, pp. 246–47.
77 Beginning in the early twentieth century, more nurses did marry. Mottus found increases of 9 and 6.7 percentage points at Bellevue and New York hospitals, respectively, between the nineteenth- and early twentieth-century graduates (*New York Nightingales*, p. 262). Comparatively, an increase of only 3.7 percent was found at Waltham. For national figures on marriage rates, see Lynn Weiner, *From Working Girl to Working Mother* (Chapel Hill: University of North Carolina Press, 1978), Tables 6 and 7, pp. 89 and 93. For comparative data on college educated women, see Barbara Miller Solomon, *In the Company of Educated Women* (New Haven, Conn.: Yale University Press, 1985), pp. 118–22.
78 Grading Committee, *Nurses, Patients and Pocketbooks*, pp. 244–46.
79 See, for example, Rama C. Patten's history in Fiske, *Waltham Training School for Nurses*, p. 178. See also Lois Scharf, *To Work and to Wed* (Westport, Conn.: Greenwood, 1980).
80 For examples see the volunteer careers of Elmira Wickenden, Agnes Turner, and Margaret Barclay in Fiske, *Waltham Training School for Nurses*, pp. 110–12, 119.
81 Grading Committee, *Nurses, Patients and Pocketbooks*, pp. 49–56.
82 Fiske, *Waltham Training School for Nurses*, pp. 97 and 105.
83 Ibid., p. 91; Grading Committee, *Nurses, Patients and Pocketbooks*, p. 257. The Grading Committee did not attempt to explain the differences in these percentages. The greater flexibility in private-duty work, which allowed a nurse to drop out when she was not on a case, may help to explain this. For a contemporary discussion of women's unpaid caring role, see Janet Finch and Dulcie Groves, eds., *A Labour of Love: Women, Work and Caring* (Boston and London: Routledge and Kegan Paul, 1983).
84 Nancy Tomes, " 'Little World of Our Own': The Pennsylvania Hospital Training School for Nurses, 1895–1907," *Journal of the History of Medicine* 33 (October 1978): 507–31.
85 These percentages were calculated from Sara Parsons, *History of the Massachusetts General Hospital Training School for Nurses* (Boston: Whitcomb and Barrows, 1922), p. 155, and George H. M. Rowe, "Historical Sketch of the Boston City Hospital

Training School for Nurses," in *A History of the Boston City Hospital,* ed. the Committee on the Hospital Staff (Boston: Municipal Printing Office, 1906), p. 389.

86 Grading Committee, *Nurses, Patients and Pocketbooks,* p. 257.

87 Fiske, *Waltham Training School for Nurses,* pp. 22–23, 131, 142.

CHAPTER 7 *Professionalization and its discontents*

1 Lavinia L. Dock, *A History of Nursing,* vol. 3 (New York: Putnam, 1912), pp. 116–236; Isabel Hampton Robb, "Presidential Address," *Proceedings of the 2nd Annual Convention 1899 of the Associated Alumnae of Trained Nurses,* p. 30; Janet James, "Isabel Hampton and the Professionalization of Nursing in the 1890s," in *The Therapeutic Revolution,* ed. Morris J. Vogel and Charles Rosenberg (Philadelphia: University of Pennsylvania Press, 1979), pp. 201–44.

2 For a somewhat similar analytic view of professionalization in nursing, see Barbara Melosh, "*The Physician's Hand*" (Philadelphia: Temple University Press, 1982), pp. 15–36.

3 Ibid., p. 22. I have expanded Melosh's categories and identified the groups and individuals holding various positions.

4 See Joyce Antler, "Women and the Professions: Emerging Historical Perspectives" (Paper presented at the Fortieth Anniversary of the Schlesinger Library Conference, Radcliffe College, March 1984). See also Melosh, "*The Physician's Hand,*" pp. 15–36. For thoughtful discussions and excellent bibliographies on the broad issue of professionalization for women, see Joan Jacobs Brumberg and Nancy Tomes, "Women in the Professions: A Research Agenda for American Historians," *Reviews in American History* 10 (June 1982): 275–96.

Race also clearly affected the process of professionalization in nursing; see Patricia Sloan, "Black Hospitals and Nurse Training Schools," and Darlene Clark Hine, "Mabel Keaton Staupers and Black Women Nurses" (Papers presented at the Fifth Berkshire Conference on the History of Women, Vassar College, Poughkeepsie, N.Y., June 1981); Darlene Clark Hine, ed., *Black Women in the Nursing Profession: A Documentary History* (New York: Garland, 1985); Adah B. Thoms, ed., *Pathfinders: A History of the Progress of Colored Graduate Nurses with Biographies of Many Prominent Nurses* (1929; reprint, New York: Garland, 1985); and Mabel Keaton Staupers, *No Time for Prejudice: A Story of the Integration of Negroes in Nursing in the United States* (New York: Macmillan, 1961).

5 See Bonnie and Vern Bullough, "Nursing as a Profession," in *Varieties of Work,* ed. Phyllis L. Stewart and Muriel G. Cantor (Beverly Hills, Calif.: Sage, 1982), pp. 213–24.

6 This does not suggest that medicine's claim for autonomy and professional power was unproblematic. See Gerald E. Markowitz and David Rosner, "Doctors in Crisis: Medical Education and Medical Reform during the Progressive Era, 1895–1915," in *Health Care in America,* ed. Susan Reverby and David Rosner (Philadelphia: Temple University Press, 1979), pp. 185–205; see also Elton Rayack, *Professional Power and American Medicine* (Cleveland: World, 1967); E. Richard Brown, *Rockefeller Medicine Men* (Berkeley: University of California Press, 1979); and Paul Starr, *The Social Transformation of American Medicine* (New York: Basic, 1982).

7 ·Susan Armeny, "Resistance to Professionalization by American Trained Nurses, 1890–1905" (Paper presented at the Fourth Berkshire Conference on the History of Women, Mt. Holyoke College, South Hadley, Mass., August 25, 1978), pp. 8–9; Dock, *History of Nursing,* vol. 3, p. 120.

8 Lyndia Flanigan, compiler, *One Strong Voice* (Kansas City: American Nurses' Association, 1976), p. 25.

9 John Shaw Billings and Henry M. Hurd, eds., *Hospitals, Dispensaries and Nursing* (1894; reprint, New York: Garland, 1984); James, "Isabel Hampton"; Celia Davies, "Professionalizing Strategies as Time- and Culture-Bound," in *Nursing*

History: New Perspectives, New Possibilities, ed. Ellen Condliffe Lagemann (New York: Teachers College Press, 1983), pp. 47–63.

10 James, "Isabel Hampton," pp. 232–33; see also M. Adelaide Nutting's letters to prospective members in the Society of Superintendents' *Letterbook,* National League of Nursing Papers, National Library of Medicine, Bethesda, Md., and Helen Munson, *The Story of the National League of Nursing Education* (Philadelphia: Saunders, 1934). The proceedings of the annual meetings of the society are the best source on the concerns of nursing leaders during the 1890s and early 1900s.

11 Flanigan, *One Strong Voice,* is the official history.

12 Ibid., p. 50. Reports of the annual conventions in the early years can be found in the *American Journal of Nursing;* see also ANA Papers, Nursing Archives, Mugar Library, Boston University.

13 See Bonnie and Vern Bullough, "The Problem of Goal Changes," *Nursing Forum* 4 (1965), Table 1, p. 86, for a compilation of ANA membership figures as a percentage of active nurses from 1920 to 1962. The highest percentage reached was 57 in 1940. See also James, "Isabel Hampton," p. 235, and Mary Roberts, *American Nursing* (New York: Macmillan, 1954), p. 46.

14 The ninety nursing leaders included the presidents of the ANA and NLNE and notable leaders listed in the following sources: Meta Pennock, ed., *Makers of Nursing History* (Buffalo, N.Y.: Lakeside, 1940); Edna Yost, *American Women of Nursing* (Philadelphia: Lippincott, 1965); Flanigan, *One Strong Voice;* Edward T. James, Janet W. James, and Paul S. Boyer, eds., *Notable American Women 1607–1950* (Cambridge, Mass.: Harvard University Press, 1971); Barbara Sicherman and Carol Green, eds., *Notable American Women: The Modern Period* (Cambridge, Mass.: Harvard University Press, 1980). Unfortunately, many of the biographies, particularly in the first sources, were very incomplete and impressionistic. On private duty as a "foundation," see entry for Laura Logan in Pennock, *Makers,* p. 90.

15 "Abolishing the Salary System," *TNHR* 3 (July 1889): 24–25; letters to the editor, ibid. (August 1889): 63–64, 75–76, and (October 1889): 153–55.

16 May 3, 1890, and reprinted in the *TNHR* 4 (May 1890): 236–39; for letters in response, see ibid. (June 1890): 286–88, and 5 (July 1890): 43–44.

17 *First Annual Meeting of the Superintendents' Society,* June 1894. JoAnn Ashley, *Hospitals, Paternalism and the Role of the Nurse* (New York: Teachers College Press, 1976), p. 22, discusses the nonpayment debate at the meeting of the American Hospital Association in 1904, but not the fact that it was of concern to the nursing superintendents as well.

18 "Effect on Discipline," *TNHR* 28 (February 1902): 103; see also "The Non-Pay System," *AJN* 2, part 2 (April 1902): 565; "Who Started It?" *TNHR* 49 (November 1912): 299.

19 Annie Goodrich to the Training School Committee, March 22, 1904; Henderson to the Training School Committee, May 29, 1907, Training School Committee Minutes, June 1902–January 1911, New York Hospital Archives. On Goodrich's attempt, and failures, to reform the training system at New York Hospital, see Esther A. Werminghaus, *Annie W. Goodrich: Her Journey to Yale* (New York: Macmillan, 1950), p. 23, and Harriet Berger Koch, *Militant Angel* (New York: Macmillan, 1951), p. 43. On June 12, 1908, Boston City Hospital nursing superintendent Lucy Drown wrote to Dr. John H. McCollum, the hospital's acting superintendent: "It is very doubtful if a sufficient number of the nurses can be obtained to go without pay, as most of them are self-supporting women." BCH Correspondence Book, Marion Parsons Papers, Nursing Archives, Mugar Library, Boston University.

20 Letter to the editor, *AJN* 2, part 2 (August 1902): 968–69.

21 Isabel Hampton Robb told the Associated Alumnae meeting in 1900: "Two things are needful – organization and legislation." See Lavinia Dock, *History of Nursing,* vol. 3, pp. 142–87, and Louie C. Boyd, *State Registration for Nurses* (Philadelphia: Saunders, 1915). For a comparison between the United States and Great Britain, see Celia Davies, "Professionalizing Strategies," in Lagemann, ed., *Nursing History,* and

"A Constant Casualty: Nurse Education in Britain and the U.S.A. to 1939," in *Rewriting Nursing History*, ed. Celia Davies (Totowa, N.J.: Barnes and Noble, 1980), pp. 102–22.

22 See Veronica M. Driscoll, *Legitimizing the Profession of Nursing: The Distinct Mission of the New York State Nurses' Association* (New York: The Association, 1976); Secretary's Minutes 1903–5, Box 10, Massachusetts Nurses' Association Papers, Nursing Archives, Mugar Library, Boston University; Anna Roth, *35 Years of the Massachusetts State Nurses' Association* (Boston: The Association, 1938); James H. Rodabaugh and Mary Jane Rodabaugh, *Nursing in Ohio: A History* (Columbus: Ohio State Nurses' Association, 1951); Carla M. Schissel, "The State Nurses' Association in a Georgia Context, 1907–1946" (Ph.D. diss., Department of History, Emory University, Atlanta, 1979); Roberta M. West, *History of Nursing in Pennsylvania* (Harrisburg: Pennsylvania State Nurses' Association, 1939); Writers Program of the Work Projects Administration in the State of Kansas, *Lamps on the Prairie: A History of Nursing in Kansas* (1942; reprint, New York: Garland, 1984).

23 Charlotte Mandeville Perry, "Raising the Standard," *TNHR* 18 (February 1897): 62–64.

24 See M. Adelaide Nutting, "Suggestions for Educational Standards for State Registration," in *Sound Economic Basis for Schools of Nursing* (1926; reprint, New York: Garland, 1984), p. 56. In recent years, the debate has been over whether a college degree is necessary for nurses. The proposal to legislate such a requirement was advocated by the New York State Nurses' Association and was known as the "1985 proposal" because of the effective date. The proposal caused an uproar in nursing circles as women who have prepared in community college and hospital diploma schools saw the requirements as downgrading their positions. See, for example, Glenn Jenkins, "1985: Closing the Door on Nurses, New York Style," *Health Pac Bulletin* no. 78 (September–October 1977): 1–7.

25 Ellen DuBois, *Feminism and Suffrage: The Emergence of an Independent Women's Movement in America, 1848–1869* (Ithaca, N.Y.: Cornell University Press, 1978), p. 15; see also her "The Radicalism of the Women's Suffrage Movement: Notes Toward the Reconstruction of Nineteenth-Century Feminism," *Feminist Studies* 3 (Fall 1975): 63–71. This is my analysis, not the nurses'. On the limitation of the legal approach from the nursing viewpoint, see Lavinia Dock, "What We May Expect from the Law," in Janet James, ed., *A Lavinia Dock Reader* (New York: Garland, 1985).

26 See Charlotte Aikens, "The Registration Movement: Its Past and Its Future," *TNHR* 44 (January 1910): 6.

27 See the state histories listed in note 22; Dock, *History of Nursing;* and Boyd, *State Registration*. See also Nancy Tomes, "The Silent Battle: Nurse Registration in New York State, 1903–1920," in Lagemann, ed., *Nursing History*, pp. 107–32.

28 See Tomes, "The Silent Battle," and Driscoll, *Legitimizing the Profession of Nursing*.

29 Vern and Bonnie Bullough, *The Care of the Sick: The Emergence of Modern Nursing* (New York: Prodist, 1978), pp. 138–39.

30 Dr. Frank Billings, letter to the editor of the *Boston Transcript* in History Volume *1905–10*, clippings, n.d. (probably 1905), Box 11, Massachusetts Nurses' Association (MNA) Papers, Nursing Archives, Mugar Library, Boston University.

31 See clippings in ibid.

32 See Tomes, "The Silent Battle," and Driscoll, *Legitimizing the Profession of Nursing*. For an analysis of the Massachusetts situation in detail, see my dissertation, "The Nursing Disorder" (Boston University, 1982), pp. 344–46.

33 "The Silent Battle," pp. 105–6.

34 Even a training school as far away from New York as one in Wheeling, W.Va., for example, tried to upgrade its program so that its graduates could register in New York State. See *Annual Report of the Ohio Valley General Hospital, 1929*, p. 11. Public Relations Office, Ohio Valley General Hospital, Wheeling, W.Va.; see also Josephine Valentine, "Report of Survey of Boston City Hospital School of Nurs-

ing, Boston, Massachusetts, June 18–19, 1937," Box 9, Folder 3, Marion Parsons Papers, Nursing Archives, Mugar Library, Boston University.

35 Tomes, "The Silent Battle," p. 106.

36 Stella Goostray, *Memoirs: Half-Century of Nursing* (Boston: Nursing Archives, 1969), p. 83. See also *Annual Report of the Board of Registration of Nurses for the Year Ending November 30, 1932,* PD no. 91 (Boston: Commission on the Administration and Finance Commonwealth of Massachusetts), p. 3.

37 See Rodabaugh and Rodabaugh, *Nursing in Ohio,* p. 101; Adda Eldredge, quoted in Goostray, *Memoirs,* p. 82.

38 See Ashley, *Hospitals, Paternalism and the Role of the Nurse,* pp. 40–51, and Philip and Beatrice Kalisch, *The Advance of American Nursing* (Boston: Little, Brown, 1978), pp. 281–84.

39 Anne Williamson, "California and the Eight Hour Law," *MH* 3 (September 1914): 183–87. In her autobiography, nursing superintendent Williamson contended that she actually supported the legislation and was forced into this position by her superiors at the California Hospital in Los Angeles (*Fifty Years in Starch* [Culver City, Calif.: Murray and Gee, 1948], pp. 83–85). Her contemporary writings, in particular her speech before the American Hospital Association, reprinted in *Modern Hospital,* suggested, however, that more was at work here than someone forced into a position to keep her job.

40 May 1, 1913, quoted in Ashley, *Hospitals, Paternalism and the Role of the Nurse,* p. 45.

41 Marie Hodden to Adelaide Nutting, October 11, 1913, quoted in ibid., p. 45.

42 "Nursing as a Profession," *MH* 8 (April 1917): 269; see also Asa Bacon, "Nurses and Factory Labor," letter to the editor, *MH* 8 (April 1917): 299.

43 "Very Like Labor Agitation," *TNHR* 22 (April 1899): 201; "Mischievous Nursing Legislation," *MH* 23 (September 1914): 176–77; "California and the Eight Hour Law," ibid.: 183–84.

By 1920, eight states had enacted eight-hour legislation. California and Utah included women hospital workers; Arizona and Nevada included hospital workers, but excluded nurses. Puerto Rico and Washington, D.C., had laws as well, but the data do not make clear if they included hospital workers. U.S. Department of Labor, Women's Bureau, *The Eight Hour Day in Federal and State Legislation,* Women's Bureau Bulletin no. 5 (Washington, D.C.: Government Printing Office, 1920), pp. 3–5. For more on changes in nursing hours, see discussion in Chapter 10.

In Illinois in 1920, two-thirds of all the training schools still required over eight hours a day of duty for their students; see Department of the Interior, Bureau of Education, *Statistics of Nurse Training Schools, 1919–1920,* Bureau of Education Bulletin no. 51 (Washington, D.C.: Government Printing Office, 1922), p. 15.

44 Roberts, *American Nursing,* p. 54, discusses the problem of the sentimentalization of nursing and the refusal of "parents" to send their daughters to nursing school. But because she does not deal with the question of class, she ignores the fact that the women from the lower middle class and working class who did enter training presumably had parents who did not think sending their daughter to training was a terrible idea.

See Everett Hughes et al., *20,000 Nurses Tell Their Story* (Philadelphia: Lippincott, 1958), pp. 186–210, for a summary of the results of surveys on the public's opinions on nurses by class. The first study of public opinion on nursing was conducted by Edward L. Bernays in 1947. For further discussion, see Leo W. Simmons, "Images of the Nurse–Studies," in Simmons and Virginia Henderson, *Nursing Research: A Survey and Assessment* (New York: Appleton-Century-Crofts, 1964), pp. 173–222.

45 The only survey of conditions for nurses were those organized by nursing groups; see further discussion in Chapter 9. See Allan Eaton and Shelby Harrison, *A Bibliography of Social Surveys: Reports of Fact Finding as a Basis of Social Action* (New York: Russell Sage Foundation, 1930). See also Department of Labor, Women's

Bureau, *Professional Nurses,* Women's Bureau Bulletin no. 203 (Washington, D.C.: Government Printing Office, 1945). The exceptions were in California and Illinois when nursing hours legislation was promulgated.

46 For a general discussion of the problem of women's boards, see Isabel Hampton Robb, "Women on Hospital Boards," *AJN* 2 (January 1902): 252–59.

47 Nancy Tomes, "A Collision of Nursing's Two Worlds: Volunteer and Professional Nurses in World War I" (Paper given at the Fifth Berkshire Conference on the History of Women, Vassar College, Poughkeepsie, N.Y., June 18, 1981). See, for example, Schissel, "The State Nurses' Association in a Georgia Context," pp. 1–66.

48 This point for medical women is made strongly in Mary Walsh Roth, *Doctors Wanted: No Women Need Apply* (New Haven, Conn.: Yale University Press, 1976), and Virginia Drachman, "*Hospital with a Heart*" (Ithaca, N.Y.: Cornell University Press, 1984).

49 The relationship between feminism and nursing needs historical exploration; see, for example, selection in James, ed., *A Lavinia Dock Reader.* For a modern discussion, see Peggy L. Chinn and Charlene Eldridge Wheeler, "Feminism and Nursing: Can Nursing Afford to Remain Aloof from the Women's Movement," *Nursing Outlook* 33 (March–April 1985): 74–77.

50 Catlin's recommendations were published as letters in *TNHR* 16 (February 1896): 96–99, and (March 1896): 155–56. The original suggestion appeared in the *Brooklyn Eagle,* December 15, 1895. On medicine in Brooklyn, see David Rosner, *A Once Charitable Enterprise* (Cambridge: Cambridge University Press, 1982).

51 The nurses' responses to Catlin can be found in the letters to the editor, *TNHR* 16 (February 1896): 97–99, and (March 1896): 156–57.

52 "Medical News," *Journal of the American Medical Association* 91 (October 27, 1928): 1296.

53 See Susan Reverby, "Starr Gazing," *Isis* 75 (Summer 1984): 559–562. For the psychological argument on male as "not female," see Nancy Chodorow, *The Reproduction of Mothering* (Berkeley: University of California Press, 1978).

54 Ashley, *Hospitals, Paternalism and the Role of the Nurse,* p. 77. The question of the misogynist attitudes and practices of physicians toward nurses is dealt with extensively in the nursing literature. Even physicians sympathetic to nursing and its efforts to professionalize shared the assumption that doctors and nurses, like men and women, had different spheres. As Dr. Richard Cabot reminded nurses in 1931, "There are two sides to the profession which we share – compassionate service and science. You are stronger on the side of compassionate service and we are stronger on the side of science" ("Christianity and Nursing," *Newsletter of the Guild of St. Barnabas,* 1931, Box IV, no. 45, Richard Cabot Papers, Harvard University Archives, Harvard University). See further discussion in Chapter 8.

55 Letter to the editor, *TNHR* 2 (April 1888): 167–68.

56 The elements of this viewpoint are culled from the letters to the editor in *TNHR* and *AJN* as well as editorials and articles in *TNHR.* This latter journal is the best source for the ideology and concerns of nurses holding these views. For excellent discussions of this issue, see Armeny, "Resistance to Professionalization by American Trained Nurses, 1890–1905," and Melosh, "*The Physician's Hand.*" I have elaborated on their analyses where relevant.

57 "The Path to Duty," *AJN* 4 (October 1904): 2.

58 J. B. S., "From a Nurse's Point of View," letter to the editor of the *Boston Transcript,* 1903, clipping in the *Massachusetts State Nurses' Association History Volume, 1905–10,* box 11, Massachusetts Nurses' Association Papers, Nursing Archives, Mugar Library, Boston University.

59 Henry C. Burdett, "A National Pension Fund for Workers among the Sick in the United States," *TNHR* 8 (July 1892): 285–300; "Do We Need this Charity?" *AJN* 6 (December 1906): 135–36.

60 Letters to the editor on the pension fund, *TNHR* 14 (June 1895): 347–49; ibid. 15

(July 1895): 37–38; Sophia A. Palmer, "The American Pension Fund," *TNHR* 14 (June 1895): 350.

61 Letters to the editor on the pension fund, *TNHR* 8 (September 1892): 448; ibid. (October 1892): 500–1; a Bellevue graduate, "The American Pension Fund for Nurses," *TNHR* 8 (June 1892): 256–57.

62 Louise Moore, "Nurses for the Poor," *TNHR* 14 (March 1895): 159; see also G. N. A., letter to the editor, *TNHR* 16 (March 1896): 157.

63 Grading Committee, *Nurses, Patients and Pocketbooks* (1928; reprint, New York: Garland, 1984), p. 311.

64 One of Them, letter to the editor, *TNHR* 10 (December 1893): 264; see also letters to the editor, *TNHR* 14 (March 1895): 158–59.

65 "Nurses and State Associations," *TNHR* 46 (January 1911): 30.

66 Clara Evelyn Watkins, letter to the editor, *TNHR* 24 (February 1900): 134.

67 Armeny, "Resistance to Professionalization."

68 Celia R. Heller, "Protective Association," *TNHR* 19 (December 1897): 334. The dispute can be followed in the pages of *TNHR* in 1897 and 1898. Armeny discusses the struggle around the NPA at length in "Resistance to Professionalization."

69 Armeny, "Resistance to Professionalization," pp. 10–14.

70 "To the Graduates of New York State," *THNR* 19 (September 1892): 156–57; Margaret G. Rutherford, "For the Protection Association," *TNHR* 19 (October 1892): 218–19.

71 Five Western Graduates, letter to the editor, *TNHR* 19 (November 1897): 276.

72 Olivia A. Grafstrom, "A Review," *TNHR* 20 (January 1898): 44.

73 "New York State Legislation," *TNHR* 24 (January 1900): 56.

74 Minnie S. Hollingsworth, speech on the Private Duty League, *Proceedings of the 16th Annual Meeting of the MSNA, 1919,* pp. 25–28; Sara E. Parsons, speech on the Private Duty League, *Proceedings of the 17th Annual Meeting of the MSNA, 1920,* pp. 9–14.

75 Hollingsworth, in *Proceedings, MSNA, 1919,* p. 26; *Proceedings, MSNA, 1920,* pp. 11–13; For other examples of the difficult relationship between private-duty nurses and the state associations, see West, *History of Nursing in Pennsylvania,* pp. 93–94, and Schissel, "The State Nurses' Association in a Georgia Context," pp. 114–17.

76 "Nurses and State Association, Why Don't Nurses Join?" *TNHR* 46 (January 1911): 30–31.

77 The development of the nursing work culture is discussed extensively by Melosh, "*The Physician's Hand.*"

78 See discussion of their position on nursing organizations in "The Beginning of Nursing Organization in America," *TNHR* 37 (October 1906): 235–37.

79 The Observer, "Organization as a Cure-All?" *TNHR* 62 (September 1920): 225–27.

80 "What Should Nursing Magazines Contain?" *TNHR* 61 (May 1919): 308.

81 "Nurses on Strike," *TNHR* 26 (February 1901): 95–96; "Nurses Strikes," 19 (September 1902): 235–36; "What Is the Remedy?" 37 (July 1906): 36–37; "The Striking Nurse," 48 (February 1912): 48; "The Striking Nurse," 51 (February 1915): 98; "A Trade or a Profession," 62 (June 1920): 529–30; "Trade Unionism and Nursing," 62 (March 1920): 240.

82 "Where We Stand on the State Registration Question," *TNHR* 24 (April 1905): 259–60; see also, "A Danger to the Profession," *TNHR* (August 1904): 111; "The War in Philadelphia," 45 (June 1910): 377–79; and "The Greater Need of Fairness," *TNHR* 51 (July 1913): 31–32.

83 "Putting Character First," *TNHR* 49 (August 1912): 96–97; "The Importance of Character" (October 1912): 232–33; "Where We Differ" 52 (January 1915): 33–34.

84 "The Character Requirement of the Nurse," *TNHR* 66 (May 1921): 433.

85 Biographical material on Fiske was obtained from her student records at Radcliffe,

her response to an alumnae survey in 1928, and her entry in Mary Hawthorne White Bunker, compiler, *Radcliffe College Class of 1894*, June 1952, pp. 78–80, all in the Radcliffe Archives, Schlesinger Library, Harvard University. I am grateful to Jane Knowles of the Schlesinger staff for making this material available to me.

86 Fiske, "Nursing as a Profession," *Radcliffe Magazine* 16 (February 1914): 94.

87 "Annette Fiske," in *A History of the Graduates of the Waltham Training School for Nurses*, compiled by Annette Fiske (Waltham, Mass.: The Waltham Graduate Nurses' Association, 1937), p. 63, and Annette Fiske, *The First Fifty Years of the Waltham Training School for Nurses* (New York: Garland, 1985).

88 Fiske, "Nursing as a Profession," p. 92.

89 Fiske, "The Need of Fairness," *TNHR* 51 (July 1913): 6.

90 Fiske, "Has the Nursing Instinct Died Out? A Plea for Genuineness of Purpose," *TNHR* 73 (November 1924): 439–49. See also, "The Future of the Private Duty Nurse," *Proceedings of the 1st Annual Convention of the New England Nurses*, June 1919, p. 48, Box 7, Massachusetts State Nurses' Association Papers, Nursing Archives, Mugar Library, Boston University.

91 Fiske, "Nursing – as a Profession, Where to Place the Emphasis?" *TNHR* 72 (March 1924): 227–28.

92 Ibid.

93 Fiske, "Importance of Training Women for Private Duty Nursing," *TNHR* 64 (January 1920): 17.

94 Fiske, "How Can We Counteract the Prevailing Tendency to Commercialism in Nursing?" *Proceedings of the 17th Annual Meeting of the MSNA, 1920*, p. 8.

95 "Charlotte A. Aikens – One of *TN*'s Own Editors," *TNHR* 123 (December 1949): 279.

96 "Report of Special Training School Committee," *TAHA* 11 (1909): 361–400; "Report of Special Committee on Nursing," 12 (1910): 101–10; "Report of Special Committee on Grading and Classification of Nurses," 15 (1913): 145–74; "Report of Special Committee on Grading and Classification of Nurses," 16 (1914): 163–88; "Report of Special Committee on Grading and Classification of Nurses," 18 (1916): 52.

97 "Report of Special Committee," *TAHA* 16 (1914): 179.

98 Mary Riddle, "The Grading of Nurses," *TAHA* 15 (1913): 139. Riddle's paper is an excellent summary of the nursing leadership's position on this at the time. Ashley (*Hospitals, Paternalism and the Role of the Nurse*, pp. 102–8) is critical of nurses' participation within the AHA without considering *why* it was politically necessary for them to be part of the debates or discussing the *content* of the debates. Furthermore, Ashley fails to discuss how much the nursing viewpoint actually prevailed since she consistently emphasizes only how nurses were victimized.

99 "Report of Special Committee" *TAHA* 18 (1916): 52. See also, "Grading of Nurses," *MH* 7 (October 1916): 310; Roberts, *American Nursing*, p. 111.

100 For a clear statement of this position, see Annie Goodrich, "The Need of Orientation," a speech she gave before the New York Academy of Medicine in 1912 and reprinted in her *The Social and Ethical Significance of Nursing* (New York: Macmillan, 1932), pp. 27–37.

CHAPTER 8 *Nursing efficiency as the link between service and science*

1 For a summary of the educational changes, see Isabel Stewart, *The Education of Nurses* (1943; reprint, New York: Garland, 1984).

2 See David Montgomery, "Whose Standards?" in his *Workers Control in America* (Cambridge: Cambridge University Press, 1979), p. 113. The literature on efficiency and scientific management is vast and has grown enormously in the last few years. The most useful studies used here, in addition to Montgomery, were Samuel Haber, *Efficiency and Uplift: Scientific Management in the Progressive Era* (Chicago: University of Chicago Press, 1964); Raymond Callahan, *Education and the Cult of Efficiency* (Chicago: University of Chicago Press, 1962); Milton Nadworny, *Scien-*

tific Management and the Unions, 1900–32 (Cambridge, Mass.: Harvard University Press, 1955); Harry Braverman, *Labor and Monopoly Capital* (New York: Monthly Review, 1974); David F. Noble, *America by Design* (New York: Oxford University Press, 1977); Daniel Nelson, *Managers and Workers* (Madison: University of Wisconsin Press, 1975); and Bryan Palmer, "Class Conception and Conflict: The Thrust for Efficiency, Managerial Views of Labor and the Working Class Rebellion, 1903–1922," *Review of Radical Political Economics* 7 (Summer 1975): 31–49.

My thinking has also been greatly influenced by the work of Susan Porter Benson; see " 'The Clerking Sisterhood': Rationalization and the Work Culture of Saleswomen in American Department Stores, 1890–1960," *Radical America* 12 (March-April 1978): 41–55; and Barbara Melosh, "*The Physician's Hand*" (Philadelphia: Temple University Press, 1982).

3 See Miss Giles, "Scientific Management in Hospitals," *SS 1912*, p. 103. For discussion of the meaning of efficiency for the professions, see Judith A. Merkle, "The Taylor Strategy: Organizational Innovation and Class Structure," *Berkeley Journal of Sociology* 13 (1968): 59–81; Robert Wiebe, *The Search for Order* (New York: Hill and Wang, 1967); Pat Walker, ed., *Between Labor and Capital* (Boston: South End, 1979); Wayne K. Hobson, "Professionals, Progressives and Bureaucratization: A Reassessment," *The Historian* 39 (August 1977): 639–58.

4 There is a growing new medical literature on the *meaning* of science for medicine. For overviews, see John Harley Warner, "Science in Medicine," in Sally Gregory Kohlstedt and Margaret Rossiter, eds., *Osiris,* 2d ser., *Historical Writing on American Science* 1 (1985): 37–58; Charles Rosenberg, "Science in American Society: A Generation of Historical Debate," *Isis* 74 (1983): 356–67; Barbara Rosenkrantz, "The Search for Professional Order in 19th Century American Medicine," in *Sickness and Health in America,* 2d ed., ed. Judith Walzer Leavitt and Ronald Numbers (Madison: University of Wisconsin Press, 1986); S. E. D. Shortt, "Physicians, Science, and Status," *Medical History* 27 (1983): 51–68.

5 See David Rosner, *A Once Charitable Enterprise: Health Care in Brooklyn and New York, 1890–1914* (Cambridge: Cambridge University Press, 1982); Morris J. Vogel, *The Invention of the Modern Hospital* (Chicago: University of Chicago Press, 1980); Charles Rosenberg, "Inward Vision and Outward Glance: The Shaping of the American Hospital, 1880–1914," *BHM* 53 (Fall 1979): 346–91. Both Rosenberg and Rosemary Stevens are completing books on the nineteenth- and twentieth-century hospital, respectively.

6 A. J. Oschner, "Hospital Growth Marks Dawn of New Era," *MH* 1 (September 1913): 1.

7 The literature on these issues is enormous. I have used, in particular, the essays by Charles E. Rosenberg, Robert E. Kohler, Gerald L. Geison, and Russell C. Maulitz in *The Therapeutic Revolution,* ed. Morris J. Vogel and Charles E. Rosenberg (Philadelphia: University of Pennsylvania Press, 1979); Edward D. Churchill, ed., *To Work in the Vineyard of Surgery: The Reminiscences of J. Collins Warren, 1842–1927* (Cambridge, Mass.: Harvard University Press, 1958); Henry K. Beecher and Mark D. Altschule, *Medicine at Harvard: The First 300 Years* (Hanover, N.H.: University Press of New England, 1977); E. Richard Brown, *Rockefeller Medicine Men: Medicine and Capitalism in America* (Berkeley: University of California Press, 1979); Martin S. Pernick, *A Calculus of Suffering: Pain, Anesthesia, and Utilitarian Professionalism in Nineteenth-Century American Medicine* (New York: Columbia University Press, 1985).

8 John Hornsby, "The Modern Hospital—A New Entity," *MH* 1 (October 1913): 112–13.

9 See, for example, Dr. Marie Zakrzewska's argument on behalf of the Medical Board to the Board of Directors of the New England Hospital, May 25, 1891, Board of Directors Records, New England Hospital Papers, folder 1890–1894, Box 6, Smith College, Sophia Smith Archives; and Charlotte Aikens, "Hospitals and Money," *TNHR* 51 (May 1914): 364. See also Vogel, *Invention of the Modern Hospital,* pp. 59–77, and David Rosner, "Business of the Bedside," in *Health Care*

in America, ed. Susan Reverby and David Rosner (Philadelphia: Temple University Press, 1979), pp. 117–31.

10 Asa Bacon, "Operating Room Economy," *TNHR* 50 (April 1913): 202–4; "Another Problem in Economy," *MH* 9 (September 1917): 230; Richard Cabot, "Suggestions for the Reorganization of Hospital Outpatient Departments, with Special References to the Improvement of Treatment," *Maryland Medical Journal,* March 1907, pp. 1–11, Item 95, Book 3, no. 10, Richard Cabot Papers, Harvard University Archives, Harvard University, Cambridge, Mass.; Vogel, *Invention of the Modern Hospital,* p. 114.

11 There is no full study of the efficiency movement in hospitals. For beginning discussion of this issue, see George Rosen, "The Efficiency Criterion in Medical Care, 1900–1920," *BHM* 50 (Spring 1976): 28–44; Rosenberg, "Inward Vision and Outward Glance"; Susan Reverby, "Stealing the Golden Eggs: Ernest Amory Codman and the Science and Management of Medicine," *BHM* 55 (Summer 1981): 156–71; Stephen J. Kunitz, "Efficiency and Reform in the Financing and Organization of American Medicine in the Progressive Era," *BHM* 55 (Winter 1981): 497–515.

12 Henry C. Wright, *Report of the Committee of Inquiry into the Departments of Health, Charities and Bellevue and Allied Hospitals in the City of New York* (New York: City of New York Board of Estimate and Apportionment, 1913), p. 11.

13 This is not to suggest that there was uniformity as to the meaning of efficiency in the private sector; see Haber, *Efficiency and Uplift;* Palmer, "Class Conception"; and the contemporary classic, Horace Bookwalter Drury, *Scientific Management: A History and Criticism* (New York: Columbia University Press, 1915).

14 Walter Morrill, "Economy and the Management of Small Hospitals," *MH* 10 (February 1918): 79–80; Aaron Waldheim, "Increasing the Efficiency of Hospital Administrators," *MH* 14 (April 1920): 298–99.

15 "The Dollar Yardstick," *MH* 3 (November 1914): 318. Although the editorial is unsigned, the language is strikingly similar to that used by *Modern Hospital* editor John Hornsby in later writings.

16 Oschner, "Hospital Growth," p. 3.

17 Charles A. Drew, "The Standardization of Hospitals," *MH* 9 (July 1918): 56; John Hornsby, "Conference on Hospital Standardization," *Bulletin of the American College of Surgeons* 3 (January 1918): 37.

18 For a discussion of the difficulties faced by such physicians, in particular Boston surgeon Ernest Amory Codman, see Reverby, "Stealing the Golden Eggs."

19 Edna Yost, *Frank and Lillian Gilbreth: Partners for Life* (New Brunswick, N.J.: Rutgers University Press, 1949), pp. 102, 240–44; A. J. Nock, "Efficiency and the High-Brow: Frank Gilbreth's Great Plan to Introduce Time-Study into Surgery," *American Magazine* 78 (March 1913): 48–50; Frank B. Gilbreth, Jr., and Ernestine G. Carey, *Cheaper by the Dozen* (New York: Crowell, 1948), pp. 101–2; Robert Latou Dickinson, "The 'New Efficiency' Systems and Their Bearing on Gynecological Diagnosis," *Transactions of the American Gynecological Society* 39 (December 1914): 43.

20 Frank Gilbreth, "Scientific Management in the Hospital," *TAHA, 1914,* pp. 483–94, and "Hospital Efficiency from the Standpoint of the Efficiency Engineer," *Boston Medical and Surgical Journal,* May 27, 1915, pp. 774–75.

21 There is no complete history of the hospital-standardization movement. Parts of the history have been told in Franklin Martin, *Fifty Years of Medicine and Surgery* (Chicago: Surgical Publishing Company of Chicago, 1934); Franklin Martin, "Genesis and Progress of the American College of Surgeons," *Surgery, Gynecology and Obstetrics* 40 (January 1925): 149–60; Loyal Davis, *Fellowship of Surgeons: A History of the American College of Surgeons* (Chicago: Thomas, 1960); Rosemary Stevens, *American Medicine and the Public Interest* (New Haven, Conn.: Yale University Press, 1971). The progress of the standardization movement can also be followed in the pages of *Surgery, Gynecology and Obstetrics,* the *Bulletin of the American College of Surgeons,* and *Modern Hospital.*

22 Hornsby, "Conference on Hospital Standardization," p. 7.

23 See correspondence files in the Ernest Amory Codman Papers, Rare Books Room, Countway Medical Library, Harvard Medical School, Boston. In particular, Dr. E. Van Hood to Codman, July 15, 1918, Box I; "Discussion of Codman Paper," n. d., 1918, Box II; and Codman to John Bowman, January 15, 1920, Box II; see also, "Report of the Efficiency Committee," March 14, 1915; "Report no. 2 of the Efficiency Committee," May 6, 1915, "Report of End Results," September 7, 1916, New England Hospital Papers, Box 6, Folder 18, Sophia Smith Archives, Smith College, Northampton, Mass.

24 Dr. Duckering, "Minutes of the Medical Board," March 4, 1915, New England Hospital Papers, Mugar Library, Boston University, Box 8, Folder 4.

25 Henry Fairfield Osborn, *Science and Sentiment* (Lancaster, Pa.: Press of the New Era Printing Company, 1907).

26 Committee on Education of the National League of Nursing Education, *Standard Curriculum for Schools of Nursing* (New York: The Committee, 1919), p. 6. For a preliminary discussion of the relationship of nursing to science, see Susan Reverby, "Legitimation, Meaning, and Science: The Constraints of the Nursing-Hospital Relationship," in *Hospitals and Communities,* ed. Diana Long and Janet Golden (Ithaca, N.Y.: Cornell University Press, in press). The history of the nursing-science link needs further attention.

27 Minnie Goodnow, "Efficiency in the Care of the Patient," *TAHA, 1914,* pp. 202–17; Harrington Emerson, *The Twelve Principles of Efficiency* (New York: Engineering Magazine, 1912).

28 Susan Armeny stresses the continued foothold in nursing until the 1920s of the definition of efficiency derived from the "frank elitism and idealization of military organization" in the tradition of the Civil War Sanitary Commission; see "Organized Nurses, Women Philanthropists, and the Intellectual Bases for Cooperation Among Women, 1898–1920," in *Nursing History,* ed. Ellen Condliffe Lagemann (New York: Teachers College Press, 1983), pp. 13–46. I do not disagree with her analysis but suggest that the shift toward a new way of understanding efficiency was being made by nursing leaders during the 1910s; see also Susan Reverby, "The Search for the Hospital Yardstick: Nursing and the Rationalization of Hospital Work," in Reverby and Rosner, eds., *Health Care in America,* pp. 206–25. See also Melosh, "*The Physician's Hand.*"

29 Harriet Berger Koch, *Militant Angel* (New York: Macmillan, 1951), pp. 19–20. See also Isabel Stewart, "Editorial: The Science and Art of Nursing," *Nursing Education Bulletin* 2 (Winter 1929): 3–4. Nurses continued to hold out hope for time studies and job analysis. In 1931, for example, the board of the National League of Nursing Education wrote to Dr. William Darrach, chairman of the Committee on the Grading of Schools of Nursing: "It is the belief of nurses that real cooperation from the medical profession will not be forthcoming until members of that profession have helped to analyze the actual work of the nurse" ("A Memorandum," Supplemental Material for Grading Committee Report, 1931, Stella Goostray Papers, Box 6, Nursing Archives, Mugar Library, Boston University). For more on the committee and this viewpoint, see Chapter 9.

30 Frank Gilbreth, "The Principles of Scientific Management as Applied to the Work of a Nurse from the Standpoint of a Patient," *SS, 1912,* pp. 108–15.

31 "The Dollar Yardstick," *MH* 3 (November 1914): 318.

32 Theresa E. Christy, *Cornerstone for Nursing Education* (New York: Teachers College Press, 1969), p. 78; Harold E. Smalley and John R. Freeman, *Hospital Industrial Engineering* (New York: Reinhold, 1966), pp. 60–65.

33 Helen E. Marshall, *Mary Adelaide Nutting* (Baltimore: Johns Hopkins University Press, 1972), pp. 111, 134, 157, 187, 192; Susan M. Strasser, "The Business of Housekeeping: The Ideology of the Household at the Turn of the Twentieth Century," *The Insurgent Sociologist* 8 (Fall 1978): 147–63; Barbara Ehrenreich and Deirdre English, *For Her Own Good: 150 Years of the Experts' Advice to Women* (New York: Doubleday, 1978), pp. 127–64. I am grateful for Delores Hayden's suggestion that I examine the home economics movement.

34 Henrietta Goodrich, quoted in Ehrenreich and English, *For Her Own Good*, p. 151.
35 Ibid., pp. 127–64; see also Carol Lopate, "The Irony of the Home Economics Movement," *Edcentric* (November 1974): 40–42, 56–57.
36 Ellen H. Richards, *Euthenics: The Science of Controllable Environment* (Boston: Whitcomb and Barrows, 1910), p. 155; Caroline L. Hunt, *The Life of Ellen H. Richards* (Boston: Whitcomb and Barrows, 1912). Nutting became a founding member of the American Home Economics Association in 1908.
37 Sue Ainslie Clark and Edith Wyatt, *Making Both Ends Meet* (New York: Macmillan, 1912), pp. 268, 270.
38 "Discussion of Robert Latou Dickinson's 'Hospital Organization' paper," *Bulletin of the Taylor Society* 3 (December 1917): 8.
39 See overviews in Sister Charles Marie Frank and Loretta E. Heidgerken, eds., *Perspectives in Nursing Education: Educational Patterns – Their Evolution and Characteristics* (Washington, D.C.: Catholic University of America Press, 1963); Stewart, *The Education of Nurses;* and JoAnn Ashley, *Hospitals, Paternalism and the Role of the Nurse* (New York: Teachers College Press, 1976).

For a view that emphasizes the importance of nursing education, as opposed to the nursing service, in the ideology of these early leaders, see Anselm Strauss, "The Structure and Ideology of American Nursing: An Interpretation," in *The Nursing Profession: Five Sociological Essays*, ed. Fred Davis (New York: Wiley, 1966), pp. 60–108.
40 "Conference on Hospital Standardization," p. 37.
41 John D. Thompson and Grace Goldin, *The Hospital: A Social and Architectural History* (New Haven, Conn.: Yale University Press, 1975); Albert J. Oschner and Meyer J. Sturm, *The Organization, Construction and Management of Hospitals* (Chicago: Cleveland Press, 1907); John Hornsby and Richard Schmidt, *The Modern Hospital: Its Inspiration, Its Architecture, Its Equipment, Its Operation* (Philadelphia: Saunders, 1913); John Elliott Benin and Edward Stevens, "A General Hospital for 100 Patients," in *Hospital Management*, ed. Charlotte Aikens (1911; reprint, New York: Garland, 1984); Wayne Andrew, *Architecture, Ambition and Americans* (New York: Free Press, 1964); David Rosner, "Social Control and Social Service: The Changing Use of Space in Charity Hospitals," *Radical History Review*, no. 21 (Fall 1979): 183–97; Charles Rosenberg, "Changing Views of Infection in the Nineteenth Century" (Lecture given in the MIT Science, Technology and Society Program, Cambridge, October 8, 1980).
42 S. S. Goldwater, "The Passing of the 'Hospital Unit,' " *MH* 2 (September 1913): 14–17; Asa Bacon, "New Plan for Efficient Hospital Proposed," *MH* 8 (May 1919): 21. See also Richard Rester, "Distinctive Type of Architecture Must Be Modern," *MH* 27 (December 1926): 70. The pages of *Modern Hospital* and *Hospital Management* are filled with drawings of the floor plans and pictures of hospitals built throughout the country.
43 Florence Nightingale, *Notes on Hospitals* (London: John W. Parker and Sons, 1850); Thompson and Goldin, *The Hospital*, pp. 153–69, 231–32.
44 Annie Goodrich, "Some Common Points of Weakness in Hospital Construction," *SS, 1903*, and reprinted in her *The Social and Ethical Significance of Nursing* (New York: Macmillan, 1932), pp. 97–104.

Nursing superintendent Minnie Goodnow worked for Edward Stevens, the first major hospital architect, for many years. See her "What a Lady Superintendent Should Know about Hospital Construction," *Hospital World* 5 (May 1914): 266–73; "Minnie Goodnow," in *Makers of Nursing History*, ed. Meta Pennock (Buffalo, N.Y.: Lakeside, 1940), p. 100.

On the importance of Edward Stevens, see E. H. L. Corwin, *The American Hospital* (New York: Commonwealth Fund, 1946), pp. 181–82; Edward F. Stevens, *The American Hospital of the Twentieth Century* (New York: Architectural Record, 1918). Goodnow's father was an architect and she spent some time working on drafting in his office until the depression of the 1890s sent her to nursing school. Perhaps because of Goodnow's urgings, Stevens wrote a series of articles on various aspects of hospital construction and equipment for nurses that appeared in the *Trained Nurse* between December 1918 and May 1919.

45 For a discussion of Gilbreth's views, see Yost, *Partners for Life*, and Ruth Cowan, "Lillian Moeller Gilbreth," *Notable American Women: The Modern Period*, ed. Barbara Sicherman and Carol Hurd Green (Cambridge, Mass.: Harvard University Press, 1980), pp. 271–73.

46 Giles, "Scientific Management in the Hospital," p. 104.

47 Charlotte Aikens, "Conserving Human Energy in Hospitals," *TNHR* 57 (December 1916): 341–42.

48 See discussion of Asa Bacon's and Edward Stevens's hospital plans in Thompson and Goldin, *The Hospital*, p. 193.

49 Dr. W. Gilman Thompson, "Efficiency in Nursing," *JAMA*, December 13, 1913, pp. 2146–49.

50 Wright, *Report of the Committee in Inquiry Into . . . Bellevue*, pp. 11, 407.

51 Elizabeth Greener, "A Study of Hospital Nursing Service," *MH* 16 (January 1921): 28–31; Blanche Pfefferkorn and Marion Rottman, *Clinical Education in Nursing* (New York: Macmillan, 1932), p. 5.

52 Pfefferkorn and Rottman, *Clinical Education*, pp. 1–5; A. Owens et al., "Some Time Studies," *AJN* 27 (February 1927): 99–101; Margaret A. Tracy, "Time Study of Nursing Procedures Used in the Care of a Variety of Surgical Cases," *Yale University School of Nursing Bulletin*, no. 1, 1928; "Looking Squarely at the Facts," *TNHR* 66 (April 1921): 337–38; E. H. Lewinski-Corwin, "The Hospital Nursing Situation," *AJN* 22 (May 1922): 603–6; Mary Roberts, *American Nursing* (New York: Macmillan, 1954), p. 117.

53 Bertha Harmer, *Methods and Principles of Teaching the Principles and Practice of Nursing* (New York: Macmillan, 1926), p. 101; Pfefferkorn and Rottman, *Clinical Education*, p. 1. For an overview of these and subsequent studies, see Myrtle Aydelotte, *Nurse Staffing Methodology* DHEW no. (NIH) 73-433 (Washington, D.C.: Government Printing Office, 1973).

54 Harmer (*Methods*, p. 101) calls it the efficiency method. More contemporary nursing administration texts refer to it as the "functional modality"; see Edythe Alexander, *Nursing Administration*, 1st ed. (St. Louis: Mosby, 1972), p. 20, and Gwen Marram et al., *Primary Nursing* (St. Louis: Mosby, 1974), p. 14.

55 Harmer, *Methods*, pp. 101–11. Harmer was also quite aware of the limitations of this method, which she noted had all the "faults of mass production–quantity at the expense of quality, skill at the expense of knowledge and understanding of the proper." As an assistant professor at Yale's nursing program in the 1920s, Harmer introduced the case study method instead, which allowed the students to plan and administer care for individual patients (Annie Goodrich, "Bertha Harmer," in Pennock, ed., *Makers of Nursing History*, p. 101).

56 "The Science and Art of Nursing," *Nursing Education Bulletin* 11 (Winter 1929): 1–4. See also Reverby, "Legitmation, Meaning, and Science."

57 Isabel Stewart, "A Search for More Exact Measures of Reliability and Efficiency in Nursing Procedures," *Nursing Education Bulletin*, n. s., no. 1 (1930): 5; see also her "Possibilities of Standardization in Nursing Techniques," *MH* 12 (June 1919): 451–54. Martha Ruth Smith, "The Variability in Existing Nursing Practices and Methods of Determining Validity," *Nursing Education Bulletin*, n.s., no. 1 (1930): 10–17.

58 For similar difficulties in medicine see Russell C. Maulitz, " 'Physician versus Bacteriologist': The Ideology of Science in Clinical Medicine," in *The Therapeutic Revolution*, ed. Morris J. Vogel and Charles E. Rosenberg (Philadelphia: University of Pennsylvania Press, 1979), pp. 91–108. Kenneth M. Ludmerer, "The Plight of Clinical Teaching in America," *BHM* 57 (Summer 1983): 218–29.

59 Minnie Goodnow, "Waste of Human Energy in Hospitals," *TNHR* 52 (February 1914): 147. For a nursing student's view on the unnecessary repetition of training, see "The Diary of Nurse Mary Clyner," Nursing Archives, Hospital of the University of Pennsylvania, Philadelphia.

60 Percy S. Brown, "A Few Facts about Scientific Management in Industry," *Proceed-*

ings of the Interim Conference of the International Council of Nurses (Geneva: International Council of Nurses, 1927), pp. 35–40, American Nurses' Association Papers, Box 229, Folder 51, Nursing Archives, Mugar Library, Boston University.

61 Quoted by Stewart, *The Education of Nurses,* p. 150.

62 Phobe Kandel, *Hospital Economics for Nurses* (New York: Harper Bros., 1930), p. 252.

63 Ibid., p. 88.

64 For a general discussion of this criticism in the culture at large, see Daniel T. Rodgers, *The Work Ethic in Industrial America* (Chicago: University of Chicago Press, 1978), pp. 51–57, and James Gilbert, *Work without Salvation* (Baltimore: Johns Hopkins University Press, 1978), pp. 44–46.

65 Meta Pennock, "Ethics and the Nurse," *TNHR* 73 (November 1924): 468.

66 "How Can We Counteract the Prevailing Tendency to Commercialism in Nursing?" *Proceedings of the 17th Annual Meeting of the MSNA, 1920,* p. 8.

67 "Report of the Committee on the State of the Training School, February 1907," MGH Nursing Records, Box 5, Folder 1, g a1, pp. 2–4; Hugh Cabot to Mrs. Whiteside, December 10, 1906, Box 5, folder 1 g a1, MGH Nursing Records, Countway Library, Rare Books Room, Harvard Medical School, Boston.

68 Stewart to Carolyn Gray, December 17, 1925, Isabel M. Stewart Papers, Cabinet VIII, Drawer 2, "Grading Committee Folder," Teachers College Archives, Columbia University, New York; Ethel Johns and Blanche Pfefferkorn, *An Activity Analysis of Nursing* (New York: Committee on the Grading of Nursing Schools, 1934), especially Chapter 1; Stewart, *The Education of Nurses,* p. 150. On Stewart's emphasis of the case study method in nursing education, see Isabel Stewart to Mary Wayland, May 27, 1937, Stewart Papers, Cabinet VII, Drawer 3, Teachers College Archives.

69 See argument by Sophia Palmer, *SS, 1909,* p. 93; May Ayers Burgess, "Grading Committee Report for 1930," p. 17, Box 6, Goostray Papers, Nursing Archives, Mugar Library, Boston University; see also Grading Committee, *Nurses, Patients and Pocketbooks,* p. 522. Burgess meant nursing and hospital superintendents, however, rather than the *entire* nursing profession. She also reiterated Palmer's 1909 comments that nurses had little knowledge or interest in improving nursing education.

70 L. R. Curtis, "Living Out vs. Living In for the Hospital Employees," *MH* 8 (April 1919): 253; "Housing the Personnel," *MH* 26 (March 1924): 205; Emma C. Webb, "Efficiency in Nurses' Homes," *TNHR* 70 (March 1923): 222–24.

71 Interview with E. M. Bluestone, New York City, October 25, 1978. Bluestone was the administrator of New York's Montefiore Hospital from the mid-1920s until 1959, and an editor of *Modern Hospital.*

72 "Welfare Work and Strikes," *MH* 8 (September 1916): 263; "Hospital Employees' Welfare," *MH* 17 (September 1921): 214. See also David Brody, "The Rise and Decline of Welfare Capitalism," in *Change and Continuity in Twentieth Century America: The 1920s,* ed. John Braeman et al. (Akron: Ohio State University Press, 1968), pp. 147–78, and Susan Reverby, "Borrowing a Volume from Industry" (Unpublished paper, 1975).

73 As a New York State nursing board inspector commented in 1925, "When the trustees of a hospital build a beautiful home for nurses and then provide them with a young, inexperienced instructor at a salary of seventy-five dollars a month, there is something wrong in their conception of nursing education" (Mary E. Gladwin, "New York State Inspection of Schools Outside the State," *AJN* 25 [August 1925]: 671).

74 Stewart, "The Science and Art of Nursing," p. 1.

75 For a general discussion of this, see Evelyn Fox Keller, *Reflections on Gender and Science* (New Haven, Conn.: Yale University Press, 1985), pp. 67–126, 158–76.

CHAPTER 9 *The limits of "collaborative relationships"*

1 See, for example, the effect of licensure laws on improvements at the Connecticut Training School in New Haven; Sister Dorothy A. Sheahan, "The Social Origins

of American Nursing and Its Movement into the University" (Ph.D. thesis, New York University, 1980), pp. 203–10.

2 Committee on the Grading of Nursing Schools, *Nurses, Patients and Pocketbooks* (1928; reprint, New York: Garland, 1984), p. 40, and *Nursing Schools Today – and Tomorrow* (New York: The Committee, 1934), pp. 30–33.

3 Gerald E. Markowitz and David Rosner, "Doctors in Crisis: Medical Education and Medical Reform during the Progressive Era, 1895–1915," in *Health Care in America,* ed. Susan Reverby and David Rosner (Philadelphia: Temple University Press, 1979), pp. 185–205; E. Richard Brown, *Rockefeller Medicine Men: Medicine and Capitalism in America* (Berkeley: University of California Press, 1979); and Mary Roberts, *American Nursing* (New York: Macmillan, 1954), p. 245.

4 Noyes to Nutting, April 8, 1917, Department of Nursing Education Archives, Teachers College, Columbia University, New York, quoted by Helen Marshall, *Mary Adelaide Nutting* (Baltimore: Johns Hopkins University Press, 1972), p. 225.
      The role of nurses during World War I has been reinterpreted by two recent historians of nursing; see Susan Armeny, "The Responses of Organized Nurses and Women Physicians to World War I" (Paper given at the Conference of Women in the Health Professions, Boston College, November 15, 1980), and "Organized Nurses, Women Philanthropists, and the Intellectual Bases for Cooperation among Women, 1898–1920," in *Nursing History: New Perspectives, New Possibilities,* ed. Ellen Condliffe Lagemann (New York: Teachers College Press, 1983), pp. 13–46; and Nancy Tomes, "A Collision of Nursing's Two Worlds: Volunteer and Professional Nurses in World War I" (Paper given at the Fifth Berkshire Conference on the History of Women, Vassar College, Poughkeepsie, N.Y., June 18, 1981).
      For the older viewpoints, see Helen Marshall, *Mary Adelaide Nutting,* pp. 223–52; Roberts, *American Nursing,* pp. 130–33; Portia Kernoodle, *The Red Cross in Action: 1882–1948* (New York: Harper and Bros., 1949), pp. 120–50; Lavinia L. Dock et al., *The Official History of Red Cross Nursing* (New York: Macmillan, 1922), pp. 229–309, 953–82.

5 See the discussion of this issue in Tomes, "A Collision of Nursing's Two Worlds." On the training of college-educated women for nursing during the war, see Gladys Bonner Clappison, *Vassar's Rainbow Division, 1918* (Lake Mills, Iowa: Graphic, 1964).

6 *Proceedings of the 24th Annual Convention, National League of Nursing Education, 1918,* p. 139 (hereinafter referred to as *Proceedings, NLNE,* and year of convention).

7 The debate can be followed in *Proceedings, NLNE, 1918,* and is discussed in detail by Tomes, "A Collision of Nursing's Two Worlds."

8 For a slightly overblown picture of Bolton's role in the whole affair, see David Loth, *A Long Way Forward: The Biography of Congresswoman Frances P. Bolton* (New York: Longmans, Green, 1957), pp. 104–8. A month before the war ended as the flu pandemic spread, aides were called up by the Red Cross. The debates can also be followed in the Red Cross Records in the National Archives, Washington, D.C.

9 Minutes of the Special Committee, Medical Board, October 3, 1918, Department of Nursing Education, Teachers College, quoted by Marshall, *Mary Adelaide Nutting,* p. 246.

10 A. A. Hoehling, *The Great Epidemic* (Boston: Little, Brown, 1961); Isabel Stewart, "Progress in Nursing Education during 1919," *MH* 14 (March 1920): 183.

11 "Wanted – 100,000 Girls for Sub-Nurses, an Answer to the Nursing Problem by Dr. Charles H. Mayo, An Authorized Interview by Genevieve Parkhurst," *Pictorial Review* (October 1921): 15 and 82; "Are Nurses Self-Seeking?" Editorial comment, *AJN* 22 (November 1921): 73–74.

12 Clara D. Noyes, "Sub-Nurses? Why Not Sub-Doctors?" *Pictorial Review* (December 1921): 28, 78–80; and Richard Olding Beard, "Fair Play for the Trained Nurse," *Pictorial Review* (February 1922): 28, 95–96.

13 Nutting to Beard, December 8, 1921. See also Beard to Nutting, November 14, 1921; Nutting to Beard, December 2, 1921; Beard to Nutting, December 3, 1921;

Beard to Nutting, December 14, 1921; Nutting Papers, Box 3, Mayo file, Nursing Archives, Teachers College, Columbia University, New York.

14   JoAnn Ashley, *Hospitals, Paternalism and the Role of the Nurse* (New York: Teachers College Press, 1976), pp. 61–63; Karen Buhler-Wilkerson, "False Dawn: The Rise and Decline of Public Health Nursing 1900–1930" (Ph.D. thesis, University of Pennsylvania, 1984), pp. 167–68; see also sporadic issues of a journal, *The Nurse,* put out by John Dill Robertson, in Division of Nursing Papers, Box 23, Nursing and Nursing Publicity–1921, Nursing Archives, Teachers College, Columbia University.

15   The necessity for the study grew out of concern over the division of labor in the public-health nursing practice field. During the 1910s, debate centered on the use of attendants to provide the bedside care for patients and health visitors to provide the teaching. Physicians returning from France, where women of "good social standing," rather than trained nurses, were used as health educators, began to press the Rockefeller Foundation to consider the training of such women. A conference to discuss this issue in December 1918 was the beginning of the Goldmark Report.
     The study was organized to solicit opinions from leading nursing and medical figures, as well as to gather in-depth information from twenty-three selected nursing schools, forty-nine public-health agencies, and a small sample of private-duty nurses. It was overseen by a nineteen-person committee of six nurses, ten physicians, and two laymen, and was chaired by public-health professor C. E. A. Winslow. The six nurses on the committee were Adelaide Nutting, Lillian Wald, S. Lillian Clayton, Mary Beard, and Helen Wood. They were all leading educators and public-health nurses. The ten physicians were a mixture of hospital superintendents, medical school leaders, public-health officials, and private practicing physicians: Hermann Biggs, Lewis Conner, David Edsall, Livingston Farrand, L. Emmett Holt, C. G. Parnall, Thomas W. Salmon, Winford Smith, E. G. Stillman, and William Henry Welch. Two laywomen sympathetic to nursing were also included: Julia Lathrop of the Children's Bureau and philanthropist Mrs. John Lowman.

16   Edwin R. Embree to Winford Smith, November 11, 1926, "Recommendations of the Conference on Nursing Education," October 20, 1925, Historical Source Materials, p. 2077, Rockefeller Foundation Archives, Tarrytown, N.Y., quoted by Sheahan, "Social Origins," p. 240. On the later contributions of the foundation to nursing, see Janet Golden and Phyllis Moore, "The Simmons-Harvard Graduate Program in Public Health Nursing, 1953–1961: A Short-Lived Success," *Public Health Nursing* (in press).

17   Goldmark's own views, as had Flexner's in the medical education study, shaped the report. A Bryn Mawr-educated feminist social investigator, she was committed to social reform through factual investigation, and the marshaling of vast amounts of qualitative and quantitative evidence. Goldmark was also a master at the weaving of a skillful argument. She had just completed work with Haven Emerson on a major health and hospital survey in Cleveland that included a study of nursing. Goldmark was thus an obvious choice to do the investigation because of her experience in surveying health facilities and her long-standing concern for women workers.
     Goldmark is perhaps best known for her monograph on women's hours of labor for her brother-in-law, Louis Brandeis, that was the basis for his winning argument before the U.S. Supreme Court in Muller vs. Oregon (1908). She was also the author of a study entitled *Fatigue and Efficiency* in 1912 and a report on factory conditions after the Triangle Shirtwaist Company fire in 1911. See Robert Bremner, "Josephine Goldmark," *Notable American Women,* vol. 2. Ed. Edward T. James et al. (Cambridge, Mass.: Harvard University Press, 1971), pp. 60–61. On Flexner's autonomy, see Daniel M. Fox, "Abraham Flexner's Unpublished Report: Foundations and Medical Education, 1909–28," *BHM* 54 (Winter 1980), 475–96.

18   Nutting to Goldmark, November 3, 1921, Nutting Papers, Box 3, Goldmark Report file; "Report of the Committee on Nursing Education," *AJN* 22 (August 1922): 878–80. See also Teresa Christy, *Cornerstone for Nursing Education* (New

York: Teachers College Press, 1969), p. 64; and Buhler-Wilkerson, "False Dawn," p. 187.

19 *Nursing and Nursing Education in the United States, Report of the Committee for the Study of Nursing Education and Report of a Survey by Josephine Goldmark* (1922; reprint, New York: Garland, 1984).

20 Smith to Goldmark, April 19, 1922, Nutting Papers, Box 3, Goldmark Report file; see also Smith to Goldmark, January 10, 1922, ibid. For a discussion of the public-health nursing response, see Buhler-Wilkerson, "False Dawn," pp. 206–8.

21 Goldmark to Nutting, September 23, 1922, Nutting Papers, Box 3, Goldmark Report file.

22 Goldmark, *Nursing and Nursing Education,* p. 177.

23 *Proceedings, NLNE, 1923,* pp. 179–84; Annie Goodrich, "The University, the School of Nursing, and the Subsidiary Group," *AJN* 23 (May 1923): 627–34; Letter to the editor, *AJN* 23 (June 1923): 786–87; Editorial, "The Training of Attendants," *AJN* 23 (June 1923): 764–65.

24 Beard succinctly summed up the nursing objection to attendants: "No tag will efficiently label her. No law will keep her within safe bounds. No economy will be realized as the Report admits, in her employ." See "The Report of the Rockefeller Foundation on Nursing Education: A Review and Critique," *AJN* 23 (March 1923): 464. Beard's article began in the February 1923 issue of the *AJN* (pp. 358–65) and continued in the April number (pp. 550–54).

By 1923 seven states had a variety of laws that licensed attendants; one state licensed practical nurses, and three others attempted, but failed, to gain attendant licensure; the remaining two prepared, but did not present, such bills. For a summary on the legislation see "Report of Sub-Committee on Recent Developments in the Training and Use of Attendants," *Proceedings, NLNE, 1922,* pp. 100–7.

25 Fox, "Abraham Flexner's Unpublished Report"; E. Richard Brown, "He Who Pays the Piper: Foundations, the Medical Profession, and Medical Education," in Reverby and Rosner, eds., *Health Care in America,* pp. 132–53.

26 Rockefeller Foundation, *Methods and Problems of Medical Education,* 21st ser., "Nursing Education and Schools of Nursing," 1932; idem, *Directory of Fellowship Awards for the Years 1917–1950* (New York: Macmillan, 1943), pp. 227–32.

27 See extensive discussion in Sheahan, "Social Origins," pp. 240–316.

28 "Report of the Acting Chair of the Education Committee," *Proceedings, NLNE, 1923,* p. 44; "Report of the Committee on the Grading of Nursing Schools," *Proceedings, NLNE, 1924,* pp. 34–35; Stewart to Beard, April 12, 1923, Isabel Stewart Papers, Box 1, Grading Committee folder, Nursing Archives, Teachers College.

29 In 1928, however, after the publication of the Grading Committee's first major report, *Nurses, Patients and Pocketbooks,* the AMA withdrew its support, although both Darrach and Smith remained on the committee as members-at-large.

30 Members of the Committee on the Grading of Nursing Schools and organizations they represented were the National League of Nursing Education: Elizabeth C. Burgess, RN, Laura R. Logan, RN; the American Nurses' Association: Helen Wood, RN, Susan C. Francis, RN; the National Organization for Public Health Nursing: Katharine Tucker, RN, Elizabeth G. Fox, RN; the American College of Surgeons: Malcolm T. MacEachern, MD, Bowman C. Crowell, MD (alternate); the American Hospital Association: Joseph B. Howland, MD, Ada Belle McCleary, RN; the American Public Health Association: Charles-Edward A. Winslow, DPH, Haven Emerson, MD (alternate); members-at-large: Mrs. Chester C. Bolton, Sister Domitilla, RN, Henry Suzzallo, Ph.D., Samuel P. Capen, Ph.D., Edward A. Fitzpatrick, Ph.D., W. W. Charters, Ph.D., William Darach, Ph.D., Winford H. Smith, MD, Nathan B. Van Etten, MD; chairman: William Darrach, MD; director: May Ayers Burgess, Ph.D.; nurse consultants: Mary M. Roberts, RN, Stella Goostray, RN, Janet Geister, RN.

On contributions, see Grading Committee, *Nursing Schools Today – and Tomorrow,* pp. 17–18.

31 Burgess had a Ph.D. in statistics from Columbia University. She had worked in the Department of Education of the Russell Sage Foundation in 1913–14 and again in 1919–20. In 1917–18, she worked with her brother, Leonard Ayers, in the statistical branch of the General Staff of the War Department. Between 1923 and 1926, she was part of Michael Davis's interdisciplinary team on the Committee on Dispensary Development in New York. As part of this work, she assisted with the statistics for a report on private-duty nursing. See "May Ayers Burgess," *Who's Who in America,* vol. 3 (Chicago: Marquis, 1960), p. 123.

32 See May Ayers Burgess's comments in Committee on the Grading of Nursing Schools, *The Second Grading of Nursing Schools,* summary part 1 (New York: The Committee, 1932), p. 154.

33 "A Program of the Grading of Schools of Nursing," *TAHA* 27 (1925): 366.

34 Strong to Stewart, December 20, 1923, Stewart Papers, Box 1, Grading Committee folder, Nursing Archives, Teachers College, Columbia University. Although not a member of the Grading Committee, Anna Strong had been a member of the NLNE's Grading Committee that had planned the larger enterprise.

35 May Ayers Burgess to Elizabeth Burgess, December 29, 1928, Stewart Papers, Box 1, Grading Committee folder.

36 *Nursing Schools Today – And Tomorrow.* See also May Ayers Burgess, "Nurses, Patients and Pocketbooks," *Proceedings, NLNE, 1928,* pp. 237–56.

37 Excerpts from the reviews of the "Red Book" (*Nurses, Patients and Pocketbooks*), Grading Committee Report for 1929, Stella Goostray Papers, Box 6, Nursing Archives, Mugar Library, Boston University.

38 Paul Keller, "The Grading Committee and Quality Nursing," *TAHA* 34 (1932): 739–45.

39 Burgess to Nutting, February 27, 1928, Nutting Papers, Box 3, Grading Folders, Nursing Archives, Teachers College, Columbia University.

40 Committee on the Grading of Nursing Schools, 1930 Report, pp. 10 and 17, Goostray Papers, Box 6, Nursing Archives, Mugar Library, Boston University. It should be noted, however, that a remarkable 74 percent, or 1,458, of schools responded to the grading requests.

41 Grading Committee, *Nurses, Patients and Pocketbooks,* pp. 390–91.

42 "Proceedings of the Grading Committee, May 1931 Meeting," pp. 27–28, Goostray Papers, Box 6. See also May Ayers Burgess, "What We Have Done and What We Might Do – Report Prepared for the Committee on the Grading of Nursing Schools, April 30, 1931," ibid.

43 "May 1931 Meeting Report," p. 7.

44 *Second Grading,* p. 154. For a devastating report on how little had really changed, see Harlan Hoyt Horner, *Nursing Education and Practice in New York State with Suggested Remedial Measures* (Albany: University of the State of New York Press, 1934).

45 "Proceedings of the Semi-Annual Meeting of the Grading Committee, November 20–21, 1931," Goostray Papers, Box 6; S. P. Capen, "A Member of the Grading Committee Speaks," *AJN* 32 (March 1932): 307–11; Laura Logan, "A Program for the Grading of Schools of Nursing," *TAHA* 27 (1925): 358–66.

46 Capen had been a U.S. Bureau of Education specialist on higher education before becoming chancellor of the University of Buffalo. During the 1930s he was considered one of the leading foes of accreditation. His speech "Seven Devils in Exchange for One," given in 1939 after the Grading Committee dissolved, is considered a major statement of the antiaccreditation forces. See William K. Selden, *Accreditation: A Struggle over Standards in Higher Education* (New York: Harper and Bros., 1960), and Selden, "The National Commission on Accrediting," in *Accreditation in Higher Education,* ed. Lloyd E. Blauch (Washington, D.C.: Government Printing Office, 1959), pp. 22–28.

47 Burgess to Nutting, March 24, 1932, Nutting papers, Box 3, Grading Committee folder, Nursing Education Archives, Teachers College, Columbia University.

48 Burgess to Frank Billings, November 12, 1926, Stewart Papers, Box 1, Grading

Committee folder, Nursing Archives, Teachers College. Shirley Titus, dean of the Nursing School at Vanderbilt University, argued that nursing was facing a "New Scutari" in its search for public acceptance and public funding; "The New Scutari," *Proceedings, NLNE, 1933,* pp. 241–45; Elizabeth Burgess, "The Principal's Dilemma," ibid., pp. 228–40; "Proceedings of the Semi-Annual Meeting of the Grading Committee," March 23, 1932, Goostray Papers, Box 7, Mugar Library, Boston University.

49 "Proceedings of the May 1931 Meeting," p. 34; Stewart, *The Education of Nurses,* p. 231; Roberts, *American Nursing,* p. 252; Margaret West and Christy Hawkins, *Nursing Schools at the Mid-Century* (New York: National Committee for the Improvement of Nursing Services, 1950). There had been informal meetings of the nurses leading the collegiate program at Teachers College since 1928. On the role and importance of the baccalaureate programs, see Sydney D. Krampitz, "The Historical Development of Baccalaureate Nursing Education in the American University, 1899–1935" (Paper presented to the Rockefeller Conference on the History of Nursing, May 22, 1981, Rockefeller Archives, Tarrytown, N.Y.).

50 This was the title of an address she gave before the American Protestant Hospital Association and reprinted in *MH* 22 (January 1929): 56–63. Burgess's reports on the Grading Committee's progress were perennials in the pages of *MH* and *AJN* during the years the committee was working.

51 "Partnership with the Public," *Proceedings, NLNE, 1932,* p. 62.

52 "Three Problems for Nurses," reprint from *The Proceedings,* Congress on Medical Education, Licensure, Public Health and Hospitals, Chicago, February 6–8, 1928 (Chicago: AMA, 1928), in Visiting Nurse Association of Boston Papers, Box 5, Folder 5, Nursing Archives, Mugar Library, Boston University.

53 "Nurses, Patients and Pocketbooks," read at the annual Convention of Nursing Organizations on June 7, 1928, and reprinted in *Bulletin of the AHA* 2 (July 1928): 300–1; see also her "Why Not Improved Training for Fewer Nurses."

54 See Nutting's notes on the margins of her copy of May Ayers Burgess's speech before the ANA in 1932; "Quality Nursing," Nutting Papers, Box 3, Grading Committee folder, Nursing Education Archives, Teachers College, Columbia University.

55 Emphasis in the original. "Program for 1932," Geister Papers, Box 10, Folder 89, Nursing Archives, Mugar Library, Boston University. For a more extensive discussion of Geister and her role, see my " 'Something Besides Waiting': The Politics of Private Duty Nursing Reform in the Depression," in Lagemann, ed., *Nursing History,* pp. 133–56.

56 Historians usually explain this transformation from private duty to staff nursing as the inevitable result of a juncture of several forces: the efforts to cope with the overproduction problem; the availability of new reimbursement mechanisms for hospital care; the rise of capital-intensive science- and hospital-based medicine; and shifting morbidity patterns in society as a whole (see further discussion in Chapter 10).

See, for example, Mary Roberts, *American Nursing;* Philip A. Kalisch and Beatrice J. Kalisch, *The Advance of American Nursing* (Boston: Little, Brown, 1978); Kathleen Cannings and William Lazonick, "The Development of the Nursing Labor Force in the United States: A Basic Analysis," *International Journal of Health Services* 5 (1975): 185–217; David Wagner, "The Proletarianization of Nursing in the United States, 1932–1946," ibid., 10 (1980): 271–90. I would also include in this viewpoint my earlier "The Search for the Hospital Yardstick: Nursing and the Rationalization of Hospital Work," in Reverby and Rosner, eds., *Health Care in America,* pp. 206–25, and "Re-forming the Hospital Nurse: The Management of American Nursing," in *The Sociology of Health and Illness, Critical Perspectives,* ed. Peter Conrad and Rochelle Kern (New York: St. Martin's, 1981), pp. 220–32. But such a transformation was inevitable in part because the advocates of reform of private duty in the community lost their struggles against the educators and public-health nurses in the nursing leadership; see Reverby, " 'Something Besides Waiting.' "

262 Notes to pages 177–78

57 Grading Committee, *Nurses, Patients and Pocketbooks*, pp. 66–86, 96–98; "The Registry Looks at the Private Duty Nurse," *AJN* 29 (December 1929): 1465; Roberts, *American Nursing*, pp. 117–24. The records of individual registries can be used somewhat as a guide to this change toward hospital specials; see, for example, *Annual Report of the Suffolk County Nurses Central Directory*, District V, Massachusetts State Nurses' Association Papers, Box 1, Nursing Archives, Mugar Library, Boston University. However, because individual registries often specialized in one type of service, these kinds of records are not a good guide to overall shifts, nor can the shift from home-based to hospital-based private duty be accurately dated.

58 C. Rufus Rorem, "Nursing–An Economic Paradox," *Proceedings, NLNE, 1933*, pp. 115–16. Rorem was citing data later published in I. S. Falk, C. Rufus Rorem, and Martha D. Ring, *The Costs of Medical Care* (Chicago: University of Chicago Press, 1933). See also Grading Committee, *Nurses, Patients and Pocketbooks*, pp. 317–61; Janet Geister, "Hearsay and Facts in Private Duty," *AJN* 26 (July 1926): 520.

59 Rorem, "Nursing–An Economic Paradox," p. 119.

60 Margaret Ashman, "The Cause and Cure of Unemployment in the Nursing Profession," *AJN* 33 (July 1933): 652–53; *20th Annual Report*, February 19, 1932, Suffolk County Nurses Central Directory, p. 4; *21st Annual Report*, February 24, 1933, ibid., p. 5; Scrapbooks, Massachusetts State Nurses' Association, District V Papers, Box 1; Ellen S. Woodward, "Federal Aspects of Unemployment among Professional Women," *AJN* 34 (June 1934): 534–38.

61 "Report of the Director at Headquarters to House of Delegates, January 1932," Geister Papers, Box 10, Folder 89, Nursing Archives, Boston University. Pearl McIver, a public-health nurse who assisted local health agencies to use unemployed nurses, estimated there were 6,000 nurses on relief during the Depression. It is impossible to check the accuracy of her count, but I suspect from other evidence that her figures are too low. "Interview with Pearl McIver," March 4, 1944, Women's Bureau Records, Record Group 86, Box 502, National Archives, Washington, D.C.

62 See, for example, "Work Sharing in Wisconsin," *AJN* 33 (March 1933): 202; "What about Our Own Catastrophe?" *AJN* 32 (January 1932): 62–63; "Unemployment Relief," *AJN* 32 (October 1932): 1053–54; Boston City Hospital Nurses' Alumnae Association, "The Newsletter," July 1932; "Our Alumnae and the 8 Hour Day," Plan to be Submitted to the Superintendents' Club of Greater Boston Introducing 8 Hour Duty for Private Duty Nurses, Marion Parsons Papers, Box 13, Folder 2, Nursing Archives, Mugar Library, Boston University. Kalisch and Kalisch (*Advance of American Nursing*, pp. 424–33) have an extended discussion on unemployment relief and nurses on federal projects in their text, but further research needs to be done on the importance of these programs in reshaping the delivery of hospital-based care and changing the careers of nurses.

63 Grading Committee, *Nurses, Patients and Pocketbooks*, pp. 311–14, 359–60, 363, 388; Geister, "Hearsay and Facts in Private Duty," p. 518.

64 For details and further discussion, see Reverby, " 'Something Besides Waiting.' "

65 Geister, "Abstract of 1933 Program, Part I, December 1932," p. 1, Box 10, Folder 88, Geister Papers, Mugar Library, Boston University.

66 "Review of Headquarters Activities for 1934 and Suggested Program for 1935," "ANA Board of Directors Minutes," January 1935, Box 42, ANA Papers, Nursing Archives, Boston University; Ella Best, *Brief Historical Review* (New York: ANA, 1940), pp. 53–54, 58–62; Lyndia Flanagan, compiler, *One Strong Voice* (Kansas City: American Nurses' Association, 1976), pp. 105–7. See also the monthly registry reports in the *AJN* and registry surveys in Box 271, ANA Papers.

67 Michael Davis, "Nursing Service Measured by Social Needs," *AJN* 39 (January 1939): 36. In an editorial comment on Davis's challenge ("Needed–More Nursing Service, A Slogan for 1939," *AJN* 39 [January 1939]: 54–55), the editors of the journal seemed to have missed the point of Davis's concern. Their editorial called

for more specialization and better preparation of nurses and applauded the move toward greater joint leadership in nursing.

68 Jonathan Grossman, *William Sylvis: Pioneer of American Labor* (New York: Columbia University Press, 1945), pp. 191–217; Philip Foner, *Women and the American Labor Movement* (New York: Free Press, 1979), pp. 88, 117–18, 155–56; Daniel Rodgers, *The Work Ethic in Industrial America* (Chicago: University of Chicago Press, 1978), pp. 40–45; John R. Commons et al., *History of Labour in the United States*, vol. 2 (New York: Macmillan, 1921); "The Girls' Co-operative Collar Co.," *Revolution* 5 (April 28, 1870), p. 267, reprinted in *America's Working Women: A Documentary History*, ed. Rosalyn Baxandall, Linda Gordon, and Susan Reverby (New York: Random House and Vintage, 1976), p. 116. Committee on the Costs of Medical Care, *Medical Care for the American People: The Final Report of the Committee on the Costs of Medical Care* (Chicago: University of Chicago Press, 1932); Rosemary Stevens, *American Medicine and the Public Interest* (New Haven, Conn.: Yale University Press, 1971), pp. 175–97.

69 For an example, see Allon Peebles et al., *Nursing Services and Insurance for Medical Care in Brattleboro, Vermont* (Chicago: University of Chicago Press, 1932); Falk et al., *The Costs of Medical Care*, pp. 476–77. On patients' continuing difficulties in paying for private-duty services, see Margaret C. Klem, "Who Purchase Private Duty Nursing Services?" *AJN* 39 (October 1939): 1069–77.

70 Grading Committee, *Nursing Schools Today – and Tomorrow*, p. 22.

71 It is also possible to speculate that there was a narrowing of focus and a less broad sense of reform among most of the second generation of women who rose to nursing leadership in the late 1920s. By then Isabel Hampton Robb was dead, and Annie Goodrich and Adelaide Nutting were still active but increasingly in the ambiguous position of senior stateswomen. Similarly, a number of early public-health nursing leaders had retired or left to pursue other interests (personal communication, Karen Buhler-Wilkerson to Susan Reverby, December 3, 1981). A study of the views of the different generations of nursing leaders would be extremely valuable for both nursing and women's history.

CHAPTER 10 *Great transformation, small change*

1 Ronda Kotelchuck, "The Depression and the AMA," *Health PAC Bulletin* no. 69 (March–April 1976): 13–18.

2 The development and importance of graduate staff nursing can only begin to be discussed in this chapter. Other historians have focused on this form of nursing. See David Wagner, "The Proletarianization of Nursing in the United States, 1932–1946," *International Journal of Health Services* 10 (1980): 271–90; Barbara Melosh, "Doctors, Patients and 'Big Nurse': Work and Gender in the Postwar Hospital," in *Nursing History*, ed. Ellen Condliffe Lagemann (New York: Teachers College Press, 1983), pp. 157–80, and *"The Physician's Hand"* (Philadelphia: Temple University Press, 1982), pp. 159–206; Marilyn E. Flood, "The Troublesome Expedient: General Staff Nursing in U.S. Hospitals in the 1930s" (Ph.D. diss., University of California, Berkeley, 1981).

3 Malcolm T. MacEachern and Carl Erickson, "Hospital Planning from Days of Nickel Plate," *MH* 51 (September 1938): 92; U.S. Bureau of the Census, *Historical Statistics of the U.S. From Colonial Times to 1957* (Washington, D.C.: Government Printing Office, 1959), Ser. B, pp. 235–36; Harry Marks, Review of Melosh, *"The Physician's Hand,"* *Technology and Culture* 26 (April 1985): 326–28.

4 C. Rufus Rorem, *The Public's Investment in Hospitals* (Chicago: University of Chicago Press, 1930), pp. 5 and 196.

5 Rosemary Stevens, *American Medicine and the Public Interest* (New Haven, Conn.: Yale University Press, 1971), p. 179; Charles Rosenberg, "The Therapeutic Revolution: Medicine, Meaning and Social Change in Nineteenth-Century America," in *The Therapeutic Revolution*, ed. Morris J. Vogel and Charles Rosenberg (Philadelphia: University of Pennsylvania Press, 1979), pp. 3–26; Edmund D. Pellegrino,

"The Socio-cultural Impact of Twentieth-Century Therapeutics," in ibid., pp. 245–66; James Borderley and A. McGehee Harvey, *Two Centuries of American Medicine 1776–1976* (Philadelphia: Saunders, 1976), p. 313; Marks, "Review of Melosh," p. 328.

6 Stevens, *American Medicine*, p. 542; Bernhard J. Stern, *American Medical Practice in the Perspective of a Century* (New York: Commonwealth Fund, 1945); Michael Davis, *Clinics, Hospitals and Health Centers* (New York: Harper and Bros., 1927); Frederick W. Washburn, *The Massachusetts General Hospital: Its Development, 1900–1935* (Boston: Houghton Mifflin, 1939); Nathaniel W. Faxon, *The Massachusetts General Hospital, 1935–1955* (Cambridge, Mass.: Harvard University Press, 1959); Shirley Titus, "The Present Position of Nursing in Hospitals in the United States," *Nosokomeion* 2 (April 1931): 288–97.

7 Iago Galdston, *Progress in Medicine* (New York: Knopf, 1940), p. 287.

8 Minnie Goodnow, *The Technic of Nursing*, 2d ed. (Philadelphia: Saunders, 1930), p. 354; for a discussion of the impact of changing medical practice on nursing see Titus, "Present Position."

9 Titus, "Present Position," p. 294; see also Ethel Johns, "Nursing Care in the Hospital from an Economic Point of View," *Nosokomeion* 2 (April 1931): 572–81. In the words of sociologist Everett Hughes, "The nurse's place in the division of labor is essentially that of doing in a responsible way whatever necessary things are in danger of not being done at all." Quoted by Ada Jacox, "Role Restructuring in Hospital Nursing," in *Nursing in the 1980's*, ed. Linda Aiken (Philadelphia: Lippincott, 1982), p. 79.

10 For an examination of occupancy rates during the Depression, see Michael Davis, *Public Medical Services* (Chicago: University of Chicago, 1937), p. 52. It should be noted that public hospitals maintained an occupancy rate of around 90 percent while the voluntary rate dropped as low as 55 percent in 1933; see also Odin Anderson, *Blue Cross Since 1929: Accountability and Public Trust* (Chicago: Ballinger, 1975), and *The Uneasy Equilibrium: Financing of Health Services in the U.S., 1875–1965* (New Haven, Conn.: College and University Press, 1968); Ronda Kotelchuck, "The Depression and the AMA."

11 Malcolm MacEachern, *Hospital Organization and Management* (Chicago: Physicians' Record, 1935), pp. 1085–1122, 1205.

12 F. V. Atwater, "A Flat Rate Plan Designed to Help Both Hospital and Patient," *MH* 41 (August 1933): 71–75.

13 Herman and Anne Sommers, *Doctors, Patients and Health Insurance* (Washington, D.C.: Brookings Institution, 1961), p. 291; see also Sylvia Law, *Blue Cross: What Went Wrong?* (New Haven, Conn.: Yale University Press, 1974), and Anderson, *Blue Cross Since 1929*.

14 "Cash or Credit," *MH* 6 (February 1931): 106.

15 William H. Spencer, "The Hospital in Modern Society," *Hospitals* 12 (June 1938): 15.

16 Frank Gilbreth, "Scientific Management in the Hospital," *TAHA, 1914*, p. 492.

17 C. Rufus Rorem, "Report of Annual Congress on Medical Education and Licensure," Chicago, February 13 and 14, 1933, *JAMA*, April 15, 1933, pp. 1180; see also his "Hospital Management" presented before a meeting of the Taylor Society, New York, December 3, 1931, and published in *Bulletin of the Taylor Society* 17 (February 1932): 23–26. Rorem, the key medical economist behind the development of Blue Cross, was also a firm advocate of hospital staff nursing by graduates.

18 Mary A. Baker, "The Employment of 3rd Year Nurses as Specials," *TAHA, 1916*, p. 277.

19 Ellen C. Daly to John Dowling, November 1, 1928, and January 11, 1929; Boston City Hospital Training School Correspondence, "Boston City Hospital Training School Scrapbook," Marion Parsons Papers, Box 1, Nursing Archives, Mugar Library, Boston University.

20 Grading Committee, *Nurses, Patients and Pocketbooks* (1928; reprint, New York: Garland, 1984), pp. 392, 416–17; H. B. J., "The Special Nurse," *AJN* 31 (January 1931): 107.
21 See, for example, Marion H. Addinton, "Cooperation between the Private Duty Nurse and the Hospital," *AJN* 31 (January 1931): 39–45; Katherine DeWitt, *Private Duty Nursing* (Philadelphia: Lippincott, 1917).
22 Subcommittee of the Joint Distributional Committee, "Institutional Nursing," *AJN* 31 (June 1931): 692; Sister Mary Paul, "Hospital Group Nursing," *TAHA, 1923*, pp. 460–64.
23 Sister Domitilla, Superintendent of St. Mary's Hospital, Rochester, Minnesota, quoted in Janet Geister, "Group Nursing," unrevised article dated September 30, 1927, Geister Papers, Box 1, Group Nursing folder, Nursing Archives, Boston University.
24 For a discussion of the different plans, see "Group Nursing," *AJN* 30 (January 1930): 32; Janet Geister, "Group Nursing and the Hospital Patient" (Unpublished article, circa 1930, Geister Papers, Box 1, Group Nursing folder, Nursing Archives, Boston University); Joseph Turner, "An Experiment with Group Nursing That Augers Success," *MH* 29 (July 1932): 49–54.
25 Geister, "Group Nursing and the Hospital Patient," p. 3.
26 "ANA Board of Directors Minutes," January 20, 1943, p. 34, ANA Papers, Box 46, Nursing Archives, Boston University.
27 Shirley Titus, "Graduate Nursing," *AJN* 31 (February 1931): 202.
28 Shirley Titus, "Group Nursing and How It Affects the Welfare of the Patient," *MH* 35 (December 1930): 128. See also her "Group Nursing," *AJN* 30 (July 1930): 845–50, and discussion in "ANA Board of Directors Minutes," June 8, 1945, p. 16, ANA Papers, Box 45, Nursing Archives, Boston University.
29 John Thompson and Grace Goldin, *A Social and Architectural History of the Hospital* (New Haven, Conn.: Yale University Press, 1975), pp. 207–25.
30 Vern and Bonnie Bullough, *The Emergence of Modern Nursing*, 2d ed. (New York: Macmillan, 1969), pp. 166–68; Anna Roth, *35 Years of the Massachusetts State Nurses' Association* (Boston: MSNA, 1938), p. 43; *Nurses, Patients and Pocketbooks*, p. 302. In 1926, Geister found that less than 2 percent of the private-duty nurses in her New York State survey worked less than a twelve-hour schedule; see "Hearsay and Facts about Private Duty," *AJN* 26 (July 1926): 520.
31 The On-Looker in Georgia, "Twelve Hour Day for Specials? The Proposition in the Affirmative," and Annette Fiske, "12 Hour Day for Specials? Individual Adaptation," *TNHR* 70 (June 1923): 516–21.
32 "The AHA Convention," *AJN* 33 (October 1933): 1004; on blanket codes, see Leverett S. Lyon et al., *The National Recovery Administration* (Washington, D.C.: Brookings Institution, 1935), and Hugh S. Johnson, *The Blue Eagle from Egg to Earth* (Garden City, N.Y.: Doubleday, Dover, 1935), esp. pp. 252–57.
33 "Report of the Joint Committee on Adjustments," Exhibit A, "ANA Board of Directors Minutes," August 25, 1933, ANA Papers, Box 41, Nursing Archives, Boston University; "Notes from Headquarters, ANA," *AJN* 33 (October 1933): 1001; "The NRA and Nursing," *AJN* 33 (September 1933): 872–73.
34 Ethel Swope, "The 8 Hour Day Makes Progress," *AJN* 33 (December 1933): 1147–52; Elizabeth S. Poupore, "Mrs. Horatio Walker Who First Introduced the Eight Hour Day for Special Duty Nurses," ibid., pp. 1154–55; Mary E. G. Bliss, "The Eight Hour Plan Makes Progress in Massachusetts," *AJN* 34 (June 1934): 571–73; Roth, *35 Years of the MSNA*, pp. 40–43.
35 Sally Johnson, "A Trial of the Eight Hour Day for Hospital Special Nurses," Memo, 1934, p. 4, MGH Nursing Records, Box 15, Folder 2T, Countway Library, Rare Books Room, Harvard Medical School, Boston, Mass.
36 "The ANA and the 8 Hour Day," *AJN* 34 (August 1934): 817.
37 Ibid; David Wagner, "The Proletarianization of American Nursing," p. 277; "The 8 Hour Day," *AJN* 37 (November 1937): 1207; See also Ronnie Steinberg, *Wages*

and Hours: Labor and Reform in 20th Century America (New Brunswick, N.J.: Rutgers University Press, 1982). Such aversion to protective labor legislation was common among professional groups.

38 Bureau of the Census, *Historical Statistics,* ser. B, pp. 235–36 and B, pp. 192–94; ANA, *Facts about Nursing* (New York: Nursing Information Bureau, 1942), p. 8; Mary Roberts, *American Nursing* (New York: Macmillan, 1954), pp. 235 and 286; Grading Committee, *Nurses, Patients and Pocketbooks;* Kathleen Cannings and William Lazonick, "The Development of the Nursing Labor Force in the United States: A Basis Analysis," *International Journal of Health Services* 5 (1975): 185–217.

Unfortunately, it is difficult to get an accurate count of where nurses were working in the country. The most reliable statistics come from the 1942 Public Health survey of nursing resources. The statistics gathered by the Grading Committee, for example, reflected nursing's ability to get information only from those hospitals where there were nursing schools. Similarly, *Facts about Nursing* reflects information on ANA *membership,* rather than all nurses. Wagner ("The Proletarianization of Nursing," p. 276) states that 800 schools closed between 1928 and 1938, but he gives no source for this figure. Since additional schools did open during the 1930s, it is possible that this number actually closed and that the final figures reflect only the net change.

39 Grading Committee, *Nurses, Patients and Pocketbooks,* pp. 290 and 435.

40 Ibid., pp. 532–34; Mary Roberts, "Are We Over-Educating Our Nurses at the Expense of the Personal Care of the Patient?" *Bulletin of the AHA* 2 (October 1928): 556–58; "Did You Ever See a Nurse Nursing?" *AJN* 38 (January 1938): 27. For a discussion of nurses' views on the *advantages* of staff nursing, see Melosh, "Doctors, Patients and 'Big Nurse,' " and "*The Physician's Hand,*" pp. 84–103.

41 Report of Ethel Swope, assistant director of headquarters, ANA, relating to special fieldwork for the year 1934, "ANA Board of Directors Minutes," January 23–25, 1935, Exhibit VI, ANA Papers, Box 42, Nursing Archives, Boston University.

42 For a discussion of Blue Cross and "reasonable costs," see Law, *Blue Cross.*

43 "Minutes of Joint Meeting of Districts 13 and 14, New York State Nurses' Association, October 8, 1934, to discuss Harlan Hoyt Horner's proposal for a Moratorium on Nursing Training," p. 12, New York Hospital Archives, Curriculum Box 1, Folder E. Horner, the assistant educational commissioner in New York State, had surveyed nursing conditions in New York in 1934 and proposed a moratorium on admissions. Nursing leaders, however, fearful that a complete closing of the schools would lower standards, did not accept his plan. See his *Nursing Education and Practice in New York State, with Suggested Remedial Measures* (Albany: University of the State of New York Press, 1934), and discussion of his findings in JoAnn Ashley, *Hospitals, Paternalism and the Role of the Nurse* (New York: Teachers College Press, 1976), pp. 67–72.

44 Marion Rottman, "Should a Hospital Close Its Nursing School? And Why?" *MH* 33 (August 1932): 77–80.

45 Adelaide Nutting to Elizabeth Burgess, January 30, 1932, Nutting Papers, Box 3, Grading Committee Folder, Teachers College Archives, Columbia University Press, New York.

46 Stella Goostray to Elnora Thomson, January 22, 1932, in "ANA Board of Directors Minutes," January 23, 1932, ANA Papers, Box 40, Mugar Library, Boston University; for press release on the letter, see "ANA Board of Directors Minutes," June 20, 1932, Exhibit V, ANA Papers, Box 40; Emilie Sargent, "The Nursing Program Works for Recovery," *AJN* 33 (December 1933): 1168.

47 "Suggestions for Trustees," *AJN* (July 1932): 782; "National Nursing Groups Appeal to Hospital Trustees," *MH* 34 (July 1932): 108.

48 "Notes from Headquarters, ANA," *AJN* 32 (December 1932): 1323.

49 Janet Geister, "Unemployment Statement, October 25, 1932," Geister Papers, Box 10, Folder 89, Nursing Archives, Boston University; Janet Geister to Adelaide Nutting, August 23, 1932, and Adelaide Nutting to Isabel Stewart, July 21, 1932,

quoted by Teresa Christy, "The First Fifty Years," *AJN* (September 1971): 1783. Christy states that the letter was sent out on July 19, 1932, but the letter was sent a month before on June 19, 1932. It is possible more replies came in later.

50 Not surprisingly, the first important discussion and estimate of the costs of a nursing service were made by Annie Goodrich in 1912. For a summary of the major studies on costs made between 1912 and 1932, see Department of Studies of the NLNE, *A Study in the Use of the Graduate Nurse for Bedside Nursing in the Hospital* (New York: NLNE, 1933), pp. 16–22. See also Blanche Pfefferkorn and Charles Rovetta, "Cost Studies and Nursing," *AJN* 37 (November 1937): 1249–53. The studies showed that the annual cost per student ran anywhere from $459 to $1,285, a graduate nurse from $1,488 to $2,000 (see *A Study in the Use*, p. 19).

51 "Standards from the April 1931 Report," p. 16, Stella Goostray Papers, Box 6, Nursing Archives, Boston University; "Proceedings of the Semi-Annual Meeting of the Committee on the Grading of Nursing Schools, March 23, 1932," pp. 5–25, Goostray Papers, Box 7; May Ayers Burgess, "What the Cost Study Showed," *AJN* 32 (April 1932): 427–32.

52 "Report of the Cost Study" by May Ayers Burgess and Phobe Gordon, quoted by Ethel Johns, "Memo Concerning Comparative Cost of Graduate and Student Nursing Service to the Hospital," April 1930, Administration School of Nursing and Nursing Service, Re: Reorganization of Above, 1929–1934, New York Hospital Archives, Box 4, Nursing Costs folder.

Despite these findings, Malcolm MacEachern, a powerful advocate of graduate staff nursing, argued that the graduate nurse needed less supervision; see, for example, his "Which Shall We Choose–Graduate or Student Service?" *MH* 38 (June 1932): 97–104. The Joint Committee on the Cost of Nursing Services and Nursing produced a study in 1938 to show that graduate nurses had fewer days of lost time due to illness than students. The study did not emphasize its other finding: that one-fourth of the hospitals surveyed had no sick leave with pay policy for graduate nurses, a policy that would affect how often any worker was "sick" (*A Study of the Incidence and Costs of Illness Among Nurses* [New York: ANA, AHA, and NLNE, 1938]).

53 "Minimal Standards for Hospital Nursing Services," *AJN* 36 (December 1936): 121–22; American College of Surgeons, *Manual of Hospital Standardization. History, Development and Progress of Hospital Standardization: Detailed Explanation of the Minimum Requirements* (Chicago: ACS, 1938).

54 Department of Studies of the NLNE, "A Study of the Nursing Service in 50 Selected Hospitals," *Report of the Hospital Survey for New York*, vol. 2 (New York: United Hospital Fund, 1937), p. 425.

55 "Graduate or Student?" *AJN* 33 (May 1933): 471–72; the editorial was commenting on an article in the same issue by A Superintendent of Nurses, "Graduate vs. Student," pp. 473–81.

56 *Boston City Hospital Alumnae Newsletter*, July 1933. For an autobiographical account of the difficulties of a returning older nurse to staff nursing, see Mary Williams Brinton, *My Cap and My Cape* (Philadelphia: Dorrance, 1950), pp. 244–62.

57 *Long Island Hospital Annual Report, 1936; New England Hospital for Women and Children Annual Reports, 1934–1938*, New England Hospital Papers, Box 1, Nursing Archives, Boston University; "Report of Survey of Boston City Hospital School of Nursing, June 18, 19, 1937"; "Report to the Board of Trustees and Medical Director, Boston City Hospital in response to 1939 Finance Commission Report," Marion Parsons Papers, Box 13, Folder 2, Mugar Library, Boston University; Patterson, Teele, and Davis, "A Study of the Yearly Expenses of the Training School for Nurses at the MGH," *Bulletin of the AHA* 6 (April 1932): 41–58; Sylvia Perkins, *A Centennial Review: The MGH School of Nursing, 1873–1973* (Boston: School of Nursing, Nurses' Alumnae Association, 1973), p. 213.

58 "ANA Advisory Council Minutes," May 12, 1940, p. 145, ANA Papers, Box 3, Nursing Archives; see also Wagner, "The Proletarianization of American Nursing."

59 This conclusion is based on statistical analysis of monthly sickness reports for nurses and students at the New England Hospital; see "New England Hospital Nursing Reports, 1938–1940," New England Hospital Papers, Box 1, Folder 2, Nursing Archives, Boston University; see also "Miss Lawler's Report at Graduation Exercises," *Johns Hopkins Hospital Nursing Alumnae* 36 (July 1937): 103.

60 "ANA Advisory Council Minutes," May 12, 1940, pp. 145–46, ANA Papers, Box 3, Nursing Archives, Boston University. This advisory council meeting has a good discussion of these problems, but these kinds of complaints can also be read in the nursing journals of the 1930s. For a general discussion of these issues, see Wagner, "The Proletarianization of American Nursing." For a 1980s analysis of similar issues, see Nancy P. Greenleaf, "Labor Force Participation by Age of Registered Nurses and Women in Comparable Occupations" (Ph.D. diss., Boston University, 1982).

61 R.N., "Letter to the Editor," *AJN* 34 (October 1934): 1011. The headline over the letter read "Is This the End Toward Which We Are Striving?"

62 "ANA Advisory Council Minutes," May 12, 1940, p. 154, ANA Papers, Box 3, Nursing Archives, Boston University. A survey of seventy-five nursing superintendents in 1936 revealed that only five believed that "adequate administration and supervision contribute to the maintenance of a satisfactory nursing group" (Emily Hicks, "Graduate Staff Nursing," *AJN* 36 [June 1936]: 595). With her characteristic humor, Janet Geister charged that nursing administrators did not understand the difference between "Snoopervision versus Supervision"; see her article with this title in *TNHR* 99 (March 1937): 240–43.

63 See E. M. Bluestone, "A Labor Program for Hospitals," *MH* 48 (April 1937): 43–45; "Labor Policies," editorial in ibid., p. 41; E. M. Bluestone, "Labor and Philanthropy," *MH* 48 (July 1937): 47–49.
    Bluestone was the administrator of Montefiore Hospital in the Bronx from 1928 to 1951. He continued to be a major consultant to hospital administrators all over the world until his death in 1980. In an interview with me on October 25, 1978, Bluestone stated that there was very little response to his proposals in *Modern Hospital* and that his suggestions were not implemented.

64 U.S. Department of Labor, "The Economic Status of Registered Professional Nurses," Bulletin no. 931 (Washington, D.C.: Government Printing Office, 1948) p. 13; *The General Staff Nurse,* Report of the Joint Committee of the ANA and NLNE to work with the AHA and CHA on the Status and Problems of the Hospital Staff Nurse (New York: The Committee, 1941); Beatrice and Philip Kalisch, *The Advance of American Nursing* (Boston: Little, Brown, 1978), p. 493.

65 "New England Hospital Nursing Reports, Report for the Year Ending May 31, 1938," New England Hospital Papers, Box 1, Nursing Archives, Boston University; Perkins, *A Centennial Review,* p. 213.

66 "Recent Hospital Association Meetings," *AJN* 34 (November 1934): 1124.

67 "ANA Board of Directors Minutes," January 24–28, 1938, p. 20, ANA Papers, Box 43, Nursing Archives, Boston University.

68 Wagner, "The Proletarianization of American Nursing," p. 280. At New York Hospital, Ethel Johns, in her 1931 memo to Dr. Canby Robinson on the comparative costs of graduate and student nursing services, noted: "Students are more amenable to discipline and often display a finer spirit of loyalty to the institution. Unfortunately, hospital authorities fail to realize that little effort has as yet been made to build up a similar esprit de corps among the graduate nursing staff." By the late 1930s, however, the nursing associations at least had realized this dimension and began to make such efforts. Ethel Johns to Canby Robinson, March 17, 1931, Administration School of Nursing and Nursing Service, Re: Reorganization of Above, 1929–1934, Box 1, Correspondence folder, Administration Robinson 10/2/19–2/6/34, New York Hospital Archives.

69 Ethel Johns, for example, expressed this in her correspondence with Dr. Canby Robinson over the changes in the New York Hospital nursing service. Johns wanted the hospital school to stay in the leadership of hospital-based nursing

schools and to continue to train women for leadership in nursing. She was arguing for more of a graduate staff with assistance from aides to free the students for classroom education. In response to Robinson's requests for time studies and the end of certain procedures on the part of the nursing staff, Johns replied, "Reductions in nursing costs can of course be made by substituting the labor of less expensive workers. To what extent this can be done with safety to the patient is a matter to be studied jointly, as you suggest, by the medical and nursing staffs."

70 One administrator claimed, for example, that 40 graduate nurses and 40 aides could replace 100 pupil nurses; see George Walker, "Calling Nurses Aides to the Rescue," *MH* 47 (September 1936): 82. The ANA House of Delegates passed a resolution from the private-duty nursing section in 1936 protesting the use of untrained nursing workers on federal nursing projects; see "The Convention," *AJN* 36 (August 1936): 800. Dorothy Johnston estimated that the WPA between 1935 and 1942 gave employment to 4,400 practical nurses and trained 5,000 ward helpers, auxiliaries, and orderlies (*History and Trends in Practical Nursing* [St. Louis: Mosby, 1966], p. 41). For further discussion of nurses' anxiety over these developments, and state-by-state surveys of the changes, see "ANA Board of Directors Minutes," January 23–27, 1939, and January 21, 1941, Box 44, and "ANA Advisory Council Minutes, May 25, 1941," ANA Papers, Box 4, Nursing Archives, Boston University.

In this period the terms "hospital helpers," "nurses' aides," "aides," and "practical nurses" were often used interchangeably. The licensed practical or licensed vocational nurse did not become a category until the mid-1940s; see Dorothy Deming, *The Practical Nurse* (1947; reprint, New York: Garland, 1985).

71 *Proceedings, NLNE, 1932–1940;* Stella Goostray, *Memoirs* (Boston: Nursing Archives, 1966), pp. 103–10; "The Convention," *AJN* 36 (August 1936): 800. For a discussion of the subsidiary worker, see "ANA Board of Directors Minutes," January 25–29, 1937, p. 94, ANA Papers, Box 43. Roberts (*American Nursing,* p. 267) states that the nursing profession "faced the issue squarely" of subsidiary workers when in 1936 the joint boards went on record recommending control by RNs. If anything, Roberts had her geometry wrong: Nursing had been circling the issue since the 1890s and only by force of circumstance finally took a position.

Wagner ("Proletarianization of American Nursing," p. 281) has argued that I have given too much weight to the role of the nursing leadership in establishing the hospital hierarchy. He suggests that the "continued disequilibrium" of the leaders on the question of subsidiary workers is an indication of this. I agree that nursing responded rather than led on this part of the rationalization question. But I think Wagner has too narrowly interpreted my understanding of the rationalization process. The question of the division of labor is only a part of this process. The nursing leadership's inability to come to terms with this narrower question of the work force reflected the divisions within nursing and their efforts to cut off the bottom of their own ranks first.

For a statement of the nursing position on subsidiary workers, see Joint Committee of the ANA, NLNE, and NOPHN, *Subsidiary Workers in the Care of the Sick* (New York: Joint Committee, 1940), and AHA and NLNE, *Manual of the Essentials of a Good Hospital Service* (1936).

On changes in the licensure laws, see Veronica M. Driscoll, *Legitimizing the Program of Nursing: The Distinct Mission of the New York State Nurses' Association* (New York: Foundation of the New York State Nurses' Association, 1976), pp. 41–58. The New York State law, however, because of continual amendments, did not become effective until 1950. Other states later followed; see *Facts about Nursing,* 1938–45.

72 See "Pressing Problems for Those in Private Duty," *TNHR* 97 (August 1936): 141–42; Louise Kieninger, "The Subsidiary Worker," *AJN* 36 (October 1936): 984–86.

On the hospital administrator's promise, see Fred Carter, "Next Call for Attendants," *MH* 48 (February 1937): 58, and A. C. Jensen, "Training Nursing Attendants," ibid., 51 (November 1938): 68.

73 "ANA Board of Directors Minutes," January 23–27, 1939, p. 64, ANA Papers, Box 44, Nursing Archives, Boston University.

74 "ANA Advisory Council Minutes," May 12, 1940, p. 114, ANA Papers, Box 3.

75 Jensen, "Training Nursing Attendants," p. 68.

76 Winifred McL. Shepler et al., "Standardized Training Course for Ward Aides," *MH* 51 (December 1938): 65–72. Key excerpts from this article have been reprinted in Carol Berkin and Mary Beth Norton, eds., *Women of America: A History* (Boston: Houghton Mifflin, 1979), pp. 311–12. It is a clear statement of the difficulties of training people for a job that had no potential for change.

77 "From Aide to Organizer: The Oral History of Lillian Roberts," interview by Susan Reverby, in *Women of America*, ed. Berkin and Norton, pp. 289–306. The full text of the interview is available through the Microfilm Corporation of America as part of "The Twentieth Century Trade Union Woman: Vehicle for Social Change," Oral History Project of the Institute of Labor and Industrial Relations at the University of Michigan–Wayne State University.

When Roberts became an official in District 37 of the American Federation of State County and Municipal Employees in New York City; she instituted an upgrading program in the New York City hospitals that made it possible for nurses' aides to train to become LPNs without going back to school and leaving their jobs. Her inability to get nurse's training despite her obvious skill at the job remained one of the most poignant disappointments of her life.

78 There is a very large literature describing both nursing conditions and the degrees of nursing "satisfaction" with work in the postwar years. See, for examples, Everett Hughes et al., *20,000 Nurses Tell Their Story* (Philadelphia: Lippincott, 1958); Temple Burling et al., *The Give and Take of Hospitals* (New York: Putnam, 1956); U.S. Department of Labor, "The Economic Status of Registered Professional Nurses"; Committee on the Function of Nursing, *A Program for the Nursing Profession* (New York: Macmillan, 1948); Susan Reverby, "Health–Women's Work," in *Prognosis: Negative*, ed. David Kotelchuck (New York: Vintage, 1976), pp. 170–83. For a theoretical discussion of professional abandonment of "hands-on" care and work, see Andrew Abbott, "Status and Status Strain in the Professions," *American Journal of Sociology* 86 (1981): 819–35, and discussion in Joan Jacobs Brumberg and Nancy Tomes, "Women in the Professions: A Research Agenda for American Historians," *Reviews in American History* 10 (June 1982): 287–88.

79 The question of whether responsibility, and even authority, means power has been discussed by others concerned with women's roles; see Rosabeth Moss Kanter, *Men and Women of the Corporation* (New York: Basic, 1977). As Kanter notes, "People who have authority without system power are powerless." For a slightly different viewpoint on this question, see Melosh, "Doctors, Patients and 'Big Nurse.' "

80 The reality of nursing shortages has been a point of political debate within the hospital industry since the early 1900s. On this question during World War II and the postwar years, see Kalisch and Kalisch, *Advance in American Nursing*, pp. 470–73, and Roberts, *American Nursing*, pp. 383–92. Franklin Roosevelt believed there was a sufficient shortage of nurses in the military to call for a draft of nurses in January 1945. Whether because of this threat and more volunteering, or a manipulation of the numbers, by April 1945 it was clear there was no shortage, either in the military or in the civilian sector.

The question of nursing shortages is the subject once again of ferment in the nursing and hospital world. See, for examples, Loretta McLaughlin, "Nurses Say Shortage Could Hurt Them," *Boston Globe*, March 2, 1981, pp. 17 and 21; Paula Span, "Where Have All the Nurses Gone?" *New York Times Sunday Magazine*, February 22, 1981, pp. 70–71, 78–79, 96, 100–1; Claire Fagin, "The National Shortage of Nurses: A Nursing Perspective," in *Nursing in the 1980's*, ed. Linda Aiken, pp. 21–39.

81 Hope Newell, *The History of the National Nursing Council* (New York: Distributed by the NOPHN, 1951).

82 Johnston, *History and Trends of Practical Nursing,* and Deming, *The Practical Nurse,* discuss these developments. The history of the use of aides in hospitals can be pieced together in part through the use of the Red Cross Records in the National Archives.

83 "Poll Shows Place for Practical Nurses in Hospitals – But with Strings Attached," *MH* 60 (August 1945): 42–43; see also E. M. Bluestone, "The Present Status of Nursing," *MH* 57 (May 1944): 54–64. Bluestone's call for a return to bedside nursing, and the necessity for decent training for practical nurses, was read at an annual symposium conducted by the United Hospital Fund of New York, the Greater New York Hospital Association, and the New York Academy of Medicine. He reported that the responses were exceedingly favorable and that after the meeting, 15,000 copies of his speech were printed in pamphlet form (E. M. Bluestone to Susan Reverby, October 26, 1978).

    See also Committee on the Function of Nursing, *A Program for the Nursing Program,* and Esther Lucille Brown, *Nursing for the Future* (New York: Russell Sage Foundation, 1948).

84 Emilie G. Sargent to Elmira Beers Wickendon, April 6, 1942, in "ANA Board of Directors Minutes," May 16–17, 1942, p. 38, ANA Papers, Box 46, Nursing Archives, Boston University.

85 Helen McDonough, "Private Duty Nurses Section Report, ANA Board of Directors Minutes," June 13–15, 1943, p. 44, ANA Papers, Box 46; Teresa Tully, "Private Duty Nurses Section Report, ANA Board of Directors Minutes," January 23, 1946, p. 45, ANA Papers, Box 45.

86 See, for example, Sue Z. McCracken, chairman of the Board of Trustees of the Ohio State Nurses' Association to Julia Stimson, president of the ANA, December 30, 1943, in "ANA Board of Directors Minutes," January 26–29, 1944, ANA Papers, Box 45.

87 For a summary of the development of nursing unionization, see Norman Metzer and Dennis Pointer, *Labor-Management Relations in the Health Services Industry* (Washington: Science and Health Publications, 1972), pp. 34–37; David R. Denton, "The Union Movement in American Hospitals, 1847–1976" (Ph.D. diss., Boston University, 1976). See also "ANA Advisory Council Minutes," April 1938, p. 24, ANA Papers, Box 3, Nursing Archives, Boston University.

88 "ANA Board of Directors Minutes," January 25–29, 1937, p. 37, ANA Papers, Box 43.

89 Editorials, "Nurse Membership in Unions," *AJN* 37 (July 1937): 766–67, and "Union Membership? No!" *AJN* 38 (May 1938): 573–74.

90 Susan Francis, "ANA Advisory Council Minutes," April 24, 1938, p. 99, ANA Papers, Box 3, Nursing Archives, Boston University.

91 Ibid., pp. 99–100.

92 Ibid., p. 93.

93 Statement by the ANA Board of Directors, January 24, 1938, in "ANA Advisory Council Minutes," April 23, 1939, p. 3, ANA Papers, Box 3.

94 "ANA Board of Directors Minutes," January 28–31, 1940, pp. 23–24, ANA Papers, Box 44. It was suggested that the ANA staff develop plans and information for state associations "as to ways in which labor union activities among nurses may be combated. It is urged that this recommendation, as such, receive no publicity and that the program be a positive program." Further, they encouraged "that, for the present, union activity be not stressed in the literature of the association, including the *AJN* and the publications of the Nursing Information Bureau, since to do so seems to give undue emphasis to unions." It also, parenthetically, makes the historian's task of uncovering this history so much more difficult.

95 The state associations historically have been reluctant to take on this bargaining role; see Betty Robinson, "Nurse Control of Nursing: The Professional Associa-

tion and Collective Bargaining" (Ph.D. diss., Boston University, 1983). See also Dennis H. Kruger, "Bargaining and the Nursing Profession," *Monthly Labor Review* 84 (July 1961): 699–75, and the more recent Andrew K. Dolan, "The Legality of Nursing Association Serving as Collective Bargaining Agents: The Arundel Case," *Journal of Health, Politics, Policy and Law* 5 (Spring 1980): 25–54; and Richard Miller, "Hospitals," in *Collective Bargaining: Contemporary American Experience,* ed. G. G. Somers (Madison, Wis.: Industrial Relations Research Association, 1979): 373–433.

96　See Roberts, *American Nursing*, pp. 465–574; The Committee on the Function of Nursing, *A Program for the Nursing Profession* (New York: Macmillan, 1948); and Esther Lucille Brown, *Nursing for the Future* (New York: Russell Sage Foundation, 1948).

97　See Claire Fagin, "Nurses' Rights," *AJN* 75 (1975): 82–85.

CONCLUSION　*Beyond the obligation to care*

1　M. Adelaide Nutting, "Apprenticeship to Duty," in *A Sound Economic Basis for Schools of Nursing and Other Addresses* (1926; reprint, New York: Garland, 1984), pp. 350–64.

2　On the relationship between duty and rights in different work settings see Eugene Genovese, *Roll, Jordan, Roll* (New York: Pantheon, 1974), pp. 146–47, and James C. Scott, *The Moral Economy of the Peasant* (New Haven, Conn.: Yale University Press, 1976), pp. 180–92.

3　See Jean Baker Miller, *Towards a New Psychology of Women* (Boston: Beacon, 1976); Nancy Chodorow, *The Reproduction of Mothering* (Berkeley: University of California Press, 1978); Carol Gilligan, *In a Different Voice* (Cambridge, Mass.: Harvard University Press, 1982); Iris Marion Young, "Is Male Gender Identity the Cause of Male Domination?" in *Mothering: Essays in Feminist Theory,* ed. Joyce Trebicott (Totowa, N.J.: Rowman and Allanheld, 1983), pp. 129–46; Author interview with Jean Baker Miller, Wellesley, Mass., January 17, 1986.

4　Estelle Freedman, "Separatism as Strategy: Female Institution Building and American Feminism, 1870–1930," *Feminist Studies* 5 (Fall 1979): 512–29; Ellen DuBois et al., "Politics and Culture in Women's History: A Symposium," *Feminist Studies* 6 (Spring 1980): 26–64; Barbara Miller Solomon, *In the Company of Educated Women* (New Haven, Conn.: Yale University Press, 1985).

5　Barbara Melosh, "*The Physician's Hand*" (Philadelphia: Temple University Press, 1982); Carroll Smith-Rosenberg, "Hearing Women's Words: A Feminist Reconstruction of History," in *Disorderly Conduct* (New York: Knopf, 1985), pp. 11–52; Gareth Stedman Jones, *Languages of Class* (Cambridge: Cambridge University Press, 1983), pp. 21–22. For a discussion of the importance of autonomy in male occupations see Eliot Freidson, "Occupational Autonomy and Labor Market Strategies," in *Varieties of Work,* ed. Phyllis L. Stewart and Muriel G. Cantor (Beverly Hills, Calif.: Sage, 1982), pp. 39–54.

6　Melosh, "*The Physician's Hand*"; Susan Porter Benson, *Counter Cultures* (Urbana: University of Illinois Press, 1986).

7　For examples see Larry Blum et al., "Altruism and Women's Oppression," in *Women and Philosophy,* ed. Carol Gould and Marx Wartofsky (New York: Putnam, 1976), pp. 222–47; Nel Noddings, *Caring: A Feminine Approach to Ethics and Moral Education* (Berkeley: University of California Press, 1984); Chodorow, *Reproduction of Mothering;* Janet Finch and Dulcie Groves, eds., *A Labour of Love: Women, Work and Caring* (London and Boston: Routledge and Kegan Paul, 1983).

8　Hilary Graham, "Caring: A Labour of Love," in Finch and Groves, eds., *A Labour of Love,* pp. 13–30.

9　Gilligan, *In a Different Voice;* see also Linda Kerber et al., "On *In a Different Voice:* An Interdisciplinary Forum," *Signs* 11 (Winter 1986): 304–33, and Owen Flanagan and Kathryn Jackson, "Justice, Care, and Gender: The Kohlberg-Gilligan Debate

Revisited," *Ethics* (in press). I am very grateful to Owen Flanagan for his help on this section.

10 Martin Benjamin and Joy Curtis, *Ethics in Nursing* (New York: Oxford University Press, 1981), pp. 21–47, and Ronald Dworkin, *Taking Rights Seriously* (Cambridge, Mass.: Harvard University Press, 1978), pp. 169–73.

11 Quoted in Lavinia L. Dock, *A History of Nursing*, vol. 3 (New York: Putnam, 1912), p. 129.

12 Benjamin and Curtis, *Ethics*, p. 40.

13 On the relationship of duty to rights, see Joel Feinberg, "Duties, Rights and Claims," in *Rights, Justice and the Bounds of Liberty* (Princeton, N.J.: Princeton University Press, 1980), pp. 130–42.

14 Claire Fagin, "Nurses Rights," *American Journal of Nursing* 75 (January 1975): 82. The American Association of Colleges of Nursing lists "altruism" as the first "essential value" for "the nurse as a professional person" (*Essentials of College and University Education for Nursing* [Washington: AACN, February 1986], p. 9).

15 Feinberg, *Rights*, p. 141.

16 For a similar argument, see Carroll Smith-Rosenberg, "The New Woman as Androgyne: Social Disorder and Gender Crisis," in *Disorderly Conduct*, p. 296.

17 Linda Aiken, "The Impact of Federal Health Policy on Nursing," in *Nursing in the 1980s*, ed. Linda Aiken (Philadelphia: Lippincott, 1982), pp. 3–20; American Nurses' Association, *Facts About Nursing 1984–85* (Kansas City: American Nurses' Association, 1985), pp. 116–21. It is interesting to note, however, that the biggest gains are in the community colleges, not the four-year programs.

18 See Patricia Benner, *From Novice to Expert: Excellence and Power in Clinical Nursing* (Reading, Mass.: Addison-Wesley, 1984), and Susan Reverby, "Health: Women's Work," in *Prognosis Negative: Crisis in the Health Care System* (New York: Vintage, 1979), pp. 170–83.

19 Reverby, "Health: Women's Work"; Boston Nurses' Group, "The False Promise: Professionalism in Nursing," *Science for the People* 10 (May-June 1978): 20–34.

20 Jennifer Bingham Hull, "Hospital Nightmare: Cuts in Staff Demoralize Nurses as Case Suffers," *Wall Street Journal*, March 27, 1985; Genrose Alfano, ed., *The All-RN Nursing Staff* (Wakefield, Mass.: Nursing Resources, 1980).

21 Margaret McClure and M. Janice Nelson, "Trends in Hospital Nursing," in Aiken, ed., *Nursing in the 1980s*, p. 63.

22 Donna Diers, "Nursing: Implementing the Agenda for Social Change" (Speech given at the Fiftieth Anniversary Symposium, "Nursing as a Force for Social Change," University of Pennsylvania School of Nursing, Philadelphia, September 20, 1985).

23 Boston Nurses' Group, "The False Promise"; Hull, "Hospital Nightmare."

24 Fagin, "Nurses' Rights"; author interview with Joan Lynaugh, University of Pennsylvania School of Nursing, January 14, 1986.

25 Bonnie Bullough, "The Struggle for Women's Rights in Denver: A Personal Account," *Nursing Outlook* 26 (September 1978): 566–67.

26 The history of the ambiguous relationship of nursing to feminism is yet to be written. On June 8–10, 1986, the Sigma Theta Tau (nursing honor society), Yale University chapter, hosted the first "Nursing and Feminism" conference. Cassandra, a radical feminist nurses' network, has been in existence since 1983.

27 For critiques of liberal feminism, see Allison M. Jagger, *Feminist Politics and Human Nature* (Totowa, N.J.: Rowman and Allanheld, 1983), pp. 27–50, 173–206; Zillah Eisenstein, *The Radical Future of Liberal Feminism* (New York and London: Longman, 1981); Juliet Mitchell, "Women and Equality," in *The Rights and Wrongs of Women*, ed. Mitchell and Ann Oakley (London: Penguin, 1976), pp. 379–99; and Rosalind Pollack Petchesky, *Abortion and Women's Choice* (Boston: Northeastern University Press, 1984), pp. 1–24.

For a similar discussion of the limits of autonomy in medical ethics, see Robert M. Veatch, "Autonomy's Temporary Triumph," *Hastings Center Report* 14 (October 1984): 38–40, and Daniel Callahan, "Autonomy: A Moral Good, not a Moral Obsession," in ibid., pp. 40–42.

28 For a parallel argument for a "multi-layered moral landscape," see Flanagan and Jackson, "Justice, Care, and Gender."

29 Miller, *Towards a New Psychology of Women;* Jane Flax, "The Conflict between Nurturance and Autonomy in Mother–Daughter Relationships and within Feminism," *Feminist Studies* 4 (June 1978): 171–91.

30 For a similar philosophical discussion, see Larry Blum et al., "Altruism and Women's Oppression."

31 On nursing as metaphor, see Claire Fagin and Donna Diers, "Nursing as Metaphor," *New England Journal of Medicine,* July 14, 1983, pp. 116–17.

Note on sources

Much of nursing's history still lies buried in attics, slowly disintegrating in forgotten hospital file cabinets, or fading in the memories of older nurses. With the continual closing of the hospital-based diploma schools, many of these records will be lost. Only an increasing awareness of the importance of these documents and recollections will arrest this process and make it possible for nursing's history to be constructed. Fortunately, this consciousness is becoming more widespread.

The single best primary source for data on nursing's history is the Nursing Archives in Mugar Library at Boston University. Their holdings include books as well as the papers of the American Nurses' Association and those of over 150 individuals, schools, and organizations. The Nursing Archives also publishes a nursing history journal. I also consulted the holdings on the National League of Nursing in the National Library of Medicine in Bethesda, Maryland; on public-health nursing in the Simmons College Archives in Boston; on various Boston programs in the Countway Library Rare Books Room at Harvard Medical School; on the Red Cross in the National Archives in Washington; and on the Teachers College leaders in the Teachers College Library, Special Collections, Columbia University.

Individual hospital and nursing school records can usually be found in the public relations, school, or administrative offices of various institutions. On occasion, the larger hospitals have their own archives. Records for public hospitals and schools are often kept in municipal and state archives. I found useful material on Boston-area institutions at Somerville, Long Island, and the Boston Lying-In hospitals (materials now in the Countway Medical Library). The Massachusetts State Archives also provided printed data on public hospitals. Other primary sources are listed in the select bibliography that follows. A useful listing of primary source holdings on nursing can be found in the January 1987 issue of *Nursing Research*.

Nursing history sources are often buried within larger medical history collections. Nursing records in the Hospital Archives at the New York Hospital in New York City and in the Massachusetts General Hospital's papers in the Countway Medical Library provided information on two more elite nursing schools. The Countway Library also has almost a complete run of the major early twentieth-century hospital, medical and nursing journals. I have edited a selected reprint series of thirty-two volumes on nursing history, which should provide a useful beginning point for research (*The History of American Nursing* [New York: Garland, 1984–85]).

Several bibliographies make the research process easier. Vern Bullough and Bonnie Bullough et al. have edited two volumes: *Nursing: A Historical Bibliography* (New York: Garland, 1981) and *Issues in Nursing: An Annotated Bibliography* (New York: Garland, 1985). An older annotated bibliography, Virginia Henderson, *Nursing Studies Index, 1900–1959,* 4 vols. (New York: Garland, 1985; reprint of Lippincott volumes from 1963, 1966, 1970, 1972), covers a wide range of issues and journals.

Nursing historians have their own organization, the American Association for the History of Nursing. The association holds annual meetings and publishes a quarterly *Bulletin.* It can be contacted at P.O. Box E 40, 210 7th Street S.E., Washington, D.C. 20003.

Sources for women's and medical history, as well as the secondary sources, are not listed here. The extensiveness of the notes should serve as a guide to the materials I found particularly helpful.

Select bibliography of primary sources

Manuscripts

Bethesda, Maryland. National Library of Medicine. History of Medicine Manuscript Collection.
    National League for Nursing Papers
Boston, Massachusetts. Brigham and Women's Hospital. Public Relations Office.
    Matron's Journals, Boston Lying-In Hospital
————. Boston University. Mugar Library. Special Collections.
    Nursing Archives. Institutional and Organizational Papers
        American Nurses' Association
        Boston City Hospital, School of Nursing
        Massachusetts Nurses' Association
        Massachusetts Nurses' Association, District V (including Central Directory for Nurses)
        New England Hospital for Women and Children
        Visiting Nurse Association of Boston
        Waltham Training School for Nurses
    Nursing Archives. Personal Papers
        Virginia M. Dunbar
        Janet M. Geister
        Annie W. Goodrich
        Stella Goostray (including Committee on the Grading of Nursing Schools)
        Elinor D. Gregg
        Virginia A. Henderson
        Marion G. Parsons
        Linda A. J. Richards
        Mary M. Roberts
        Emilie G. Sargent
        Effie J. Taylor
        Shirley C. Titus
        Jane Van de Vrede
        Theresa Wolfson
————. Harvard University Medical School. Countway Medical Library. Rare Books Room.
    Institutional Papers

Boston Medical Library Directory for Nurses
Children's Hospital
Long Island Hospital
Massachusetts General Hospital
Personal Papers
Ernest Amory Codman
Robert Latou Dickinson
————. Harvard University. Harvard University Archives.
Richard Cabot Papers
————. Radcliffe College. Schlesinger Library.
Home for Aged Women Collection
————. St. Margaret's Hospital. Nursing Director's Office.
Nursing School and Student Records
New York, New York. Columbia University. Teachers College. Nursing Education Archives.
M. Adelaide Nutting Papers
Isabel M. Stewart Papers
————. New York Hospital. Hospital Archives.
Administration School of Nursing and Nursing Service Reorganization Records
Board of Governors Records
Conference Committee Records
Training School Committee Records
Secretary-Treasurer's Papers
Visiting Committee Records
Northampton, Massachusetts. Smith College. Sophia Smith Archives.
New England Hospital for Women and Children Papers
Somerville, Massachusetts. Somerville Hospital. President's Office and Nursing School Office.
Hospital History Papers
Nursing School and Student Records, Nursing School Director's Office
Squantum, Massachusetts. Long Island Hospital. Nursing Director's Office.
Nursing School and Student Records
Washington, D.C. National Archives.
Federal Mediation and Conciliation Service Records
Red Cross Records
Women's Bureau Records

Proceedings and annual reports

American Hospital Association. *Transactions of Annual Conferences, 1908–45.*
American Society of Superintendents of Training Schools for Nurses. *Proceedings and Reports of Annual Conventions, 1894–1912.*
Association of Hospital Superintendents of the United States and Canada. *Transactions of Annual Conferences, 1900–07.*
Boston City Hospital. *Annual Reports,* 1865–1945. Boston.
Boston Lying-In Hospital. *Annual Reports,* 1875–1940. Boston.
Boston Medical Library. *Annual Reports,* 1880–1914. Boston.

Long Island Hospital. *Annual Reports,* 1898–1938. Boston.
The reports are filed as part of:
Annual Reports of the Pauper Institutions, City of Boston, 1898–1908
Annual Reports of the Boston Infirmary Department (Pauper Institutions Department) of the City of Boston, 1909–21
Annual Reports of the Institutions Department of the City of Boston, 1921–38
Massachusetts General Hospital and McLean Asylum. *Annual Reports,* 1890–96. Boston.
Massachusetts State Nurses' Association. *Proceedings of the Annual Conferences,* 1904–40.
National League of Nursing Education. *Proceedings of the Annual Conventions,* 1912–50.
New England Hospital for Women and Children. *Annual Reports,* 1862–1945. Boston.
Ohio Valley General Hospital. *Annual Reports,* 1915–30. Wheeling, W.Va.
Somerville Hospital. *Annual Reports,* 1896–1935 (scattered reports). Somerville.
Suffolk County Nurses Central Directory. *Annual Reports,* 1913–40. Boston.
Waltham Training School for Nurses. *Annual Reports,* 1886–1937. Waltham.

Journals

American Journal of Nursing, 1900–45.
Bulletin of the American College of Surgeons, 1916–45.
Bulletin of the American Hospital Association, 1920–29.
Hospital Management, 1916–45.
Hospitals, 1927–45.
Johns Hopkins Hospital Nurses' Alumnae Magazine, 1937–42.
The Modern Hospital, 1913–45.
National Hospital Record, 1897–1910.
The Nurse, 1892–1917.
The Nurses Journal of the Pacific Coast, 1905–1907.
The Nursing World, 1895–99.
Pacific Coast Nursing Journal, 1908–30.
The Trained Nurse, 1888–93.
The Trained Nurse and Hospital Review, 1894–1945.

Interviews

Bird, Virginia. Waltham Graduate Nurses' Association. Waltham, Mass., October 21, 1976, June 5, 1977.
Bluestone, E.M. Former Administrator, Montefiore Hospital, Bronx, New York, and editor of *Modern Hospital.* New York City, October 25, 1978.
McLaughlin, Mary Elizabeth (pseud.). Waltham Graduate Nurses' Association. Somerville, Mass., January 27, 1980.

Government statistical documents

Massachusetts, Bureau of Statistics of Labor. *The Working Girls of Boston,* by Carroll D. Wright. Boston: Wright and Potter, 1884.

United States, Bureau of Education. *Educational Status of Nursing,* by M. Adelaide Nutting. Bureau of Education Bulletin 7, no. 475. Washington, D.C.: Government Printing Office, 1912.

———. *The Inception, Organization and Management of Training Schools for Nurses, 1882.* Circulars of Information of the Bureau of Education. Washington, D.C.: Government Printing Office, 1882.

———. *Training Schools for Nurses, 1879.* Circulars of Information of the Bureau of Education. Washington, D.C.: Government Printing Office, 1879.

United States, Department of Commerce and Labor, Bureau of the Census. *Benevolent Institutions, 1904.* Washington, D.C.: Government Printing Office, 1905.

United States, Department of Commerce, Bureau of the Census. *Benevolent Institutions, 1910.* Washington, D.C.: Government Printing Office, 1913.

———. *Comparative Occupation Statistics for the United States, 1870–1940,* by Alba M. Edwards. Washington, D.C.: Government Printing Office, 1943.

———. *Historical Statistics of the United States from Colonial Times to 1957.* Washington, D.C.: Government Printing Office, 1959.

———. *Statistics of Women at Work, 1900.* Washington, D.C.: Government Printing Office, 1907.

———. *Women in Gainful Occupations, 1870–1920,* by Joseph Hill. Washington, D.C.: Government Printing Office, 1929.

United States, Department of Interior, Bureau of Education. *Developments in Nursing Education Since 1918,* by Isabel Stewart. Bureau of Education Bulletin no. 20. Washington, D.C.: Government Printing Office, 1921.

———. *Statistics of Nurse Training Schools, 1919–1920.* Bureau of Education Bulletin no. 51. Washington, D.C.: Government Printing Office, 1922.

United States, Department of Labor, Bureau of Labor Statistics. *The Economic Status of Registered Professional Nurses, 1946–47.* Bureau of Labor Statistics Bulletin no. 931. Washington, D.C.: Government Printing Office, 1947.

United States, Department of Labor, Women's Bureau. *The Eight Hour Day in Federal and State Legislation.* Women's Bureau Bulletin no. 5. Washington, D.C.: Government Printing Office, 1921.

———. *Handbook on Women Workers.* Washington, D.C.: Government Printing Office, 1975.

———. *Professional Nurses.* Women's Bureau Bulletin no. 203. Washington, D.C.: Government Printing Office, 1945.

———. *Women's Occupations through Seven Decades,* by Janet Hooks. Women's Bureau Bulletin no. 218. Washington, D.C.: Government Printing Office, 1947.

Index

Post bellum hospital as moral universe, nurse as woman, caring & little responsibility. cheap students as labour

Early 1900s, bid for clearly defined role for nurses, not just subordinate to phys^ns but equal before hosp trustees — rejecting U medical role.

Expan^n of need for nursing, plus availability of alternative career opportunities, → 1900-1970, ↑ difficulty in finding recruits, less "womanly" candidates & more clearly "work".

Graduates
→ ↗ private nursing — predominante
→ Admin^n of smaller charitable hospitals
→ ↘ Public health nursing
→ independence, choice, but uncertainty.

Profess^alisation vs work — contradictory ideologies → probs of identity &
— this as central chapter — note not recognised as self-reg^d work needing reform by general public — identific^n & problems of nurses not made.
— urge not just of image of nursing, but of constraints on working nurses preventing them seeking such improvements — profess^al^n inappropriate

Efficiency as poss means to clearer defin^n of nurses' work, but note uncertainty over task vs care.

Bid for higher standards explicitly meant to excluding working class women.

Growth of hospital care, & depression, → collapse of private nursing

Massive overprod^n of graduate nurses by depress^n years → ↑graduate employment